Essential Readings in Rehabilitation Outcomes Measurement

Application, Methodology, and Technology

Edited by

Edward A. Dobrzykowski, MHS, PT, ATC

Director of Development
Focus On Therapeutic Outcomes, Inc.
Knoxville, Tennessee

AN ASPEN PUBLICATION®
Aspen Publishers, Inc.
Gaithersburg, Maryland
1998

Library of Congress Cataloging-in-Publication Data

Essential readings in rehabilitation outcomes measurement:
application, methodology, and technology/
[edited by] Edward A. Dobrzykowski.
p.   cm.
Includes bibliographical references and index.
ISBN 0-8342-1194-7
1. Medical rehabilitation—Evaluation.
2. Outcome assessment (Medical care)   I. Dobrzykowski, Edward A.
[DNLM: 1. Rehabilitation—organization & administration collected works.
2. Outcome and Process Assessment (Health Care)—methods collected works.
WB 320 E78 1998]
RM930.E86   1998
617'.03—DC21
DNLM/DLC
for Library of Congress
98-20405
CIP

Orders: (800) 638-8437
Customer Service: (800) 234-1660

About Aspen Publishers • For more than 35 years, Aspen has been a leading professional publisher in a variety of disciplines. Aspen's vast information resources are available in both print and electronic formats. We are committed to providing the highest quality information available in the most appropriate format for our customers. Visit Aspen's Internet site for more information resources, directories, articles, and a searchable version of Aspen's full catalog, including the most recent publications: **http://www.aspenpublishers.com**
Aspen Publishers, Inc. • The hallmark of quality in publishing
Member of the worldwide Wolters Kluwer group.

Editorial Services: Kathy Litzenberg
Library of Congress Catalog Card Number: 98-20405
ISBN: 0-8342-1194-7

Printed in the United States of America

1   2   3   4   5

Table of Contents

Contributors

Hussein Abdel-Dayem, MD
Professor of Radiology
St. Vincent's Medical Center
New York, New York

Alphonso L. Amato, MBA, PT
President
Focus On Therapeutic Outcomes, Inc.
St. Louis, Missouri

Mark J. Ashley, MS, CCC-SLP, CCM
Executive Director
Centre for Neuro Skills
Bakersfield, California

John D. Banja, PhD
Associate Professor
Department of Rehabilitation
   Medicine
School of Medicine
Emory University
Atlanta, Georgia

Stephen N. Berk, PhD
Neuropsychologist
Good Shepherd Rehabilitation
   Hospital
Allentown, Pennsylvania

Rita Bode, PhD
Postdoctoral Fellow
Rehabilitation Institute of Chicago
Chicago, Illinois

Susan Braun, MLS, OTR/L
Director
WeeFIM Services
Uniform Data System for Medical
   Rehabilitation
Buffalo, New York

Velda L. Bryan, PT
Senior Clinical Specialist
Centre for Neuro Skills
Bakersfield, California and Irving,
   Texas

David F. Cella, PhD
Director of Psychosocial Oncology
Rush Cancer Institute
Rush-Presbyterian-St. Luke's Medical
   Center
Chicago, Illinois

Lea Chiaromonte, MS, CCC-S
Vice President of Clinical Services
South Coast Rehabilitation Services
Laguna Hills, California

Kristine C. Cichowski, MS
Director of Outcomes Management
Rehabilitation Institute of Chicago
Chicago, Illinois

Nancy Claiborne, MSW, ACP
Social Worker
Spinal Treatment Evaluation Process
Texas Orthopedic Hospital
Houston, Texas

Janet Cockburn, PhD
Psychologist
University of Reading
Reading, England

Anne Pas Colborn, EdD, OTR/L
Associate Investigator and Clinical
   Research Consultant
Occupational Therapy Section
Rehabilitation Medicine Department
National Institutes of Health
Bethesda, Maryland

Michael A. Counte, PhD
Professor and Chair
Department of Health Administration
School of Public Health
St. Louis University
St. Louis, Missouri

Anne Deutsch, RN, MS, CRRN
Doctoral Student
Department of Social and Preventive
   Medicine
State University of New York
Buffalo, New York

Edward A. Dobrzykowski, MHS, PT, ATC
Director of Development
Focus On Therapeutic Outcomes, Inc.
Knoxville, Tennessee

Teresa L. Elliott-Burke, MHS, PT
Vice President
Clinical Services
PeakCare
Lake Zurich, Illinois

Randall W. Evans, PhD
President and Chief Operating Officer
Learning Services Corporation
Durham, North Carolina
Clinical Associate Professor of
    Psychiatry
School of Medicine
University of North Carolina
Chapel Hill, North Carolina

Judith A. Falconer, PhD, OTR
Professor of Health Sciences
University of Wisconsin
Milwaukee, Wisconsin

Arthur M. Gershkoff, MD
Clinical Director
Stroke and Neurological Diseases
    Program
MossRehab Hospital
Philadelphia, Pennsylvania

Marian Gillard, MS, OTR/L
Assistant Professor
Department of Occupational Therapy
Temple University
Philadelphia, Pennsylvania

Gary Goldberg, MD
Attending Physiatrist
Drucker Brain Injury Center
MossRehab Hospital
Philadelphia, Pennsylvania

Carl V. Granger, MD
Professor of Rehabilitation Medicine
State University of New York
Director
Center for Functional Assessment
    Research
Buffalo, New York

Stephen M. Haley, PhD, PT
Associate Dean for Research
Sargent College
Boston University
Boston, Massachusetts

Karyl Hall, EdD
Director of Rehabilitation Research
Santa Clara Valley Medical Center
San Jose, California

Daniel P. Harris, PhD
Director of Clinical Information
    Services
Healthcare Rehabilitation Center
Austin, Texas

Dennis L. Hart, PhD, PT
Director
Research and Consulting Services
Focus On Therapeutic Outcomes, Inc.
Knoxville, Tennessee

Dennis R. Hays
Vice President
Centre for Neuro Skills
Bakersfield, California and Irving,
    Texas

Allen W. Heinemann, PhD
Professor
Department of Physical Medicine and
    Rehabilitation
Rehabilitation Institute of Chicago
Northwestern University Medical
    School
Chicago, Illinois

Patricia Larkins Hicks, PhD
President
Outcomes Management Group, Ltd.
Columbus, Ohio

Michael Hutchinson, DPhil, MD
Assistant Professor of Neurology
New York University Medical
    Center
New York, New York

Shawn Johns, MS, CCC-S
Director of Clinical Projects
South Coast Rehabilitation Services
Laguna Hills, California

Edward Kan, BS
Research Assistant
Rehabilitation Institute of Chicago
Chicago, Illinois

Jeffrey Kozak, MD
Spinal Surgeon
Fondren Orthopedic Group
Houston, Texas

Trudy Millard Krause, DrPH
Director
Spinal Treatment Evaluation Process
Texas Orthopedic Hospital
Houston, Texas

**David K. Krych, MS, CCC-SLP,
    CCM**
Executive Director
Centre for Neuro Skills
Irving, Texas and Bakersfield,
    California
Adjunct Professor
Rehabilitation Institute of the College
    of Education
Southern Illinois University
Carbondale, Illinois

Jin-Shei Lai, PhD, OTR
Senior Research Specialist
College of Health Professions
University of Illinois at Chicago
Chicago, Illinois

J. Scott Ling, PsyD
Executive Director
Midwest Region
Learning Services
Madison, Wisconsin

Daniel Luciano, MD
Assistant Professor of Neurology
New York University Medical Center
New York, New York

Cecelia M. Lux, MA, CCC-S
Vice President
Sun Quest Consulting, Inc.
Cypress, California

Mary Jo Marino, MS, PT
President
The Therapy Center, Inc.
Knoxville, Tennessee

Alireza Minagar, MD
Resident in Neurology
New York University Medical Center
New York, New York

Malcolm H. Morrison, PhD
President and Chief Executive Officer
Morrison Informatics, Inc.
Mechanicsburg, Pennsylvania

Terri Nance, MS
Director of Operations
Focus On Therapeutic Outcomes, Inc.
Knoxville, Tennessee

Paul C. Nystrom, PhD
Manegold Professor in Management
School of Business Administration
University of Wisconsin
Milwaukee, Wisconsin

Michael A. O'Hearn, BSc, PT
Physical Therapist
Lakeland Rehabilitation Center
St. Joseph, Michigan

Rolland S. Parker, PhD
Adjunct Professor of Clinical
  Neurology
New York University Medical Center
New York, New York

Adele Patrick, PhD
Associate Director
Human Services Management Institute
University of Georgia
Athens, Georgia

Craig S. Persel, BA
Director
Department of Research and
  Development
Centre for Neuro Skills
Bakersfield, California

Lori Pothast, PT
Private Practitioner
Wanconda, Illinois

Susan C. Robertson, MS, OTR/L
Primary Investigator and Senior
  Occupational Therapist
Occupational Therapy Section
Rehabilitation Medicine Department
National Institutes of Health
Bethesda, Maryland

Richard R. Schall, PhD
Director of Psychology
Good Shepherd Rehabilitation Hospital
Allentown, Pennsylvania

Nancy D. Schmidt, MS
Vice President
Clinical and Professional Services
Prism Health Group
Boston, Massachusetts

John D. Schultz
Vice President
Centre for Neuro Skills
Irving, Texas and Bakersfield, California

Mary E. Segal, PhD
Research Scientist
Moss Rehabilitation Research Institute
MossRehab Hospital
Assistant Professor
Department of Physical Medicine and
  Rehabilitation
Temple University
Philadelphia, Pennsylvania

Sidney I. Silverman, DDS
Adjunct Professor of Clinical Neurology
New York University Medical Center
New York, New York

Steven E. Simon, PhD
Chief
Vocational Rehabilitation and
  Counseling Program
Florida Region
Department of Veterans Affairs
St. Petersburg, Florida
Adjunct Lecturer
Rehabilitation Services Program
DePaul University
Chicago, Illinois

Teresa M. Steffen, PhD, PT
Program Director of Physical Therapy
Concordia University Wisconsin
Mequon, Wisconsin

Meri Beth Stegall, PhD
Assistant Professor
Program in Healthcare
  Administration
College of Biological Sciences
University of Osteopathic Medicine
  and Health Sciences
Des Moines, Iowa

Scott Stegall, PhD
Assistant Professor
Program in Healthcare
  Administration
College of Biological Sciences
University of Osteopathic Medicine
  and Health Sciences
Des Moines, Iowa

Dale C. Strasser, MD
Assistant Professor of Rehabilitation
  Medicine
School of Medicine
Emory University
Chief of Rehabilitation Medicine
Wesley Woods Geriatric Hospital
Atlanta, Georgia
Medical Co-Director
Rehabilitation Research and
  Development Center
Atlanta Veterans Affairs Medical
  Center
Decatur, Georgia

Barbara Tate Unger, RN, FAACVPR
Department of Cardiovascular
    Services
Itasca Medical Center
Grand Rapids, Minnesota

Craig A. Velozo, PhD, OTR
Associate Professor
Department of Occupational Therapy
College of Associated Health
    Professions
University of Illinois at Chicago
Chicago, Illinois

George J. Wan, MPH
Doctoral Student
Health Services Research
School of Public Health
St. Louis University
St. Louis, Missouri

Thomas T.H. Wan, PhD, MHS
Professor and Chair
Department of Health Administration
Medical College of Virginia
Virginia Commonwealth University
Richmond, Virginia

Barbara A. Wilson, PhD
Senior Scientist
Applied Psychology Unit
Medical Research Council
Addenbrookes Hospital
Cambridge, England

Preface

It has been said that the only constant today is change. The health care industry and, more specifically, rehabilitation practice is not an exception. As rehabilitation providers evolve from a market-driven, cost-based model to one based upon an outcomes paradigm, a need is created for practical and pragmatic methods, applications, and uses of technology for outcomes measurement.

Clinicians, administrators of quality and performance measurement, and researchers alike are struggling with questions, such as:

- What outcomes are most important to our customers?
- How does one measure outcomes and manage the process of data collection, analysis, and reporting?
- What measures are available for the variety of patient diagnoses in the rehabilitation continuum of care?
- In comparisons of programs and benchmarking results, what methods have been implemented for risk adjustment and patient variability?
- How can effectiveness and efficiency be linked?
- How can outcomes information be applied in practice improvement, marketing, sales, accreditation, and research?

This book contains thirty-eight articles that address such questions. The work is presented in eight topical sections: (I) The State of Rehabilitation Outcomes Measurement; (II) Patient Satisfaction; (III) Orthopedic Rehabilitation Outcomes; (IV) Stroke and Brain, Spinal Cord, and Head Injury Rehabilitation Outcomes; (V) Speech-Language Outcomes; (VI) Cardiac Rehabilitation Outcomes; (VII) Technology in Rehabilitation Outcomes Measurement; and (VIII) Rehabilitation Outcome Measures.

Many of the articles were selected from the *Journal of Rehabilitation Outcomes Measurement*, which was created to promote the dissemination of current and timely information pertaining to the development of validated new and existing rehabilitation outcome scales, the methodology and process of outcomes measurement used in rehabilitative care, the analysis and interpretation of data, and applications of outcome information. Articles from two other journals, *Journal of Head Trauma Rehabilitation* and *Topics in Stroke Rehabilitation*, supplement the selection.

PART I

The State of Rehabilitation Outcomes Measurement

1

The Methodology of Outcomes Measurement

Edward A. Dobrzykowski

THE GROWING IMPORTANCE OF OUTCOMES MANAGEMENT

Outcomes management in health care, broadly defined as the process of data collection, analysis, and interpretation of the effectiveness and efficiency of patient treatment, probably garners as much attention as health care industry reform efforts during the 1990s. More precisely, Ellwood[1] defines outcomes management as a "technology of patient experience designed to help patients, payers, and providers make rational medical-care related choices based on better insight into the effect of these choices on the patient's life. Outcomes management consists of a common patient-understood language of health outcomes; a national database containing information and analysis on clinical, financial, and health outcomes that estimates as best we can the relation between medical interventions and health outcomes, as well as the relation between health outcomes and money; and an opportunity for each decision maker to have access to the analyses that are relevant to the choices they must make." In other words, outcomes management is the determination of the results of health care intervention through a reliable measurement methodology, ascertaining the most efficient manner in which to achieve the desired result, and improving results over time.

Outcomes research has attempted to understand and elucidate provider "economic" variation, as reflected in the variable costs of similar conditions seen in billing data without benefit of accompanying patient health status, satisfaction, and clinical data. Why does it cost $1,000 for an episode of rehabilitation care for a patient with a low back disorder from one health care professional, and $1,500 for an episode of rehabilitative care for a patient with a low back disorder from another health care professional? Why does it cost $10,000 for an inpatient episode of care for a patient with a stroke in one rehabilitation unit, and $13,500 for an inpatient episode of care for a patient with a stroke in another rehabilitation unit? Can the variation be "explained" statistically by differences in patient acuity (time from onset of condition) levels, severity of the disorder, socioeconomic status, insurance reimbursement level, geographic area, or other undiscovered confounding variables? Was the patient's functional outcome result and health status improved to a greater extent in the higher cost examples, which resulted in less recidivism? In other words, did spending more money "up front" result in a more durable outcome and save health care dollars over the long term?

In order to more fully understand and study these apparent differences of outcomes, the standardization of measures and the process for data collection, analysis, and reporting is necessary. The "industry" of rehabilitation as a whole, with one notable exception the use of the functional independence measure in inpatient rehabilitation, has not reached an agreement on standardized measures. Many areas in the rehabilitation continuum of care are practicing bereft of reliable and valid outcome measures. Even in situations where measures are available, the administrative burden far surpasses their practical implementation and resultant value of the information. Fortunately, research is under way to develop outcome measures with sound psychometric properties, carefully balancing the need for comprehensiveness and responsiveness in a measure with the logistics of health care delivery. There is consideration of productivity implications of clinicians and staff, and the cost to administer and process data. Present technological barriers become the outcome data collection facilitators, as data are collected without duplication and processed in more user-friendly and "real time" environments.

J Rehabil Outcomes Meas, 1997, 1(1), 8–17

RATIONALE FOR COLLECTION OF OUTCOMES DATA

The purpose of outcomes management includes the measurement of the effectiveness (assessing the impact of treatment programs on a population) and the efficiency (assessing outcomes in conjunction with the resources used) of health care. The rationale for collection of outcomes data includes reducing unexplained variation in the results of clinical care, improving quality, and lowering cost.

There is a variety of customers with a need for outcomes information. For many years, the Rehabilitation Accreditation Commission has required the measurement of outcomes for several types of rehabilitation services through its program evaluation standards. The Joint Commission on Accreditation of Healthcare Organizations (Joint Commission) has required performance measurement in its accreditation process, and has recently defined attributes for performance measurement system data collection instruments[2] (see box entitled "Attributes of Conformance"). Other purposes for outcomes management may be continuous quality improvement, benchmarking, management reports, and marketing.

Attributes of Conformance

1. Performance measure characteristics: The characteristics of the performance measures submitted by measurement systems for use in the ORYX initiative*
2. Database (measurement system technical capabilities): The operational characteristics of measurement systems
3. Performance measure accuracy: The extent to which performance measures correctly identify the events they were designed to identify
4. Risk adjustment/stratification: A process for reducing, removing, or clarifying the influences of confounding patient factors that differ among comparison groups
5. Performance measure related feedback: Performance measure related information that is available, on a timely basis, to health care organizations participating in the measurement system, for use in the organization's ongoing internal efforts to improve patient care and organizational performance
6. Relevance for accreditation: The extent to which performance measurement systems are useful and relevant in the accreditation process
7. Technical reporting requirements: The requirements related to the transmission of accredited health care organization data to the Joint Commission by performance measurement systems

*For further information on the ORYX initiative, contact the Joint Commission Internet site or call (630) 792-5085.

Source: Joint Commission on the Accreditation of Healthcare Organizations, 1998. Reprinted with permission.

Much of the rationale and impetus recently for the outcomes movement has originated from the actual or perceived influence of managed care. Cost containment efforts result in quality differences becoming more and more perceptible by the consumer, with the delivery of health care every day becoming more commodity-like. The attainment of "optimal" outcomes with a minimal acceptable quality level will become a means of service differentiation.

There are few markets in the United States today where the measurement of outcomes remains an option; rather, it is an essential part of clinical practice and survival. The time to gather outcomes information is *before* your customers ask.

OUTCOMES DATA FROM START TO FINISH

The collection, analysis, and management of outcomes data are arduous tasks. What are the measures needed for inclusion in a minimum dataset that demonstrates predictive power in rehabilitation outcome? Fortunately, research is under way to measure outcomes and define measurement systems comprising minimum datasets, backed by unparalleled growth in supportive technology and information systems infrastructure. There are profound and thought-provoking implications for management decision making assisted by the use of outcomes data. In the daily practice of patient care, clinicians in rehabilitation have begun to case manage and accurately predict outcomes at the start of rehabilitation of their patients.

Many providers and organizations involved in the delivery of rehabilitation services have begun or are planning a system of outcomes measurement. It is not the intent of this article to provide a discussion of a standardized outcome system such as the Uniform Data System for Medical Rehabilitation (UDSMR^{SM})[3] for inpatient rehabilitation outcomes measurement. The purpose of this article is to provide an overview of the methodology to consider in the development of a process for outcomes management in rehabilitation. Guidelines are provided in order to plan and initiate an outcomes measurement system for your clinical practice or organization. The basic steps of an effective outcomes measurement system that are described apply in any type of rehabilitation practice.

Key Questions: Methodology of Outcomes Management

- What is your practice location in the health care continuum?
- What are the prevalent patient diagnoses?
- Who are the customers seeking outcome information?
- What are the questions that customers are asking?
- Which outcomes do you wish to measure?
- What outcome measures or systems are available?
- What is the data collection protocol?

- How will you train the staff?
- How will you process the data?
- How will you analyze and interpret the results?

What Is Your Practice Location in the Health Care Continuum?

In the selection of outcome measures and reporting of results, the location in the health care continuum and the type of program are considered, such as a rehabilitation unit based in a hospital or a skilled nursing facility. The precise definition of the practice location and program type is crucial, in order to classify outcome data and provide a valid comparison of outcomes between similar facilities. In rehabilitation, the type of practice includes acute care, subacute care, rehabilitation unit, skilled nursing, transitional care, assisted living, long-term care, home care, and outpatient. These services are provided in acute care hospitals, nursing homes, rehabilitation hospitals, homes, and outpatient facilities.

Presently, outcomes databases are segmented by program type and practice location. In the future, this classification scheme will become less relevant to the payers of services. The health care continuum is evolving rapidly with advances in medical treatment, blurring the boundaries and episode classification. Increasingly, vertically integrated health care providers perform patient case management and are or will be accountable for the outcome from onset of the patient's condition to completion of rehabilitation in home or outpatient services.

What Are the Prevalent Patient Diagnoses?

The practice of rehabilitation includes neurology, orthopedics, pediatrics, geriatrics, cardiopulmonary, sports, and others. Within your area of clinical practice, whether generalized or specialty, what are the most prevalent patient diagnoses? For example, does your neurology practice include patients with diagnoses such as stroke, traumatic brain injury, and spinal cord injury? In orthopedic practices, are the prevalent diagnoses spinal disorders, knee joint replacements, and knee reconstructions? In pediatric practices, are the prevalent diagnoses cerebral palsy and spina bifida? In cardiopulmonary practices, are the prevalent diagnoses myocardial infarction and chronic obstructive pulmonary disease?

After the identification of prevalent diagnoses, begin research for outcome measures and systems that have previously been validated in that particular patient population. The more useful measures should parallel frequently occurring patient goals and be responsive to change.

Essential strategy 1

When initiating an outcomes management process, begin with the identification of the most prevalent diagnoses.

Who Are the Customers Seeking Outcome Information?

The potential customers of outcome information include managed care organizations and other payers of rehabilitation services, including Medicare and Medicaid; employers; patients; patients' families; clinicians; referral sources; management; board members; and accreditation agencies such as CARF . . . The Rehabilitation Accreditation Commission, the Joint Commission, and the National Committee for Quality Assurance (NCQA).

What Are the Questions that Customers Are Asking?

In the development of an outcomes management system, ponder carefully the questions from each of these customer groups. There will of course be some potential for overlap. Do not neglect questions from your own perspective. The box entitled "Customer/Questions" lists sample questions pertaining to outcomes management from customers.

Once the questions have been determined, compile a list of potential outcome measures and descriptive indicators. For example, if the measurement of patient health status is deemed essential for the assessment of treatment results, what health status questionnaires should be considered? Careful and deliberate selection of each measure improves the quality and utility of the information.

The total number of measures in an outcomes management system should be kept to the absolute minimum. One of the more frequent errors in design is the assimilation of too many measures, resulting in a high level of cost and adminis-

---

Customer/Questions

Managed Care Organizations: What are the resource use, level of patient satisfaction, and cost to rehabilitate this patient?

Patients: What result of treatment can I expect, and what is the level of patient satisfaction?

Patient's Family: What result and prognosis are expected? What will be the capabilities of the patient?

Clinicians: Which processes of treatment lead to the best or optimal outcomes?

Referral Sources: What are the results of treatment and patient satisfaction?

Management: What are our program outcomes? How do we compare with others?

Board Members: What are our program and facility outcomes? How do our outcomes compare with other programs?

Accreditation: What are the program and facility doing as a process to measure and improve outcomes? What action steps for improvement have been taken?

trative burden. There are, of course, productivity implications for the staff. The only exception is in those rare practice situations that are automated in data collection methods, and outcomes management is integrated with computerized methods of documentation and billing.

Essential strategy 2

The total number of measures must be an absolute minimum.

What Outcomes Do You Wish to Measure? What Measures Are Available?

Outcomes can be categorized into the following: patient-reported, quality of life (i.e., health status) and satisfaction; clinician-reported (i.e., function, motivation, treatments); and a descriptive dataset (i.e., demographics, diagnosis, employment status). Let's explore each of these categories in more detail.

Outcome Measures: Patient Reported

The patient's perspective on the result of his or her health care experience and the measurement of this perception are essential to a valid outcomes management system. The patient's view of his or her quality of life and health status is at least as important, and maybe even more important, than the viewpoint of the clinician. Patient-reported outcomes have focused on the measurement of satisfaction and more recently on quality of life (see box entitled "Sample Research Questions").

Health status surveys

There are several general health status surveys available that assess the perceived quality of life from the patient's perspective. Two of the more frequently used and valid health status

---

Sample Research Questions

Quality of Life
- What is the present health status of the patient, and does the health status of the patient improve as a result of treatment intervention?
- What is the prolonged treatment effect and outcome durability over time?

Satisfaction
- Is the patient satisfied? If so, to what extent?
- If the patient was not satisfied, what were the reasons?
- What elements of health care delivery are important to patient satisfaction?
- How can health care providers improve patient satisfaction?

---

questionnaires are the MOS SF-36 or Short Form-36[4] and the Health Status Questionnaire 2.0 or HSQ 2.0.[5] The surveys are 36 and 39 questions, respectively. The SF-36 and the HSQ 2.0 are derivatives of more comprehensive health status surveys and were abbreviated following delineation of item questions within each of the domain categories, which explained significant portions of their variance. Both the SF-36 (Medical Outcomes Trust, Boston, Massachusetts) and HSQ 2.0 (Health Outcomes Institute, Bloomington, Minnesota) are available for a nominal licensing fee.

The development of patient health status surveys has focused on a questionnaire that measures many of the domains indicative of quality of life, is psychometrically sound, and has the ability to quantify a patient's quality of life perspective longitudinally over time and through movement within the health care continuum. Other desirable features are fewer items in each domain of the survey, ease in scoring, and simplified management reporting.

The domains measured in these surveys include the following eight of the most frequently represented health concepts: mental health, physical health, role limitations (physical), role limitations (emotional), social functioning, pain, energy/fatigue, and health perceptions. The SF-36 and HSQ 2.0 questionnaires are essentially identical, and differ only in that the HSQ 2.0 offers an additional three questions for the assessment of depression. The scoring and analysis of these health status surveys result in an individual score for each of the representative domains. Fortunately, published work by McHorney et al.[6] has simplified scoring methodology for the SF-36, with the demonstration of two distinct constructs and summary scores from the eight domains: a physical component summary scale and a mental component summary scale.

The use of health status surveys in ambulatory care has been validated for use by those patients a minimum of 14 years of age with normal cognitive abilities.[7] The data are typically gathered from the patient via questionnaire, personal interview, or over the telephone. The survey is not intended for or valid for proxy completion, such as a spouse or caregiver.

In rehabilitation, the health status survey is most often administered upon initiation/admission into the program and at conclusion/discharge. These questionnaires are sensitive to change and can be utilized as often as weekly. The survey has also been incorporated in postdischarge outcomes assessment, usually at 90 days. Postdischarge outcomes assessment is important for the measurement of outcomes durability, particularly in meeting requirements for programs that are accredited through CARF . . . The Rehabilitation Accreditation Commission, and the Joint Commission.

Research is under way to translate and validate the SF-36 into other languages, along with norm development for use in other countries, through the auspices of the International Quality of Life Assessment (IQOLA) Project.[8–10] There is a

Spanish language test version of the HSQ 2.0 available from the Health Outcomes Institute.[11]

Limitations in the use of health status surveys include the number of questions and the time for completion, particularly when coupled with other information normally required for patient intake and assessment at the time of initiation of treatment. In response to the need for more brevity in health status instrumentation, in early 1996 an abbreviated version of the SF-36 health status survey became available, known as the Short Form-12 or SF-12.[12] In any reduction of survey items, there can be a compromise in the level of information. The SF-12 retained 90 percent of the variance explained in the physical and mental components of the SF-36, while reducing self-administration time to two minutes.

There are disease-specific patient-reported measures available. These questionnaires are brief and may be more sensitive than the general health status measures. For this reason, disease-specific measures have been used in conjunction with general health status measures.

In orthopedic rehabilitation, examples of disease-specific measures include the Oswestry Low Back Disability Questionnaire,[13] the Lysholm Scale,[14] the Neck Disability Index (NDI),[15] and the Shoulder Pain and Disability Index (SPADI).[16] The Self-Report Questionnaire provides a measure for patients with rheumatoid arthritis in eight areas of daily living.[17]

In earlier unpublished work at Focus On Therapeutic Outcomes, Inc. (FOTO), an outcomes research and database company, significant correlations were demonstrated among the Oswestry, NDI, and Lysholm scales and the SF-36. As a result, the FOTO outpatient orthopedic outcome measurement system no longer includes disease-specific questionnaires.

Patient satisfaction

Patient satisfaction was one of the earliest generally accepted measures included in a process of outcomes management. Patient satisfaction began, however, in the 1970s, largely as a marketing ploy. In the 1980s, patient satisfaction evolved and became an integral part of quality improvement. Today it would be difficult to find a health care provider or organization *not* using a method of patient satisfaction. However, due to the lack of survey and method standardization, it is impossible to provide valid comparisons and differences among organizations.

There has been interest in the measurement of patient satisfaction and identification of factors that correlate to improved satisfaction levels. Some of the factors that have been demonstrated to correlate to satisfaction include the quality of patient interactions with the clinician and staff; the appearance of the treatment facility; the overall rehabilitation results; and the timeliness of initiation of treatment following onset of condition. It is imperative as a clinician to fully comprehend the quality of patient interaction, which goes well beyond contact with the clinician. An unfavorable first impression with a harried receptionist on the telephone could result in a canceled visit even before treatment is initiated! Some patients do not return after the first visit, when their initial impression has been unfavorable. Remember that patients do not segment their experiences into the myriad factors that influence satisfaction; rather, patients view their entire health care experience homogeneously and may frequently "rate" their impressions according to the least satisfied element.

Experienced clinicians are cognizant of the positive value attributable to patient motivation in contributing to a successful outcome. The challenge to the researcher is in the quantification of patient motivation and measurement of predictive influence on outcome. One innovative approach has been to develop measures to evaluate patient motivation both from the perspectives of the patient *and* the clinician, and assessing any potential differences.[18] Another approach has evaluated patient expectations of eventual outcome, both from the patient's and clinician's viewpoints.[19]

In the measurement of worker physical capacities and perceptions, outcome measurement instruments are available that evaluate both the patient's own perspective of his or her physical capabilities and perception and the clinician's measurement of the worker physical capacities and perceptions.[18] For example, consider the assessment of worker capabilities in tasks related to job function, such as lifting, sitting tolerance, standing tolerance, handling, etc. When quantification of worker capacity and perceptions from the worker perspective is achieved, comparisons can be made with presumably more objective measurement of worker physical capacities by the clinician. These differences in worker and clinician perspectives can be discerned and recognized early in the rehabilitation process, which should lead to improved treatment regimens and outcomes.

Outcome Measures: Clinician Reported

Astute clinicians have known for some time the importance of documented improvement in patient function versus improvements demonstrated in impairments such as strength, range of motion, endurance, and edema. Impairment ratings may be important for clinical progression of treatment; however, changes in impairments may have little relevance or correlation to changes in patient function. As a result, reimbursement of clinical services by many payers has been increasingly predicated on documentation of improved patient function and outcomes.

A proliferation of outcome measures, including the functional independence measure (FIM[SM]),[20] level of rehabilitation scale (LORS-III),[21] the patient evaluation conferencing system (PECS),[22] and the Rehabilitation Institute of Chicago functional assessment scale (RIC-FAS),[23] provide precise and sensitive measures for the evaluation and documentation of functional outcomes. The measurement of patient function in multidisciplinary inpatient rehabilitation facilities was a premise in design. These outcome instruments include standardization of measures, operational definitions, data collection procedures, scoring, and training. The goal of a standardized outcome measurement system is to promote data interrater and intrarater reliability, of particular importance in the development and promulgation of outcome databases.

The functional independence measure consists of 18 items in a minimum valid dataset to measure function in activities of daily living, locomotion, transfers, sphincter control, communication, and cognition. The results in each of the 18 items evaluated can be reported individually, but are usually consolidated and reported in two components: an ADL/self-care scale and a communication/cognitive scale.[24,25] Following an initial measurement in the patient assessment process at admission to the program or facility, the functional independence measure is utilized at the conclusion of rehabilitation or discharge from the facility. The measure can also be used at periodic intervals during rehabilitation for the assessment of progress. The outcome reflects the change in score from admission to discharge.

A promising new method of outcome assessment in a clinician-reported measure in orthopedic rehabilitation has been developed as part of the Medirisk, Inc. Orthopedic Rehabilitation Outcomes Scale.[26] The measure includes common impairments routinely utilized and familiar to clinicians. Upon beginning the rehabilitation program, an assessment is made by the clinician of the patient's impairment level, such as in the areas of strength and range of motion, and is followed by the designation of a functional goal for the patient. The distance or "interval" between the assessment and the functional goal is measured and quantified on a standardized scale.

Other clinician-reported measures include the functional assessment measure (FAM),[27] designed specifically to be a complement to the functional independence measure and more sensitive in the measurement of outcomes in brain injury. In pediatrics, two promising clinician instruments include the WeeFIM[28] and the Pediatric Evaluation of Disability Index (PEDI).[29] In home care, the standardized Outcome and Assessment Information Set (OASIS)[30] is presently in development. In 1995, the functional communication measures became available through the American Speech-Language-Hearing Association.[31] In future issues of this journal, these and other measurement systems will be discussed in more detail.

The relative paucity of outcome measures in some specialty areas of rehabilitation has resulted in occasional inappropriate and invalid use of existing functional outcome measures. The reader is cautioned and advised against the use of any outcome measure that has not been validated in a cohort of patients similar to the reader's own. Even in those practice situations where suitable measures exist, there may be overwhelming administrative burden in their application and use.

Population Descriptive Indicators

In any measurement system of patient outcomes, it is necessary to describe in some detail aspects of the patient population. These indicators include the age, gender, ethnicity, income, and education level of the patient. Information on the payer such as source of insurance (Medicare, Medicaid, etc.) and the type of plan (fee for service, preferred provider organization, etc.) is gathered. Diagnostic information is also included, such as the primary diagnosis and one or more secondary diagnoses, comorbidities, and the episode (number of occurrences) of the condition.

Risk Adjustment

In any valid and credible outcomes management system, a mechanism must exist to help account for factors beyond the control of the clinician that can influence outcomes. These factors, known as confounding variables, include the patient's age, gender, number of prior episodes, comorbidities, severity of the condition, and acuity level (the time from onset of the patient's condition to the initiation of rehabilitation). The patient's location within the country and mechanism for reimbursement can also influence outcome results, particularly on lengths of stay (inpatient) or visits (outpatient) and costs.

There are likely other yet undiscovered factors and confounding variables that influence practice variation and outcome results. In one noteworthy example, Velozo reported that although he could explain 40 percent of the variance seen in outcome of stroke patients, a sizable 60 percent of the variance remained unexplained by present measures contained in the system.

What Time Intervals Will Be Used?

The determination of time intervals for data collection at the initiation of any outcome measurement system is essential. At a minimum, the prototypical format includes collection of data at admission or initiation of the rehabilitation program and at discharge or conclusion. There must be at least two data points for the measurement of outcome, in order to calculate the outcome. Optional data collection points include designated intervals during the episode of care, and at 90 days postdischarge.

The use of interval measures becomes important in those episodes of care longer than two weeks in duration. When visits or patient encounters are limited, the measurement of outcomes is even more crucial! For example, if only one visit or treatment session is authorized for reimbursement with a referral for evaluation and a "home program," a method should be developed to collect outcome information postdischarge.

Postdischarge assessment of outcome durability is continuing and expanding from today's standard of 90 days to one year. In the future, it is possible that partial reimbursement of provider services may be withheld pending outcome success longer-term. In this scenario, it is hoped that more efficient and effective providers will be recognized and rewarded with enhanced patient volume and reimbursement levels by the payers of health care services.

Essential strategy 3

The minimum data collection points are admission, discharge, and at 90 days postdischarge.

How Will Data Be Collected?

Outcomes data can be collected in a variety of ways. The recommended initial method is paper-based forms for use during the pilot phase for several months. This process will provide an opportunity to evaluate the selected measures and operational definitions within your system design. A popular method in outcomes data collection today, particularly in the proprietary outcome systems, is the use of optical scan forms. Other methods include keying or touch-screen data entry into software. The important reminders are the careful considerations of the customers entering data, including patients, clinicians, clerical staff, medical records, and others. In rehabilitation programs with computer programming resources and information systems available, a portion of outcomes data may be collected from existing input sources, minimizing data gathering redundancies.

Essential strategy 4

Carefully consider the data collection interface for customers entering data, and minimize data gathering redundancy when feasible.

How Will Staff Be Trained?

It is imperative that all individuals involved in the outcomes management effort be thoroughly trained, not only in the operational definitions of measures and the data collection protocol, but also, perhaps more importantly, in the "vision" for the research. The entire team within a service program environment must be well informed and firmly committed to the research. Training goes beyond the clinician level and is particularly recommended for nonclinical staff with roles essential to the administration of patient-reported measures such as health status questionnaires, and the population descriptive information required. Retraining

should occur on an annual basis, or sooner if substantive changes are made in staffing or in the outcome measurement system.

There is an expectation that exists for the training and testing of clinicians on their knowledge in standardized system's outcome measures, purportedly for enhancement of data reliability. The Uniform Data System for Medical Rehabilitation requires users of the functional independence measure to be credentialed through a training and testing process. Medirisk, Inc. also requires users to verify competency through a process of certification testing. Periodic retraining is also recommended.

The testing process adds cost to these systems, both directly from facilitation of training, and indirectly through lost staff productivity during the training time. Newer creative adult education and testing methods may reduce administrative burden and cost. In the future, statistical analyses of clinician rating patterns and outcome databases may prove more useful than training for identifying those programs and clinicians that are not rating reliably, albeit from incorrect or incomplete knowledge of the measure or purposeful "manipulation" of ratings.

Essential strategy 5

Provide a method to train all staff members involved in your outcomes management process.

How Will Data Be Processed and Analyzed?

The processing and analysis of outcome data into information for decision making are formidable tasks. Outcome data processing and analysis require individuals with experience and knowledge in programming and statistics. The programming and management report writing can take a considerable amount of time. At this point in the design of an outcomes management process, many providers contemplate outsourcing this work to a consultant or consider the use of an external outcomes database service vendor.

Essential strategy 6

The data processing and analysis of outcomes information require individuals with expertise in statistics and computer programming.

How Will Data Be Interpreted?

Outcomes information may bring some intriguing revelations about your practice. One of the purposes of outcomes management is to minimize unexplained variation in the results of health care and stimulate cost reduction through improved efficiencies. It is recommended that providers trend their outcome results for a minimum of one year before planning and implementing changes in the delivery of services. A quarter with lower than expected results may simply be a statistical anomaly. However, four consecutive quarters of higher than expected utilization and charges, or less than expected health status results, indicate the need for an in-depth review of both the program structure and the service delivery process.

The modification of a clinician's or a program's outcome results should be approached in a nonpunitive fashion. It is not uncommon to review an outcomes management report with a mixture of satisfactory and unsatisfactory results. For example, consider the outcome results in an orthopedic outpatient rehabilitation practice for both low back and neck patients, as shown in Table 1. Assume that the results have been risk adjusted.

The low back outcome results appear less than satisfactory, while the neck outcome results appear to be satisfactory. One interpretive strategy would be to examine the process of treatment of patients with these disorders. Should clinical pathways be developed, or if available, modified? Are there algorithms needing development or monitoring to promote more efficiencies in the delivery of care? Is continuing education and inservicing of clinicians in these conditions in order? Are patients possibly taking more time as the result of delayed referral to rehabilitation? Are the patients more chronic in nature (this should be accounted for in the risk adjustment of the outcomes data)?

Essential strategy 7

Outcomes information should be examined and monitored for a minimum of one year prior to definitive changes in the planned delivery of health care services.

WHAT ARE THE BUDGET IMPLICATIONS?

There will be both direct and indirect expenses to consider and budget for in a process of outcomes management. According to Doyle,[32] costs fall into three main categories: start-up, technology development, and ongoing operations.

Start-up costs include the design and planning in the outcomes management system, the research of measures and indicators, the development of data collection forms, pilot testing of the prototype outcomes system, and training of the clinicians and support staff. Technology development costs include the potential purchase of hardware and software, plus expenses for programming, data analysis, and management report generation. Ongoing operations costs include the cost per patient, purchase or copying of data collection forms, productivity impact of both clinicians and support staff, data processing, and reports.

Table 1 Outcome Results in an Orthopedic Outpatient Rehabilitation Practice

Low back disorders	Facility	Database
Visits	11.2	8.1
Charges	$1350	$877
Health status gain	34%	38%
Neck disorders	Facility	Database
Visits	9.3	9.5
Charges	$962	$1054
Health status gain	28%	27%

WHAT MECHANISM EXISTS FOR DATA QUALITY CONTROL?

An outcomes management process provides a valid picture of your program results with reliable measures and complete datasets. Unless the facility dutifully randomizes its patients, which is *not* recommended, one of the continual challenges to the process will be the collection of complete data. A quality indicator should be developed to monitor data collection efforts. A benchmark to use for complete patient-reported data for outpatient services is 70 percent, with a goal of 100 percent of clinician- and staff-reported data. Of course, in the cognitively impaired patient, health status information will not be collected.

The issue of reliability in outcomes management is essential. The reliability of health status questionnaires reported by patients has been established.[33,34] The reliability of clinician-reported data in the absence of clear operational definitions is suspect. Pilot testing of your outcome measurement system should address and test interrater and intrarater reliability for any measure in the absence of previously conducted research and documentation of acceptable reliability.

• • •

The implementation of an outcomes management process should be well planned prior to execution. A series of key questions has been devised as a guide through the developmental stages. A technologically advanced organization with sophisticated information system capabilities may facilitate the collection and analysis of multiple measures and indicators for outcomes management, but is no guarantee of success. It is highly recommended that a concerted effort be made to gather only a few measures of substance, keeping in mind the concept of a minimum dataset. Begin with a paper-based system until all desirable measures and indicators are thoroughly defined before moving to a more automated system. Provide program results for a minimum one-year period prior to reengineering of your care delivery processes. Share the results with your staff on a regular basis.

Begin an outcomes management process now! Don't wait until the "perfect system" arrives, or until customers ask for the information. The methodology of outcomes measurement may seem muddled initially, but with persistent leadership and perseverance quickly becomes an integral and essential process of health care management.

REFERENCES

1. Ellwood, P.M. "Shattuck Lecture—Outcomes Management." *New England Journal of Medicine* 318 (1988): 1549–59.

2. Joint Commission on Accreditation of Healthcare Organizations. Oakbrook Terrace, IL: 1996.

3. *Uniform Data System for Medical Rehabilitation.* Buffalo, NY: State University of New York at Buffalo.

4. *Medical Outcomes Study Short Form-36.* Boston, MA: Medical Outcomes Trust.

5. *Health Status Questionnaire 2.0.* Bloomington, MN: Health Outcomes Institute.

6. McHorney, C.A., Ware, J.E., and Raczek, A.E. "The MOS 36-Item Short-Form Health Status Survey (SF-36): II. Psychometric and Clinical Tests of Validity in Measuring Physical and Mental Health Constructs." *Medical Care* 31 (1993): 247.

7. McHorney, C.A., et al. "The Validity and Relative Precision of MOS Short- and Long-Form Health Status Scales and Dartmouth COOP Charts: Results from the Medical Outcomes Study." *Medical Care* 30, suppl (1992): MS253.

8. Sullivan, M., Karlsson, J., and Ware, J.E. "The Swedish SF-36 Health Survey: I. Evaluation of Data Quality, Scaling Assumptions, Reliability, and Construct Validity across Several Populations in Sweden." *Social Science in Medicine* 41, no. 10 (1995): 1349–58.

9. Bullinger, M. "German Translation and Psychometric Testing of the SF-36 Health Survey: Preliminary Results from the IQOLA Project." *Social Science in Medicine* 41, no. 10 (1995).

10. McCallum, J. "The SF-36 in an Australian Sample: Validating a New General Health Status Measure." *Australian Journal of Public Health* 19, no. 2 (1995): 160–66.

11. Health Outcomes Institute, Bloomington, MN. Personal correspondence, 1996.

12. Ware, J.E., Kosinski, M., and Keller, S.D. "A 12-Item Short-Form Health Survey: Construction of Scales and Preliminary Tests of Reliability and Validity." *Medical Care* 34 (1996): 3220–33.

13. Fairbank, J.C.T., et al. "The Oswestry Low Back Pain Disability Questionnaire." *Physiotherapy* 66 (1980): 66.

14. Tegner, Y., and Lysholm, J. "Rating Systems in the Evaluation of Knee Ligament Injuries." *Clinical Orthopaedics and Related Research* 198 (1985): 43–48.

15. Vernon, H., and Mior, S. "The Neck Disability Index: A Study of Reliability and Validity." *Journal of Manipulative and Physiological Therapeutics* 14 (1991): 409–15.

16. Williams, J.W., et al. "Measuring Shoulder Function with the Shoulder Pain and Disability Index." *Journal of Rheumatology* 22 (April 1995): 4727–32.

17. Pincus, T., et al. "Self-Report Questionnaire Scores in Rheumatoid Arthritis Compared with Traditional Physical, Radiographic and Laboratory Measures." *Annals of Internal Medicine* 110, no. 4 (1989): 259–66.

18. *Occupational Outcomes Measurement System.* Chicago, IL: Medirisk, Inc. (formerly Formations in Health Care, Inc.), 1995.

19. Focus On Therapeutic Outcomes, Inc. (FOTO), Knoxville, Tennessee, 1996.

20. *Uniform Data System for Medical Rehabilitation,* SUNY Buffalo.

21. *Level of Rehabilitation Scale.* Chicago, IL: Medirisk, Inc.

22. *Patient Evaluation and Conferencing System.* Wheaton, IL: Research Foundation.

23. Rehabilitation Institute of Chicago, Chicago, Illinois.

24. Silverstein, B., et al. "Applying Psychometric Criteria to Functional Assessment in Medical Rehabilitation: II. Defining Interval Measures." *Archives of Physical Medicine and Rehabilitation* 73 (1991): 507–18.

25. Heinemann, A.W., et al. "Relationships between Impairment and Physical Disability as Measured by the Functional Independence Measure." *Archives of Physical Medicine and Rehabilitation* 74 (1993): 566–73.

26. Medirisk, Inc., *Occupational Outcomes Measurement System.*

27. *Functional Assessment Measure.* San Jose, CA: Santa Clara Valley Medical Center.

28. *Uniform Data System for Medical Rehabilitation,* SUNY Buffalo.

29. PEDI Research Group, Department of Rehabilitation. *The Pediatric Evaluation of Disability Inventory (PEDI).* Boston, MA: New England Medical Center Hospitals.

30. Shaughnessy, P.W., Crisler, K.S., and Schlenker, R.E. "Medicare's OASIS: Standardized Outcome and Assessment Information Set for Home Health Care." Washington, D.C.: National Association for Home Care, 1995.

31. *Functional Communication Measures.* Rockville, MD: American Speech Language and Hearing Association.

32. Doyle, A. Personal communication, Health Outcomes Institute seminar, Minneapolis, Minnesota, 1994.

33. McHorney et al., "The Validity and Relative Precision of MOS."

34. Ware, Kosinski, and Keller, "A 12-Item Short-Form Health Survey."

2

Risk Adjustment in Rehabilitation

Edward A. Dobrzykowski

THE NEED FOR RISK ADJUSTMENT IN REHABILITATION

Rehabilitation and medical effectiveness researchers, who develop methods to assess, evaluate, and compare the results of health care provider services, are keenly interested in explaining and achieving optimal outcomes. Outcome differences (variation in results), both real and perceived, have largely been identified through analyses of financial databases derived from bills supplied by providers to the payers of health care services. As a result, purchasing decisions for health care are made increasingly upon incomplete knowledge of the differences in heterogeneous patient populations experiencing countless varieties of conditions.

Observed differences in outcomes can largely be explained through four factors: differences in whether available data sources are true (reliability); differences in patient risk factors (i.e., age, health status, comorbidity); severity/acuity; other variations, including chance, that cannot be explained; or differences in the effectiveness of health services provided or the process of care.[1] Feinstein[2] described sources of variation seen as input variability (data entry, medical record), procedure variability (risk adjustment process), and user variability (rater error). The method for rehabilitation outcomes management must provide a mechanism for the measurement and consideration of these sources of risk and outcome variation largely outside of the control of the provider.

The term risk adjustment, for purposes of this discussion, will include the effects of case-mix (population demographics), severity, sickness, intensity, complexity, comorbidity, and health status of the patient.[1] *Risk adjustment considers factors other than the health care intervention itself or the*

J Rehabil Outcomes Meas, 1997, 1(2), 11–15
© 1997 Aspen Publishers, Inc.

process of care that helps to explain variation in patient outcomes.[1] As the outcomes movement grows in momentum and sophistication, and providers, consumers, and payers become more knowledgeable in the reporting and comprehension of outcomes information, there will be a corresponding need for classification of the available measures and preferred statistical methods for risk adjustment.

The types of outcomes routinely gathered in rehabilitation programs include measures of effectiveness such as functional status, health status ("quality of life"), satisfaction, and discharge disposition (return to home, employment); and corresponding measures of efficiency such as length of stay (inpatients), visits (outpatient), cost, and resource utilization. Patient and clinician reported measures are typically recorded at the initiation and at the conclusion of treatment intervention, and increasingly postdischarge for an assessment of outcome durability. Data collection at multiple points during treatment is optional during the episode of care. Demographic and descriptive information concerning the population is also collected, such as data pertaining to patient age, gender, socioeconomic status, diagnosis(es), comorbidities, and the acuity of the condition. For a detailed description of specific measures and methods commonly used in rehabilitation outcomes measurement, the reader is referred elsewhere.[3]

Health care clinicians have seen the promulgation of outcome measures and systems in rehabilitation and the development of national outcomes databases. A primary reason for this proliferation has been the need to reduce variation in observed financial outcomes while maintaining quality outcomes, provide benchmarking for quality improvement, and drive efficiencies in the delivery of services. The purveyors of outcomes database services provide periodic management reports to health care "subscribers." These reports deliver important information to clinicians and administrators regarding the overall effectiveness and efficiency of their rehabilitation programs and services through direct comparisons and "predictions" made by the database.

In order to fairly and equitably compare rehabilitation programs and clinicians, and provide for an "apples to apples" comparison; a method for risk adjustment that encompasses identifiable patient groups similar in terms of major characteristics is essential. For example, an outcomes management report reveals that a program's outcomes appear to be worse than predicted by the database (Figure 1). However, further investigation and analysis reveals that the facility does in fact treat more patients who have conditions that are of a more chronic nature, are older, experience more extensive medical comorbidity, and are of lower socioeconomic status. As a result, after "adjustment" for these factors, which clearly lie beyond the control of the clinician, the program's same outcomes are actually *better* than predicted by the database (Figure 2).

Outcomes that have not been appropriately risk adjusted are at best misleading, and at worst may abate the viability of rehabilitation providers who treat a higher proportion of severely impaired or medically complicated patients.[4] In a retrospective analysis of nearly 38,000 patients within 52 physician practices in a large staff model HMO, Salem-Schatz[5] reported that failure to adjust for case mix factors can result in overestimation of the extent of variation and misidentification of (provider) outliers. Indeed, after adjustment for patient characteristics in this study, there was a decline in greater than 50 percent of the observed outcome variation.

The process of risk adjustment within the confines of outcomes research attempts to mitigate and control for the influence of the confounding and variable risk factors seen in a heterogeneous patient population. Risk adjustment is of par-

Functional Health Status

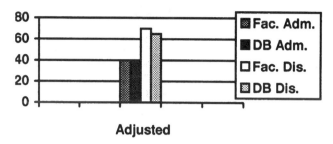

Adjusted

Figure 2. Facility outcomes compared to database, risk adjusted. Key: Fac. Adm. = facility admission. DB Adm. = database admission. Fac. Dis. = facility discharge. DB Dis. = database discharge. *Source:* Adapted with permission of Formations in Health Care, Inc., Chicago, IL, a subsidiary of Medirisk, Inc.

ticular importance in the analysis leading to comparison and prediction of provider outcomes in rehabilitation effectiveness research. There is a distinct difference from research methods employing randomized controlled trials, which meticulously monitor and attempt to account for these population factors.

The methodology of risk adjustment is complicated by the fact that no consensus exists for a standard risk adjustment measure or mechanism.[6] Despite this situation, rehabilitation outcome measurement systems both in existence and in development must consider and account for the presence (or absence) of many patient factors beyond the provider's control that affect outcome variance. These factors can include the number and type of medical comorbidities, the severity and chronicity of the condition, the age of the patient, the baseline functional and cognitive health status, and the length of elapsed time from onset of the patient's condition to the initiation of rehabilitation. Additional factors that may contribute to risk include utilization restrictions, the level of family support, patient motivation and expectations, and the availability of a preferred discharge location.

A research challenge exists in the identification and measurement of the factors contributing to risk, translating clinically relevant concepts into variables that can be measured reliably and validly.[1] Many risk factors can involve sensitive information that is difficult to obtain and measure reliably from the patient.[1]

In each rehabilitation diagnosis, the degree to which various risk factors are correlated with particular outcomes can vary with the outcome being assessed. Age may be an important predictor of functional outcome in stroke but may not predict as much variance as admission functional health status. Greenfield et al.[7] reported in a cohort of 283 patients who had undergone total hip replacement that the presence

Functional Health Status

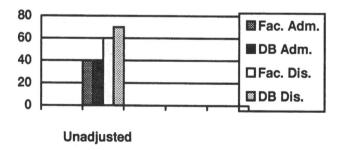

Unadjusted

Figure 1. Facility outcomes compared to database, not risk adjusted. Key: Fac. Adm. = facility admission. DB Adm. = database admission. Fac. Dis. = facility discharge. DB Dis. = database discharge. *Source:* Adapted with permission of Formations in Health Care, Inc., Chicago, IL, a subsidiary of Medirisk, Inc.

and amount of coexistent disease were significant predictors of postoperative complications.

Stineman et al.[8,9] reported on a case-mix classification system for medical rehabilitation. The functional related groups (FRGs), a method devised to classify multiple diagnoses of rehabilitation patients into 53 groups (analogous to DRGs), were developed with an inclusion of risk adjustment methods; altogether 31.3 percent of the variance in length of stay was explained.[8,9] The model included patient age, diagnosis, and admission motor and cognitive functional status subscales of the functional independence measure.

OUTCOMES MANAGEMENT REPORTING

The reporting and comparisons of outcome results among providers, programs, and organizations is developing rapidly. In order to more fairly and equitably compare outcomes of providers, there must be methods in place to both accurately describe and measure population risk factors. Methods of reporting outcomes data to providers must consider and statistically "adjust" for the influence of the confounding risk factors. When risk adjustment is considered in situations of more recent onset of patient conditions and treatment, the acute clinical stability and acute attributes of the principal diagnosis and coexisting conditions are most important in assessment and measurement. In more chronic situations and longer-term disability, physical functioning and various nonclinical factors are more effective in risk adjustment methods.[1]

Consider, for example, the "risk" of a patient presently in rehabilitation status poststroke. Although the diagnosis and primary pathology is the stroke itself with resultant left hemiplegia, the patient has had a past history of diabetes, osteoarthritis in both knees, and hypertension. These medically related conditions, all too common in rehabilitation, affect the plan of care and may affect outcome variation by altering the intensity and type of services provided. Additionally, the severity, location of the stroke insult, extent of hemiparesis, and number of prior occurrences all contribute to the eventual demonstrated outcome.

There are statistical methods normally used in evaluating for risk and predicting outcomes, through analysis of relatively large patient data sets that are statistically representative of patient parameters. Some of the more common methods are: multiple regression analysis (MR); structural equation modeling (SEM); classification and regression trees (CART); and artificial neural networks.[10] Although detailed explanation of these methods is beyond the scope of this article, the reader is encouraged to explore sources elsewhere.[1,11] These statistical procedures are designed to assess the impact of each risk factor and measure the contributing influence and "weight" of each factor upon the observed outcomes.

Even if the statistical methods used in risk adjustment to produce outcome predictions are considered state of the art, further work is often necessary to fully interpret risk-adjusted data and to clarify how the predictions demonstrate quality of care and cost effectiveness of provider treatment.[12] The fact that risk-adjusted data are used does not assume quality care or cost-effective service provision.

QUALITY OF RISK MEASURES

Measurement tools used in risk adjustment, as with the use of clinician and patient reported measures, must be psychometrically sound. The essential qualities of a quality measure, such as validity, are further described by Daley and Iezzoni[6] (see box).

• • •

At this point in the evolution of outcomes analysis, risk adjustment models exist that can be both costly and time-consuming because of the real need for retrospective data abstraction from patient records. There are some sophisticated computer programs available for performing risk adjustment, but most are used in intensive care or acute hospital treatment. These analytical programs are generally designed for predicting mortality, and do not predict rehabilitation outcomes such as length of stay and functional status at discharge. Velozo[13] and Stineman[8,9] have proposed that

---

Dimensions of Validity

Validity dimension	Definition
Face validity	A measure contains the types of variables that will allow it to do what it aims to do.
Content validity	A measure contains all relevant concepts.
Construct validity	A measure correlates with actual indicators of risk in the expected way.
Convergent validity	A measure has a positive correlation with other indicators of actual risk.
Discriminant validity	A measure has a stronger correlation with indicators specific to its purpose rather than with other indicators.
Criterion validity	A measure correlates with the "gold standard" measure.
Predictive validity	A measure explains variations in outcomes.
Attributional validity	Findings using the measure permit one to make statements about the causes of what is observed.

Source: Adapted with permission from *Risk Adjustment for Measuring Health Care Outcomes,* second edition by Lisa I. Iezzoni (Chicago: Health Administration Press, 1997) 336.

rehabilitation outcomes prediction should be based on admission age, diagnosis, comorbidity, severity, and functional status. Evidence exists that these variables can account for a significant amount of variation in outcomes.

Standardized methods for using risk adjustment technology to predict outcomes are promising. A model for case-mix adjustment of long-term rehabilitation outcomes, proposed by Segal and Whyte,[10] includes specific diagnoses, certain demographic variables, admission "triage" into rehabilitation, and measures of functional status, mortality, morbidity, and timing of admission after onset of patient condition as predictor variables.

As patient documentation of services is automated, with computerization of medical records and linkages to billing, cost accounting, and patient data repositories rapidly becoming the norm, the measurement of risk factors contributing to outcome variations will expand and become more simplified. Further research is needed to measure population risk factors, the process of care delivery, and treatment interventions. The need for additional measures and statistical methods for risk adjustment should not preclude use of current methodologies to measure and explain outcome variance. At the same time, resources are needed to support development of new measures and methods for risk adjustment that are more effective in explaining medical rehabilitation outcomes.

REFERENCES

1. Daley, J., and Shwartz, M. "Developing Risk-Adjustment Methods." In *Risk Adjustment for Measuring Health Care Outcomes,* ed. L. Iezzoni. Ann Arbor, MI: Health Administration Press, 1994.

2. Feinstein, A.R. *Clinimetrics.* New Haven, CT: Yale University Press, 1987.

3. Dobrzykowski, E. "The Methodology of Outcomes Measurement." *Journal of Rehabilitation Outcomes Measurement* 1, no. 1 (1997): 8–17.

4. Turpin, R.S., and Ratner, D.H. "A Method to Risk Adjust Rehabilitation Outcomes Using Functional Related Groups." *American Journal of Physical Medicine and Rehabilitation* 76, no. 2 (1997): 138–143.

5. Salem-Schatz, S., et al. "The Case for Case-Mix Adjustment in Practice Profiling." *Journal of the American Medical Association* 272, no. 11 (1994): 871–74.

6. Daley, J. "Validity of Risk Adjustment Methods." In *Risk Adjustment for Measuring Health Care Outcomes,* ed. L. Iezzoni. Ann Arbor, MI: Health Administration Press, 1994.

7. Greenfield, S., et al. "The Importance of Co-existent Disease in the Occurrence of Postoperative Complications and One-Year Recovery in Patients Undergoing Total Hip Replacement." *Medical Care* 31, no. 2 (1993): 141–54.

8. Stineman, M.G., et al. "A Case-Mix Classification for Medical Rehabilitation." *Medical Care* 32, no. 4 (1994): 366–79.

9. Stineman, M.G., et al. "Functional Gain and Length of Stay for Major Rehabilitation Impairment Categories." *American Journal of Physical Medicine and Rehabilitation* 75, no. 1 (1996): 68–78.

10. Segal, M.E., and Whyte, J. "A Model of Case Mix Adjustment of Long Term Rehabilitation Outcomes." *Archives of Physical Medicine and Rehabilitation* (in press).

11. Hall, G.H., and Pound, A.P. "Logistic Regression-Explanation and Use." *Journal of the Royal College of Physicians of London* 28, no. 3 (May–June 1994): 242–46.

12. Iezzoni, L.I., and Greenberg, L.G. "Risk Adjustment and Current Health Policy Debates." In *Risk Adjustment for Measuring Health Care Outcomes,* ed. L. Iezzoni. Ann Arbor, MI: Health Administration Press, 1994.

13. Velozo, C.A. "Limitations of Traditional Approaches for Severity Adjustment." Presented at First International Outcome Measurement Conference, Chicago, IL, 1996.

3

A Framework for Organizing Health-Related Quality of Life Research

George J. Wan, Michael A. Counte, and David F. Cella

THE CHALLENGE OF DEFINING HRQL

There is no single, universally accepted approach to defining health-related quality of life (HRQL). Furthermore, the operationalization and measurement of HRQL as a patient health care outcome is partially dependent on the contrasting perspectives of authors who have attempted to define HRQL. Three distinctive schools of thought have emerged from the literature: 1) the Social Science School, 2) the Health Indicators School, and 3) the Medical Ethics School.[1] The social scientists focus on developing indicators for social progress, such as a society's performance of specific functions (crime prevention, operation of the economy), in addition to the level of general well-being or life satisfaction of its population. The Health Indicators School emphasizes the development of health status measures as well as the evaluation of health care outcomes. The Medical Ethicists are primarily concerned with defining the meaning or importance of quality in an individual's life. These three models of HRQL have created multiple perspectives for conceptualizing HRQL. Hence, a systematic approach is needed to integrate the growing information that is available concerning HRQL.

HRQL instruments can also be used as either discriminant, predictive, or evaluative measures.[2] A discriminant index is used to classify individuals into underlying categories when no gold standard is available. A predictive index is used to distinguish between individuals with respect to a set of predetermined dimensions when an external criterion is available. An evaluative index is used to quantify the importance of temporal change in individuals.

HRQL Defined

HRQL can be conceptualized as either a multidimensional[3–8] or unidimensional[9–11] construct. It is generally agreed, however, that HRQL is subjective. Thus it should be viewed as a multidimensional construct that includes an individual's physical, functional, emotional, and social well-being relative to their actual and anticipated levels of functioning.[8,12–14] The conceptualization of HRQL as the gap or disparity between an individual's expectations and achievements was first proposed by Calman[15,16] and later studied by Wan et al.[13] The latter group of authors found that personal expectations influenced both overall HRQL and the dimensions of HRQL (satisfaction with treatment, physical, social, emotional, and functional well-being). Personal expectations remained important even after adjusting for the effects of sociodemographic and clinical characteristics such as age, gender, race/ethnicity, socioeconomic status, disease site, ratings of activity level, and disease stage. However, more research is still needed to identify factors that account for the large amount of unexplained variance in HRQL.

Purpose

Since there is no normative criteria or gold standard for measuring HRQL, differences in conceptualizing HRQL continue to exist. Thus, the primary objective of this article is to present a framework for organizing conceptual issues re-

Support for this project was provided in part by Grant #5 R01 CA61679 from the National Cancer Institute, David F. Cella, PhD, Principal Investigator. The authors acknowledge Steve Lloyd, Elizabeth A. Hahn, Chih-Hung Chang, and Maria Corona from the Rush-Presbyterian-St. Luke's Medical Center for preliminary review of the manuscript as well as data support.

J Rehabil Outcomes Meas, 1997, 1(2), 31–37

garding HRQL. This framework is adapted from those presented by Cameron[17,18] and Cameron and Whetten.[19] For purposes of this paper, HRQL is examined at the service delivery/treatment evaluation level as opposed to the organizational level. HRQL can be assessed in terms of the dimensions, perspective, unit of analysis, data source, referent, and timeframe utilized by the individual performing the evaluation (see Figure 1).

DIMENSIONS OF HRQL

It is imperative that the dimensions of the construct be clearly defined when appraising HRQL. Since a person's HRQL rating is subjective and assessed at the individual level, multiple dimensions for measuring HRQL likely should be considered. Aaronson[5] argues that HRQL is a multidimensional construct with four core domains: 1) physical functional status, 2) disease and treatment-related physical symptoms, 3) psychological functioning, and 4) social functioning. Additional aspects of HRQL include sexuality and body image, health perceptions, functional morbidity, cognitive impairment, and fear of disease recurrence.[5,20]

Other studies utilized factor analysis to estimate psychometric characteristics of HRQL instruments.[11,21,22] Cella and Tulsky[23] performed a literature synthesis of 24 studies and found 10 distinct properties of HRQL: 1) physical conditions, 2) functional ability or activity, 3) family well-being, 4) emotional well-being, 5) spiritual beliefs, 6) satisfaction with treatment, 7) future orientation/hope, 8) sexuality/intimacy, 9) social functioning, and 10) occupational functioning. Cella[24] contends that single-dimension measures such as pain scales, activity of daily living measures, and ratings of activity level are not acceptable measures of HRQL because they are by design unidimensional and limited in scope.

Factor analysis studies of three commonly used HRQL instruments demonstrated the replicability of four primary dimensions (functional, emotional, physical, and social well-being).[3,6,8,25,26] All four of the dimensions can be aggregated to form a single, global multidimensional index of HRQL.[3] These four domains are considered by many to be the core dimensions of HRQL. Functional well-being refers to an individual's mobility or current level of functioning. Functional activities of daily living include mobility, self-care, and ability to carry out one's usual activities.[24] Emotional well-being relates to the existence of psychological distress or symptoms such as depression, anger, or anxiety. Physical well-being refers to the presence of physical distress or symptoms such as pain, nausea, or fatigue. Social well-being includes participation in social activities, family relationships, and sexuality.[27] Cella and Tulsky[28] state that sexuality, leisure activity, and spirituality may be related to these four core dimensions. However, factor analytic or multitrait scaling studies have not consistently established the independence of these three factors as separate entities of HRQL.

PERSPECTIVE AND UNIT OF ANALYSIS

HRQL can be appraised objectively by use of a health provider or proxy (nonpatient) evaluation or subjectively via a patient's self-rating of their HRQL since the unit of analysis is at the individual level. The subjective (patient) perspective is clearly preferred since HRQL is usually self-reported. Studies have clearly indicated that demographic differences such as age, gender, and ethnicity influence the reporting of HRQL.

Age Differences

Numerous studies demonstrate that older adults tend to report higher levels of HRQL than younger adults.[13,29–32] Nevertheless, these variations may be restricted to differences on only certain dimensions of HRQL. For example, Wan and colleagues[14] identified lower physical and emotional well-being scores among younger adults.

Gender Differences

Many studies, particularly in patients with chronic disease, report differences in HRQL dimension scores among males and females.[33–37] Women tend to report lower scores on certain HRQL dimensions than men. These discrepancies may be largely related to gender differences in the reporting of emo-

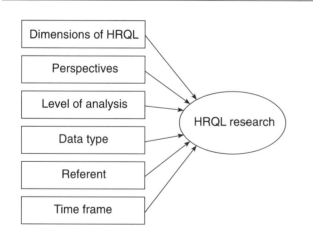

Figure 1. Framework for organizing HRQL research. *Source:* (1) Cameron, K.S. "Critical Questions in Assessing Organization Effectiveness." *Organizational Dynamics* 9, no. 2 (1980): 66–80. (2) Cameron, K.S. "The Enigma of Organizational Effectiveness." In *New Directions in Program Effectiveness: Measuring Effectiveness,* ed. D. Baugher. San Francisco: Jossey Bass, 1981. (3) Cameron, K.S., and Whetten, D.A. "Some Conclusions about Organizational Effectiveness." In *Organizational Effectiveness: A Comparison of Multiple Models,* ed. K.S. Cameron and D.A. Whetten. Orlando, FL: Academic Press, 1983.

tional[13,37] or functional well-being.[14] Another possible explanation is that men may be less likely to report extreme ratings (high or low) of distress than women.[38] In any event, multiple regression analyses indicate no significant differences between men and women in overall HRQL, after adjusting for other demographic factors.[13,14,38]

Racial/Ethnic Differences

It is uncertain whether ethnic or racial differences really exist in the reporting of HRQL. However, Wan et al.[14] found that Hispanics and black non-Hispanics reported lower scores of satisfaction with treatment and overall HRQL compared to whites. In addition, these racial/ethnic groups reported lower social and functional well-being after adjusting for clinical factors (i.e., cancer site, ratings of activity level) and sociocultural factors (i.e., socioeconomic status, survey method, religious affiliation, spiritual beliefs). However, these differences may actually be due to selection bias, interviewer bias, language of respondent, and comprehension levels. The adoption of cross-culturally sensitive instruments for assessing HRQL among special populations is necessary to sort out the relative importance of these variables.

DATA TYPE

The type of data employed is dependent on the dimensions defined, the perspective, and the level of analysis used.[39] Since HRQL is usually subjectively assessed from an individual's perspective, the most appropriate type of data is obtained from self-reports or interviews. The two approaches for measuring HRQL include generic instruments, which summarize overall HRQL, and component-specific instruments, which evaluate problems related to multiple areas of functioning.[40] Respondents with low comprehension levels often require assistance from the interviewer when completing these questionnaires. Specifically, numerous methodological issues are encountered when developing HRQL surveys for culturally and linguistically diverse individuals. These problems include the need for idiomatic translations, unfamiliarity with the questionnaires, potential lack of cultural relevance, and low literacy skills.[41]

REFERENT

The referent being used must be clearly established when assessing HRQL. Thus far, our review has concluded that: (1) HRQL is multidimensional and (2) it is based on an individual's self-rating of HRQL. The next question to ask is, against what standard do we measure HRQL?[42] Calman[15,16] explains that individuals perceive HRQL in terms of their hopes, dreams, and aspirations. At the treatment evaluation level, the referent for measuring HRQL can

be defined as the gap between a respondent's expectations and reality.[42] Thus the smaller the gap between these two reference points, the higher the HRQL (see Figure 2). HRQL can therefore be enhanced by either changing a person's expectations to reflect more realistic goals or improving the end results or outcome.[13]

However, altering an individual's expectations to reflect more realistic goals presents several measurement concerns. First, attempting to change a participant's expectations in a controlled environment such as a hospital or a randomized clinical trial (RCT) may promote a biased assessment of HRQL. In other words, the validity and reliability of the data obtained from the respondents may be suspect. For example, since the respondents in a controlled environment are essentially "captive subjects," and although they purportedly consent to participate, they may inaccurately recall key events during the evaluation process. The individual may also be reluctant to report valid impressions of what actually occurred. When HRQL is assessed in clinical trials, it may be inappropriate for practitioners to alter an individual's expectations, since this could be perceived as "tinkering with the data." Interrater reliability must also be estimated if several interviewers administer an instrument in one clinical trial.[43] These problems may be alleviated by eliminating potential sources of bias in the design or data collection stage of an HRQL study. For example, one way to reduce potential bias with respect to the administration of the data collection instrument is to maintain confidentiality of the study subjects as well as the interviewer. Another means is to implement a comprehensive training program for study personnel.

Nevertheless, Calman[16] contends that reducing a person's expectations does not necessarily deny hope but may actually permit an individual to construct appropriate goals. For example, it may be unrealistic for individuals who are in

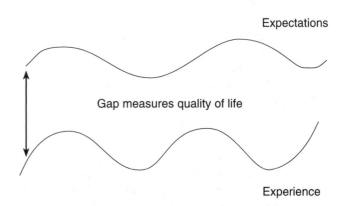

Figure 2. Improving HRQL. *Source:* (1) Calman, K.C. "Guest Editorial: Quality of Life in Cancer Patients." *Current Concepts in Oncology* 6, no. 4 (1984): 2–3. (2) Calman, K.C. "Quality of Life in Cancer Patients—An Hypothesis." *Journal of Medical Ethics* 10 (1984): 124–27.

very poor health to believe that their health will improve. Nonetheless, maintaining hope for a cure may be positively associated with higher HRQL in some individuals. Calman[16] offers nine basic principles to help understand HRQL in the context of individual expectations: (1) HRQL can only be evaluated by the individual, (2) it must take into account many dimensions of life, (3) it must be associated with a person's aims and goals, (4) improvement is related to the ability to achieve these goals, (5) illness and treatment may alter the goals, (6) the goals must be realistic, (7) action is needed to narrow the disparity between expectation and actual experience, (8) the gap between expectation and experience may be a strong influence for some individuals, and (9) the gap continually changes when a goal is reached and a new one is identified.

TIME FRAME

In contrast, different respondents may have varying perspectives about their own condition over a period of time.[44] The selection of an appropriate time frame is essential because a person's appraisal of their current functioning likely varies over time. For example, as a respondent's rating of their activity level worsens, individuals tend to report lower overall HRQL.[13,14] Unfortunately, current instruments usually measure an individual's assessment of HRQL cross-sectionally or at one single point in time.[40] On the other hand, evaluative instruments assess longitudinal changes in HRQL within individuals over time.[40] Temporal trends need to be considered when evaluating the impact of certain factors on HRQL. Accordingly, a respondent's assessment of their satisfaction with treatment, overall HRQL, physical, social, functional, and emotional well-being may also vary over time.

The importance of time frame in the context of HRQL and treatment is clear. An individual's assessment of HRQL can be measured at multiple time intervals such as prior to treatment to determine baseline information, during the middle of therapy, at the conclusion of the treatment, and some time after the end of the therapy.[45] A follow-up period is recommended in order to evaluate individuals who have achieved some distance from the acute diagnostic and treatment phase and may thereby add a valued perspective on the impact of treatment on HRQL.

Other factors that are commonly thought to influence HRQL reports over time include clinical factors such as disease site, ratings of activity level and disease stage,[45] treatment choice such as surgery or pharmacotherapy,[45] and demographic characteristics including age.[46,47]

DISCUSSION AND CONCLUSION

Conceptual and measurement issues regarding HRQL have been addressed in this article. As noted by Calman,[44]

HRQL encompasses all areas of life and experience as well as the influence of illness and treatment. Moreover, HRQL can be related only in individual terms and it is dependent on personal past experiences and future expectations.[44] It is important to identify the appropriate dimensions, perspectives, levels of analysis, data types, referents, and time frames when conducting HRQL studies. The dimensions of HRQL reflect the multiple domains that conceptualize the construct of HRQL. There are four primary dimensions: physical, social, emotional, and functional well-being. The perspective and unit of analysis are by necessity subjective since they are based on an individual's appraisal of HRQL. The source of data that is commonly used for HRQL measurement usually comes from self-administered surveys or interviews. The referent is defined as the reference point used for assessing HRQL. In this case the referent is the gap or disparity between a person's expectations of function and actual functioning. The time frame refers to the recommended point in time for assessing HRQL. (It is also important to recognize the limitations and differences between discriminative and evaluative HRQL instruments.)

Implications for Research

Since there is no single approach to defining HRQL, the considerations discussed serve as a useful frame of reference for patients, health service researchers, clinicians, and policy makers. Furthermore, this approach can be applied when assessing HRQL, formulating definitions of HRQL, and implementing studies that propose to improve measurement of HRQL. It is also important to note that these guidelines serve only as frameworks for assessing HRQL and should not be considered as absolute criteria.

Implications for Practice

As suggested by Calman,[15,16,44] to improve HRQL, an individual's expectations regarding treatment should reflect realistic goals. Thus, the disparity between a person's expectations regarding illness or treatment and actual experience should ideally be narrowed. In addition, individuals should set goals that are achievable. One need is for clinicians or policy makers to accurately inform the public concerning the risks, benefits, alternatives, and end results of a treatment regime or therapy.[13]

Suggestions for Future Study

HRQL measures are widely viewed as pertinent outcomes of medical and surgical interventions.[48–50] At the individual patient level, information pertaining to HRQL outcomes is often used to improve the quality of that person's treatment.[43] Although HRQL is evaluated at the treatment service level, there is also a need for researchers and clinicians to assess HRQL at the organizational or even system level. At this level, the information that is obtained from HRQL instruments may be compared within health care organizations (improvement evaluation), across institutions (comparative evaluation), or against some ideal criteria or gold standard (normative evaluation).[19] In other words, there is a need to evaluate HRQL as an indicator of organizational performance. However, data are usually gathered based on the participants' self-assessment of HRQL. Thus, this data source is subject to the advantages and disadvantages of self-reported data.

HRQL can also be used to measure the impact of pharmaceutical interventions on health outcomes. For instance, at the drug or therapy level, HRQL outcomes can be used to differentiate between two therapies with marginal differences in survival or morbidity.[43] Pharmaceutical companies are already using HRQL outcomes as a means of demonstrating value in terms of health outcomes and the expenditures associated with developing or adopting new medical treatments.[51,52] These medical treatments may include pharmaceutical, surgical, or other health care interventions. In addition, HRQL outcomes and pharmacoeconomics can be used to compare the medical costs and health outcomes related with new medical interventions compared with existing medical treatments.[53,54]

Perhaps in the future, HRQL data will be collected by insurers, consumers, government agencies, managed care organizations, integrated delivery networks, and other health care organizations to assist assessing internal effectiveness, improving the allocation of health care resources, evaluating competitors, measuring community benefit, and as a marketing tool for consumers and employers.

REFERENCES

1. Lerner, D.J., and Levine, S. "Health-Related Quality of Life: Origins, Gaps, and Directions." *Advances in Medical Sociology* 5 (1995): 43–65.
2. Guyatt, G.H., et al. "Measurements in Clinical Trials: Choosing the Right Approach." In *Quality of Life and Pharmacoeconomics in Clinical Trials*, ed. B. Spilker. New York: Lippincott-Raven Publishers, 1996.
3. Stewart, A.L., Ware, J.E., and Brook, R.H. "Advances in the Measurement of Functional Status: Construction of Aggregate Indexes." *Medical Care* 19 (1981): 473–88.
4. Schag, C.A., Heinrich, R.L., and Ganz, P.A. "Cancer Inventory of Problem Situations: An Instrument for Assessing Cancer Patients' Rehabilitation Needs." *Journal of Psychosocial Oncology* 1, no. 4 (1983): 11–24.
5. Aaronson, N.K. "Quality of Life Assessment in Clinical Trials: Methodologic Issues." *Controlled Clinical Trials* 10 (1989): 195S–209S.
6. Hays, R.D., and Stewart, A.L. "The Structure of Self-Reported Health in Chronic Disease Patients." *Psychological Assessment: American Journal of Consulting Clinical Psychologists* 2, no. 1 (1990): 22–30.
7. Ganz, P.A., et al. "The CARES: A Generic Measure of Health-Related Quality of Life for Patients with Cancer." *Quality of Life Research* 1 (1992): 19–29.
8. Cella, D.F., et al. "The Functional Assessment of Cancer Therapy Scale: Development and Validation of the General Measure." *Journal of Clinical Oncology* 11, no. 3 (1993): 570–79.
9. Karnofsky, D.A., and Burchenal, J.H. "The Clinical Evaluation of Chemotherapeutic Agents in Cancer." In *Evaluation of Chemotherapeutic Agents*, ed. C.M. McCleod. New York: Columbia University Press, 1949.
10. Bradburn, N.M. *The Structure of Psychological Well-Being*. Chicago: Aldine, 1969.
11. Ferrans, C.E., and Ferrell, B.R. "Development of a Quality of Life Index for Patients with Cancer." *Oncology Nursing Forum* 17, no. 3 (suppl) (1990): 15–21.
12. Cella, D.F., and Bonomi, A.E. "The Functional Assessment of Cancer Therapy (FACT) and Functional Assessment of HIV Infection (FAHI) Quality of Life Measurement System." In *Quality of Life and Pharmacoeconomics in Clinical Trials*. New York: Lippincott-Raven Publishers, 1996.
13. Wan, G.J., Counte, M.A., and Cella, D.F. "The Influence of Personal Expectations on Cancer Patients' Reports of Health-Related Quality of Life." *Psycho-Oncology,* in Press.
14. Wan, G.J., et al. *A Cross-Cultural Analysis of Reports of Health-Related Quality of Life*. Unpublished manuscript, 1996.
15. Calman, K.C. "Guest Editorial: Quality of Life in Cancer Patients." *Current Concepts in Oncology* 6, no. 4 (1984): 2–3.
16. Calman, K.C. "Quality of Life in Cancer Patients—An Hypothesis." *Journal of Medical Ethics* 10 (1984): 124–27.
17. Cameron, K.S. "Critical Questions in Assessing Organization Effectiveness." *Organizational Dynamics* 9, no. 2 (1980): 66–80.
18. Cameron, K.S. "The Enigma of Organizational Effectiveness." In *New Directions in Program Effectiveness: Measuring Effectiveness.* ed. D. Baugher. San Francisco: Jossey Bass, 1981.
19. Cameron, K.S., and Whetten, D.A. "Some Conclusions About Organizational Effectiveness." In *Organizational Effectiveness: A Comparison of Multiple Models*, ed. K.S. Cameron and D.A. Whetten. Orlando, FL: Academic Press, Inc., 1983.
20. Testa, M.A., and Nackley, J.F. "Methods for Quality-of-Life Studies." *Annual Review of Public Health* 15 (1994): 535–59.
21. Bliss, J.M., et al. "A Method for Assessing the Quality of Life of Cancer Patients." *British Journal of Cancer* 65, no. 6 (1992): 961–66.
22. Ferrans, C.E., and Powers, M.J. "Psychometric Assessment of the Quality of Life Index." *Research in Nursing & Health* 15 (1992): 29–38.
23. Cella, D.F., and Tulsky, D.S. "Measuring Quality of Life Today: Methodological Aspects." *Oncology* 4, no. 5 (1990): 29–38.
24. Cella, D.F. "Quality of Life: The Concept." *Journal of Palliative Care* 8, no. 3 (1992): 8–13.
25. Schipper, H., et al. "Measuring the Quality of Life of Cancer Patients: The Functional Living Index—Cancer: Development and Validation." *Journal of Clinical Oncology* 2 (1984): 472–83.
26. Yancik, R., Edwards, B.K., and Yates, J.W. *Quality of Life Assessment: A Pilot Study Report*. Washington, DC: National Cancer Institute, Division of Cancer Prevention and Control, 1987.
27. Revicki, D.A. "Health-Related Quality of Life in the Evaluation of Medical Therapy for Chronic Illness." *Journal of Family Practice* 29, no. 4 (1989): 377–80.
28. Cella, D.F., and Tulsky, D.S. "Quality of Life in Cancer: Definition, Purpose, and Method of Measurement." *Cancer Investigation* 11, no. 3 (1993): 327–36.
29. Sackett, D.L., and Torrance, G.W. "The Utility of Different Health States as Perceived by the General Public." *Journal of Chronic Disease* 31 (1978): 697–704.

30. Cassileth, B.R., et al. "Psychosocial Status in Chronic Disease: A Comparative Analysis of Six Diagnostic Groups." *New England Journal of Medicine* 311 (1984): 506–11.

31. Ganz, P.A., Schag, C.A., and Heinrich, R.L. "The Psychosocial Impact of Cancer on the Elderly: A Comparison with Younger Patients." *Journal of the American Geriatric Society* 33 (1985): 429–35.

32. Rodin, J. "Aging and Health: Effects of the Sense of Control." *Science* 233 (1986): 1271–76.

33. Schag, C.A., and Heinrich, R.L. *Cancer Rehabilitation Evaluation System (CARES) Manual*. Los Angeles: CARES Consultants, 1988.

34. Ganz, P.A. "Age and Gender as Factors in Cancer Therapy." *Clinical Geriatric Medicine* 9 (1993): 145–55.

35. Schag, C.A., et al. "Quality of Life in Adult Survivors of Lung, Colon and Prostate Cancer." *Quality of Life Research* 3, no. 2 (1994): 127–41.

36. Ferrell, B.R., et al. "Quality of Life in Long-Term Cancer Survivors." *Oncology Nursing Forum* 22, no. 6 (1995): 915–22.

37. Myken, P., et al. "Similar Quality of Life after Heart Valve Replacement with Mechanical or Bioprosthetic Valves." *Journal of Heart Valve Disease* 4, no. 4 (1995): 339–45.

38. Hadorn, D.C., and Uebersax, J. "Large-Scale Health Outcomes Evaluation: How Should Quality of Life be Measured? Part I—Calibration of a Brief Questionnaire and a Search for Preference Subgroups." *Journal of Clinical Epidemiology* 48, no. 5 (1995): 607–18.

39. Bedeian, A.G., and Zammuto, R.F. "Organizational Effectiveness." In *Organizations: Theory and Design*, eds. A.G. Bedeian and R.F. Zammuto. Chicago: The Dryden Press, 1991.

40. Guyatt, G.H. "A Taxonomy of Health Status Instruments." *Journal of Rheumatology* 22, no. 6 (1995): 1188–90.

41. Canales, S., Ganz, P.A., and Coscarelli, C.A. "Translation and Validation of a Quality of Life Instrument for Hispanic American Cancer Patients: Methodological Consideration." *Quality of Life Research* 4 (1995): 3–11.

42. Schipper, H., Clinch, J., and Powell, V. "Definitions and Conceptual Issues." In *Quality of Life Assessments in Clinical Trials*, ed. B. Spilker. New York: Raven Press, 1990.

43. Spilker, B. "Introduction." In *Quality of Life Assessments in Clinical Trials*, ed. B. Spilker. New York: Raven Press, 1990.

44. Calman, K.C. "Definitions and Dimensions of Quality of Life." In *The Quality of Life of Cancer Patients*, eds. N.K. Aaronson and J. Beckman. New York: Raven Press, 1987.

45. Cella, D.F., and Cherin, E.A. "Quality of Life During and After Cancer Treatment." *Comprehensive Therapy* 14, no. 5 (1988): 69–75.

46. Ganz, P.A., et al. "Exploring the Influence of Multiple Variables on the Relationship of Age to Quality of Life in Women with Breast Cancer." *Journal of Clinical Epidemiology* 45, no. 5 (1992): 473–85.

47. Sarna, L. "Women with Lung Cancer: Impact on Quality of Life." *Quality of Life Research* 2, no. 1 (1993): 13–22.

48. Eisenberg, J.M. "Clinical Economics: A Guide to Economic Analysis of Clinical Practices." *Journal of the American Medical Association* 262 (1989): 2879–86.

49. Patrick, D.L., and Erickson, P. *Health Status and Health Policy: Allocating Resources to Health Care*. New York: Oxford University Press, 1992.

50. Revicki, D.A. "Health Care Technology Assessment and Health-Related Quality of Life." In *Health Care Technology and Its Assessment: An International Perspective*, eds. H.D. Banta and B.R. Luce. New York: Oxford University Press, 1993.

51. Baker, A.M. "Practical Aspects of Designing and Conducting Pharmacoeconomic Studies." In *Quality of Life and Pharmacoeconomics in Clinical Trials*, ed. B. Spilker. New York: Lippincott-Raven Publishers, 1996.

52. Revicki, D.A. "Relationship of Pharmacoeconomics and Health-Related Quality of Life." In *Quality of Life and Pharmacoeconomics in Clinical Trials*, ed. B. Spilker. New York: Lippincott-Raven Publishers, 1996.

53. Drummond, M.F., Stoddart, G.L., and Torrance, G.W. *Methods for the Economic Evaluation of Health Care Programmes*. New York: Oxford University Press, 1987.

54. Banta, H.D., and Luce, B.R. *Health Care Technology and Its Assessment: An International Perspective*. New York: Oxford University Press, 1993.

4

Outpatient Rehabilitation Outcomes: The Cost-Effectiveness Challenge

Malcolm H. Morrison

The growth of managed care and the increasing use of outpatient treatment is resulting in a major challenge to demonstrate and maintain cost-effectiveness in health services delivery.[1] Traditionally, medical rehabilitation has been in the forefront in developing and using functional measures for documenting treatment effectiveness.[2] The influence of rehabilitation has been so successful that functional measurement is now used extensively for assessing the health status of patients receiving treatment in all types of settings—inpatient, skilled nursing, outpatient, home health, assisted living, and so forth.[3]

Despite extensive use of functional measurement in rehabilitation including numerous outpatient outcomes measures,[4,5] determining and documenting both costs and effectiveness of treatment remain problematic. Progress in developing cost-effectiveness measurement has been slow because of factors including multiple accreditation requirements, inconsistent measurement instruments, lack of databases and standard benchmarks, inadequacy of information systems, and the narrow focus of managed care decision making.

First, the number and complexity of accreditation requirements in outcomes/program evaluation and quality management, and their limited focus on costs, have not encouraged providers to address the cost-effectiveness of treatment. In addition, accreditation has addressed individual treatment venues, rather than the multiple levels of treatment frequently provided in post–acute care episodes. This has not encouraged development of comprehensive cost-effectiveness analysis techniques. Second, although functional measurement is in widespread use, measurement tools and variables are not consistent and costs are rarely measured

similarly by providers. National databases for outpatient outcomes are still being developed and refined and there are, therefore, very few reliable standards and benchmarks for comparison purposes.[4] This means that when providers perform cost-effectiveness analysis, the results can only rarely be generalized, although major provider networks may be an exception to this conclusion. Third, billing and cost-accounting systems are usually not linked with clinical data, and therefore, obtaining cost-effectiveness information is often difficult and sometimes impossible. And fourth, despite considerable discussion about managed care concern with quality, the current reality is that the price of services is the most important determinant in managed care decision making.

Despite these difficulties, there is agreement that in the future, managed care will want information on (1) short and longer term outcomes, (2) total case costs, (3) patient satisfaction, (4) post-treatment health care use, (5) provider quality, and (6) a measure of cost-effectiveness and/or cost and quality advantages to managed care. At some point, and perhaps quite soon, managed care organizations will want data on cost-effective continuum-of-care approaches for persons having chronic illnesses. How these requirements will affect specialty treatment such as medical rehabilitation is not yet clear. At present, usually the existence of a "standard" outcomes measurement system (preferably including patient satisfaction) and competitive pricing satisfy most managed care requirements. This is particularly the case for short-term outpatient treatment of orthopedic, cardiac, pulmonary, and neurologic conditions, where relatively rapid progress is expected and where "inappropriate" use of treatment is monitored. However, these initial, limited information requirements will soon be inadequate for providers who want to maintain their competitive positioning. As cost-reduction pressure increases, providers will have to manage treatment more cost-efficiently and effectively and this will mean up-

J Rehabil Outcomes Meas, 1997, 1(2), 43–47

grading their information systems to produce management reports combining cost, resource use, and treatment effectiveness data.

While there is general agreement that rehabilitation treatment must become "accountable" and more cost-effective, the methods, measurement tools, data, analysis, and information reporting needed to accomplish this objective are still being developed and are subject to change. For this reason, the response by both providers and payers to the cost-effectiveness challenge must be flexible and creative, so that today's information needs are met while preparing for tomorrow's more extensive reporting requirements influenced by managed care.

This article provides practical guidance in developing and implementing outcomes and cost-effectiveness systems for outpatient rehabilitation that will meet today's needs and be adaptable for future requirements. The discussion and recommendations presented here are not a substitute for a more comprehensive description of accreditation requirements or a more complete review of outcomes, program evaluation, and quality management issues. Rather, this article critically evaluates, selects, and clarifies outcomes evaluation and cost-effectiveness analysis, so that the reader has a sound basis for deciding how to proceed. This discussion also is designed to provide guidance in meeting the accreditation requirements listed in the box.

While it would be very helpful if there were a set of "gold standard" outcomes and cost-effectiveness measures, analytical methods, and reporting techniques, these do not yet exist for outpatient medical rehabilitation treatment. Therefore, some uncertainty will remain even after systems are developed and implemented.

While price continues to be the dominant factor in managed care contract decision making, most managed care organizations are requiring outcome and quality data from providers. And many are using profiling methods to evaluate providers, methods that include use of some limited outcomes and quality data. To some degree, managed care responds (sometimes very quickly) to changes in medical practice patterns when these result in greater efficiency of treatment and lower cost of care. If, for example, outpatient and/or home health treatment can be substituted for inpatient care with similar results, or if similar results can be achieved with fewer treatment visits, these will be preferred or mandated by managed care.

No matter how the debate about outcomes maximization versus optimization under managed care is resolved, "providers should be prepared to address the outcomes expectations of managed care entities: qualifications and expertise of providers, injury/re-injury prevention, medical complications, long-term outcomes, total case costs and reduction of future health care usage."[4(p.112)] To do this, providers need up-to-date information systems that effectively link cost and effectiveness (outcomes) information, a focus on efficiency in treatment, and recognition that health care delivery will continue to evolve toward even more outpatient treatment, an emphasis on prevention, and systems that efficiently and effectively manage the overall health care of patients whether on an episodic or chronic care basis. Meeting the cost-effectiveness challenge will therefore require use of outcomes management in outpatient rehabilitation.

OUTLINE OF OUTCOMES MANAGEMENT

Outcomes management is a term frequently used to indicate that a provider is using results of treatment to assist in managing patient care; that is, care is managed to produce the desired results. Sometimes, outcomes management is also assumed to mean that cost-effective and efficient care is provided. But this assumption is not necessarily correct if costs, effectiveness, and efficiency are not being measured, analyzed, and compared to benchmarks.

A comprehensive outcomes management program is generally used for five purposes:

1. marketing of programs and services,
2. quality management, including risk management, outcomes and patient satisfaction reporting, and case management reporting,
3. benchmarking for internal and external use,
4. accreditation of providers and to meet managed care requirements, and

---

Accreditation Requirements

*CARF . . . The Rehabilitation Accreditation Commission**
- Measures of effectiveness
- Measures of efficiency
- Measures of customer satisfaction
- Characteristics of persons served
- Interpretation of results

Joint Commission on the Accreditation of Healthcare Organizations†
- Efficacy of procedure/treatment
- Appropriateness of test/procedure/service
- Timeliness of test/procedure/treatment/service
- Effectiveness of test/procedure/treatment/service
- Efficiency of treatment

*Source: "Program Evaluation Management Reports," *1995 Standards for Medical Rehabilitation.* Tucson, AZ: Commission on Accreditation of Rehabilitation Facilities, 1995.

†Source: "Quality Performance Dimensions," *Accreditation Manual for Hospitals.* Oakbrook Terrace, IL: Joint Commission on the Accreditation of Healthcare Organizations, 1995.

5. request for proposal (RFP) requirements of managed care organizations.

Although information is presented differently in meeting these purposes, often a basic data set (including data on outcomes, quality, and risk incidents) can be used to satisfy many types of reporting requirements.

In addition to the above purposes, there are five new areas that soon may be included in outcomes management programs:

1. New accreditation requirements
   - National Committee on Quality Assurance indicators for Medicare patients in health maintenance organizations
   - Joint Commission on the Accreditation of Healthcare Organizations Quality Measurement Program (including approved software for measuring provider quality and outcomes)
2. Improved patient satisfaction measurement and reporting
3. Patient-centered care initiatives
   - self-knowledge/self-care
   - patient compliance
   - prevention
   - outcomes measurement
4. Disease management for chronic conditions
   - interventions
   - outcomes
   - patient tracking
5. Clinical pathways
   - describe treatment process
   - establish and chart goals
   - monitor and report outcomes

The timing and extent to which these new areas will be included in an outcomes management program will vary, depending on the extent and nature of managed care contracting, the speed of establishing new accreditation standards, the types and duration of treatment provided (changes in health care delivery), and the demonstrated effectiveness of these new techniques. Irrespective of current outcomes reporting, in the future, more complete information on patient results over time will be required by managed health care payers and health systems. In addition, there will be major competitive advantage in presenting cost-effectiveness information to payers.

IMPLEMENTING OUTCOMES MANAGEMENT

Outcomes management is basically focused on just three questions:

1. What treatment is effective (outcomes)?
2. What is the cost?
3. What is the value of the treatment?

Answering these questions requires information on patient functional improvement (focused on the presenting problem or problems, not just on overall health status), return to work or home environment, patient satisfaction with the process and results of treatment, length and intensity of treatment, and costs. Determining whether treatment is cost-effective also requires norms for costs and outcomes. If providers use many different measures of effectiveness and do not report costs in a standard and consistent manner, it will not be possible to objectively and comparatively evaluate the cost-effectiveness of treatment. Pending the development of nationally representative databases, providers can report their own information on results achieved and costs incurred. But, this information is of only limited value as a measure of cost-effectiveness, because it cannot be compared to normative data. It is likely that managed care organizations will use information from multiple providers to perform their own cost-effectiveness evaluations and then use the norms produced to profile providers. There may well be lack of comparability in these managed care analyses, but unless providers agree to use standard and consistent data collection tools, methods, and analyses, they will not be able to assemble a database large enough to use when negotiating with managed care organizations. In these circumstances, managed care can compare providers based on the limited information available (whether accurate or not) and base decisions and negotiation on that information alone. Thus, provider survival and competitive success will depend on having valid and reliable data and information to use in managed care contract negotiations as well as in quality improvement efforts.

To be useful, therefore, an outcomes management program must at a minimum collect data on patients, length of treatment, amount of treatment, and key outcomes achieved. A comprehensive program requires additional data on treatment programs, case management and patient progress, payers, costs, patient satisfaction, and follow-up results. In fact, only this more complete data can be used to evaluate costs and effectiveness, review internal quality, and identify quality improvement targets. Thus, to more completely respond to internal and external information requirements, data on patients, their treatment, and payers are needed (see the box).

Although these data requirements seem to be substantial because they involve cost-accounting, billing, clinical, and patient reported data, information technology now available can significantly reduce the work required to produce, analyze, and report the information needed. The use of electronic patient records, data repositories, and decision support analytical tools are several technology-based solutions to the increasing requirements for information.[6]

Establishing an outcomes management program requires decisions and action steps including choosing appropriate outcomes measurement instruments (or having these developed for specialty treatment programs), deciding on whether to

**Patient, Treatment, and
Payer Data Requirements**

Patient data
- Demographics
- Diagnoses
- Admission status
- Progress
- Discharge status
- Patient satisfaction
- Follow-up

Treatment data
- Type(s) of treatment
- Length
- Intensity
- Costs/charges
- Staffing (resource use)

Payer data
- Payment provisions
- Case management reports
- Patient outcomes
- Cost-effectiveness data
- Treatment length and intensity
- Internal provider analysis of payer rates (margin analysis)

program. While in most instances, some additional investment in information technology and services will be required to develop the program, this will often have only minor budget impact because of other technology requirements already being addressed. The focus of the investment should be on information production and reporting to meet internal and external requirements.

Benefits of proceeding with outcomes management include improved software for data collection and analysis, including software for clinical pathways, protocols, and outcomes tracking, improved information presentation and reporting tools, and faster electronic communication methods. While these new technologies are not yet in widespread use, reliance on paper records is decreasing, as are long delays in access to performance data. The major challenge is to organize, interpret, and report information on the cost-effectiveness and efficiency of treatment, and to be able to compare these data with credible national, regional, or local performance norms. Providers should prepare to meet this challenge and continue to expect requirements for greater accountability for the costs and results of health care treatment.

adopt a proprietary outcomes system provided by a vendor, deciding on a patient satisfaction measurement instrument, establishing links between cost and clinical data (and assuring that cost or expense data are reliable and valid), developing analytical and reporting methods for internal and external communication, determining the information needed to internally review costs, resource use, process quality, patient outcomes, and satisfaction and compliance with accreditation requirements and having that information reported, developing a method for consistently reporting cost-effectiveness of treatment, and establishing a process to monitor changes in provider, payer, and patient information needs.

Since these decisions are interrelated, it is crucial to establish a "general plan" that, although subject to change, can guide the process of developing an outcomes management

REFERENCES

1. Lansky, D.L. "Overview: Performance Measures—The Next Generation." *Journal of Quality Improvement* 22, no. 7 (1996): 439–42.
2. Fuhrer, M.J., ed. *Rehabilitation Outcomes: Analysis and Measurement.* Baltimore: Brookes Publishing, 1987.
3. Dijkers, M. "Measuring Quality of Life," in *Assessing Medical Rehabilitation Practices,* ed. M.J. Fuhrer. Baltimore: Brookes Publishing, 1997, 153–80.
4. Forer, S. *Outcomes Management and Program Evaluation Made Easy: A Toolkit for Occupational Therapy Practitioners.* Bethesda, MD: American Occupational Therapy Association, 1996.
5. Jette, A.M., and Jette, J.U. "Assessing Health Status Outcomes in Rehabilitation," in *Assessing Medical Rehabilitation Practices,* ed. M.J. Fuhrer. Baltimore: Brookes Publishing, 1997, 181–207.
6. Morrison, M.H. "Information Technology for Medical Rehabilitation." *Journal of Rehabilitation Outcomes Measurement* 1, no. 3 (1997, in press).

5

Evaluating National Outcomes Data Systems: Which One Meets My Needs?

Patricia Larkins Hicks

Survival in today's competitive health care environment is in part contingent upon rehabilitation professionals measuring and managing outcomes data. To effectively negotiate contracts, demonstrate quality to consumers, payers, and regulators, and maintain quality services, rehabilitation professionals must know the outcomes of their services. It is equally important that they know how their outcomes compare with other providers.

There are at least three nationally recognized outcomes database systems currently available in the market place: Focus On Therapeutic Outcomes (FOTO), Medirisk, Inc. (formerly Formations in Health Care), and Uniform Data System for Medical Rehabilitation (UDSMR). Given the increasing provider demands for outcomes data, other outcome database systems are beginning to emerge. It is essential that rehabilitation professionals know how to evaluate these systems so that they can select and invest in an outcomes system that best meets their needs.

FACTORS TO EVALUATE

When evaluating a national outcomes data system, there are at least 10 factors that should be assessed to assist in selecting an appropriate system:

1. subscribers
2. database size
3. outcomes scales/measures
4. data collection methods
5. data integrity
6. reports
7. training and support services
8. rater reliability
9. contractual requirements
10. costs.

The following describes each of these factors and questions that need to be addressed.

SUBSCRIBERS

Subscribers are the number of program participants who submit data to the outcomes database system. They may represent a variety of health care settings including rehabilitation inpatient, subacute, outpatient, home, and acute. Additionally, subscribers are located in various geographic locations.

To determine if there is an adequate number of subscribers that will allow for meaningful comparisons of data and to determine if the subscribers are similar to your practice, ask: "How many subscribers are submitting data?" "What health care settings do they represent?" "Where are they located?" Selecting a system based upon answers to these questions will begin to facilitate an "apples to apples" versus "apples to oranges" database comparison.

DATABASE SIZE

Database size represents the number of patient assessments and/or episodes that have been submitted to the outcomes system.

An adequate database size is necessary in order to provide outcome comparisons. Also, size affects the subscribers' ability to advocate effectively with payers, regulators, and accrediting agencies. To understand the systems' database size, you need to ask: "How many patient assessments and/or episodes does the outcomes database represent in each measurement system?"

J Rehabil Outcomes Meas, 1997, 1(2), 38–42

Selecting a system based upon answers to this question will assist you in awareness of systems that may be unable to provide meaningful data comparisons.

OUTCOMES SCALES/MEASURES

Outcomes scales/measures are commonly used in rehabilitation to assess patient acuity, medical improvement, functional gain, patient satisfaction, and quality of life.

When considering scales/measures and the determination of what they measure, ask: "What is this scale/measure designed to measure?" Answers to this question will facilitate selection of a scale/measure that will provide data able to meet your needs. Of course, this means that before you begin analyzing scales/measures, your data needs have been defined. That is, you have answered the question: "How do you plan to use outcomes data?" Understanding your data needs thoroughly will help define for you the data elements that should be collected. Additionally, it will help clarify for you the type of scales/measures needed.

When selecting a scale/measure, it is important that you determine the reliability and validity of the data collection instrument. Reliability helps to assess the reproducibility of the results. In other words, if you are administering a questionnaire, and you gave it to the same patient twice in a short period of time, the patient would give very similar answers.

Validity ensures that the instrument measures what it is designed to measure. For example, if you administer a scale to five patients who function independently and your results indicated that they were dependent in their ability to function, you should question the validity of the scale.

Remember to ask: "What are the results of reliability and validity studies on this scale/measure?" The measures must be reliable to be valid. Answers to this question will help facilitate the selection of a scale/measure that has been tested for reliability and is valid in specific patient populations.

When examining scales or measures, do not forget to determine how easy the scale/measure is to administer, and ask: "How long does it take to administer this scale/measure?" Answers to this question will focus you on the efficiency of the data collection instrument.

DATA COLLECTION METHODS

Data collection methods are the formats and processes by which data are collected and submitted for analysis.

These formats vary and may include: optical scan forms, data entry software, bar coded forms, paper/pencil forms, and standard billing forms. Examples of data collection processes being used include: completing optical scan forms, shipping to the outcomes database, and having the data scanned into the outcomes system; completing optical scan forms and faxing to a central database where the data are automatically entered into the system; submitting results through software by which the data are transferred into the outcomes system via modem or diskette.

Given the technological advances, other alternative ways of collecting and transferring data are being explored including the Internet, interfacing with existing clinical documentation and financial accounting software, touch screen and pen-based hardware, and integrated voice technology.

Data collection format will impact efficiency and staff productivity. For example, formats that require computer technology may or may not be more efficient than use of forms. To determine the potential impact upon the efficiency of your data collection and submission, ask: "What data collection format and process is required for participation?" "How much time is involved in collecting and submitting data?"

Some formats may not impact efficiency of data collection, but may impact the efficiency by which reports will be generated. For example, data that are submitted using a paper/pencil format that must then be keyed into the system after the data have been submitted will require a longer response time for reports than data that are transferred directly into a system via software. Another question that will provide useful information about the system's efficiency is: "How long will it take for reports to be generated once data have been submitted to the outcomes system?"

DATA INTEGRITY

Data integrity refers to the accuracy and completeness of data submitted to the outcomes system.

Systems have different processes for ensuring the integrity of their data. For example, in one system, database engineers clean, analyze, and standardize all transactions before they are entered into the database, ensuring that data-entry errors and statistical outliers do not skew the validity of the results. All new data passes through multiple screens that capture inconsistencies. Records are marked that fall outside predetermined tolerance parameters, and descriptive statistics and standardized variables are calculated.

Another example of data integrity is provided for through a data entry software program that allows for error detection by the subscriber prior to data transmission.

To guarantee that you select a system that ensures data integrity, ask: "What precautions are taken to ensure that data entered into the system are complete and accurate?" Additionally, to ensure efficiency, ask: "Are precautions taken to ensure data integrity prior to or after data submission?" "If precautions are taken after data have been submitted, what is the responsibility of the subscriber and timeline to correct problems identified by the system?" Answers to this question will provide useful information about the system's efficiency.

REPORTS

Reports are the presentation of the analysis of data submitted. Information can be presented in either tabular or graphic format. Reports presented in graphic format are generally more easily understood and more readily used.

Each system has its own reporting requirements, that is, what reports will be generated, when, and how often. To ensure that you select a system that will provide you with the types of reports that you need and within your timeline, ask: "What type of reports are provided subscribers?" "When are these reports provided?" "How often will reports be received?"

Because you may have needs unique from other subscribers that are participating in the outcomes system, you will need to ask: "Are custom reports available?" "What is the process for receiving customized reports?" Answers to these questions will indicate the extent of flexibility of the outcomes system.

TRAINING AND SUPPORT SERVICES

Training and support services are the assistance provided by the outcomes system to ensure that subscribers can meet requirements to participate and that all questions are answered in a timely manner.

The amount, type, and focus of training varies among outcomes systems. Current training include self-study manuals, videotapes, and one-day training workshops for staff and "train the trainer" sessions. To assist you in selecting a system that will provide the type of training that will meet your needs, ask: "What type of training is available to subscribers?" "How long will it take to be trained?" "When is training provided?" "How is training managed?" Answers to these questions will provide useful information about the ease with which employees within your organization will be able to use the system, that is, "How quickly will your organization be able to have meaningful data?"

A variety of support services are provided including an 800 number, newsletters, and various consultative and research services. To assess the level of support services, ask: "What type of support services are offered?" "When are support services provided?" "How often?" Answers to these questions will assist you in determining whether the support provided by the system is what you need and will be provided in a timely manner.

RATER RELIABILITY

Various methods of credentialing (training) clinicians and others providing ratings who will be submitting data have been developed. These processes are designed to improve the reliability of the data within the outcomes system.

To assist in evaluating the system's mechanisms to determine the reliability of persons submitting data, you should ask:

"What rater credentialing process is required for participation in the outcomes system?"

Because staff may be changing positions within organizations, or moving from one organization to another, it is important to participate in systems that have efficient credentialing processes. Useful information can be obtained by asking: "How much time is involved in the credentialing process?" Answers to this question will assist you in determining how quickly persons within your organization can be credentialed.

Additional information on the credentialing and training processes is provided in the section on cost, which follows.

CONTRACTUAL REQUIREMENTS

Contractual requirements are the agreed-upon expectations of both the provider and the database system to participate in the outcomes measurement effort.

Prior to selecting a system, it is essential that you have obtained a copy of the contract and reviewed it with legal counsel. In determining an appropriate system, you should ask: "What is expected of the subscriber to participate?" Equally important is to ask: "What does the outcomes system agree to provide the subscriber?" Answers to these questions will assist you in determining whether the outcomes system requirements are realistic for your organization. If not, you will want to ask: "Can this contract be modified to meet our needs?" The answer to this question will indicate the outcomes system's flexibility.

COST

Cost is the financial investment necessary to participate in an outcomes system. This includes both tangible and intangible expenses.

A subscriber generally pays a predetermined fee to participate in a national outcomes data system. This fee entitles the subscriber to predetermined benefits. To determine the fee required to participate in an outcomes system, ask: "What is your subscriber fee?" "What does that fee entitle a subscriber to obtain?"

Both data collection format and processes may impact cost of participation. For example, if a system requires a specific software program, subscribers will need the appropriate hardware support. If this hardware does not currently exist within the organization, then additional costs will be incurred. To assist you in determining all expenses associated with resources needed to support data collection and submission, ask: "What resources are required to collect and submit outcomes data?" Be sure to review costs associated with postage, copying information, and telephone costs.

Examine your human resource needs. Will you need additional staff to manage your participation in a national outcomes data system? If the answer is affirmative, then you will need to determine the costs associated with adding additional staff.

If the maintenance of data integrity is a part of the subscriber's responsibility, then you need to make sure these costs are calculated and included in your total costs to participate. For example, in the data integrity section, it was mentioned that some systems screen for errors after data are submitted. Subscribers then must assume some responsibility for correcting data. The estimated time and effort that will be involved in data integrity activities needs to be calculated so that these costs are included in the total cost for participation.

Sometimes there are additional costs associated with optional database services. If a system will flex to meet your individual needs, then there is a need to determine these additional costs, if any. To obtain information like this, an example of one question you might ask is: "Are there additional costs for customized reports?" If there are other ways in which the outcomes system is flexing to meet your needs, be sure and ask: "Are there additional costs?"

Depending upon the type and amount of training provided there will be additional costs. To determine training costs, ask: "How much does training cost?" If workshops are provided, be sure and ask: "What other costs must the subscriber incur other than trainer costs (e.g., travel and related expenses)?" If products are available, ask: "What costs are associated with the products (eg., manual, videotape)?"

In order to be trained, some persons may need to spend time away from their normal job responsibilities. In order to account for these intangible expenses, be sure to ask: "How much time will each person spend in training?" This information will help you calculate these intangible expenses.

If support services are provided by the outcomes system, determine the costs to the subscriber for use by asking: "If I utilize your support services, will there be additional costs?" "Are these costs contingent upon the frequency of use?"

Some outcomes systems have elaborate credentialing processes. If you choose to participate in a system that credentials raters, be sure to determine associated costs by asking: "How much does it cost to participate in your credentialing process?"

If legal assistance is needed to review contracts, the costs associated with these reviews need to be determined. These will represent additional costs to participate in the outcomes system.

When you have determined the actual costs to participate in the outcomes data system, you will then need to compare those costs with your budget. Comparing costs to budget will facilitate selecting an outcomes system that is affordable.

• • •

Before subscribing to any national outcomes data system, it is essential that you thoroughly evaluate the system and your own requirements. An in-depth analysis is required. Failure to complete an assessment across the 10 factors identified previously may result in your participation in an outcomes system that costs too much in time and productivity, provides information that has little value, and in general does not meet your needs. Investing significant time will prove to be cost-effective and beneficial in the long term.

Further information regarding the three nationally recognized outcomes database systems mentioned in the beginning of this article may be obtained by contacting them directly:

- Focus On Therapeutic Outcomes (FOTO), Inc.
  P.O. Box 11444
  Knoxville, TN 37939
  800-482-FOTO (3686)
  423-450-9484 (fax)
  http://www.fotoinc.com (Internet)
- Medirisk, Inc.
  155 North Wacker Drive, Suite 725
  Chicago, IL 60606
  312-849-4200
  312-849-3060 (fax)
  http://www.medirisk.com
- Uniform Data System for Medical Rehabilitation
  82 Farber Hall, SUNY
  Main Street
  Buffalo, NY 14212
  716-829-2076
  716-829-2080 (fax)
  http://www.udsmr.com

SUGGESTED READING

"Instrument Review Criteria." *Medical Outcomes Trust Bulletin,* September 1995.

Reynolds, J.P. "Are Your Ready To Join an Outcomes Database?" *PT Magazine* 4, no. 10 (1996): 36–42, 67.

Rothstein, J.M., and Echternach, J.L. *Primer on Measurement: An Introductory Guide to Measurement Issues.* Alexandria, VA: American Physical Therapy Association, 1993.

6

Outcomes Management:
A New Paradigm for Leadership

Mary Jo Marino

THE MANAGEMENT CHALLENGE

The management of a rehabilitation service has always presented challenges when the need arose to distinguish and differentiate the quality of patient care services. These challenges occur when the manager is motivating a clinician to improve their results, marketing the service, appealing an insurance claim that has been denied, or negotiating on a contract with a managed care organization. The inclusion of outcomes information into The Therapy Center, Inc.'s (TTC) facilities for nearly three years has added several new dimensions to our armamentarium of management activities. The purpose of this article is to discuss the vision of our outcomes philosophy, review specific applications of outcomes information, and to share insights gleaned from our past experiences.

RECOGNIZING THE NEED FOR OUTCOMES QUANTIFICATION

In 1994, TTC, a multispecialty, privately owned rehabilitation practice with six locations in eastern Tennessee, began the inculcation of an additional vision into its facilities: the measurement and management of outcomes information. The vision focused on the incorporation of a process of outcomes measurement into daily practice management activities, including the delivery of patient care and marketing. The rationale for this change evolved gradually from a paucity of treatment effectiveness and efficiency information when marketing to physicians and payers over several years.

With the onset of health care reform in the early 1990s, a startling wake-up call ensued when a large workers' compensation insurance carrier requested a meeting. I diligently prepared for the session with data from our practices regarding fees and the average number of visits with this particular payer. Unfortunately, I had mistakenly assumed that the topic of discussion would be price (level of reimbursement) negotiation. A large employer, one of the insurance carrier's primary customers, had noted that one of their employees seen in our practice resulted in excessive utilization of services and cost. Upon my later investigation the patient was clearly a statistical anomaly due to an outlier case, and I had minimal evidence to rebut this case and to demonstrate that the majority of patients seen in our practices did not result in similar outcomes. I experienced the painful realization that I had little information to talk objectively and functionally about my outcomes of care. I was literally at the mercy of the insurance company and their data. As a result of this case, I lost the confidence of the insurance carrier and the employer and subsequently lost a sizable book of business.

Prior to 1992, there was minimal motivation or incentive for provider change in our market. Patient utilization was largely driven by the experience of the clinician, the patient's relationship with the clinical team, and the extent of the patient's insurance reimbursement. We began our "outcomes" process with an internal quality assurance audit that identified and reviewed all patient cases that exceeded 10 visits. This case-by-case review evaluated the achievement and continuation of documented functional improvement by the patient. However, there was no tool or system available at the time that more objectively quantified functional progress and provided evidence of effectiveness in outpatient orthopedic rehabilitation, with the ability to compare our outcome results within and external to TTC. The managed care and reimbursement environment as well as rehabilitation practice consolidation was moving so fast that I became convinced that a new paradigm of practice was necessary to both survive and thrive. The vehicle to drive the

J Rehabil Outcomes Meas, 1997, 1(3), 58–62

new model and change for TTC clinical practice became the process known as outcomes management.

LEARNING OUTCOMES MANAGEMENT

In the fall of 1994, The Therapy Center contracted with Focus On Therapeutic Outcomes, Inc. (FOTO™), an outcomes database company, for participation in FOTO's standardized method of outcomes measurement for outpatient musculoskeletal rehabilitation practice. The FOTO process includes the use of the health-related quality of life (HRQL) measure known as the SF-36™ (Medical Outcomes Trust, Inc., Boston, MA); patient satisfaction measures; and additional indicators of effectiveness and efficiency. Quarterly outcomes management reports are provided for subscribers with several ad hoc reporting capabilities. The FOTO outcome reports are risk-adjusted for age, impairment category (low back, neck, shoulder, arm/hand, hip/leg, other, and total) and admission health status score of the patient. With the implementation of the FOTO process, I would have relational data on practice effectiveness, satisfaction, utilization, cost, referral sources, and so on, with a comparison to national norms. I enhanced and solidified my marketing and clinical practice improvement efforts.

The FOTO management reports list each practice location and provide patient outcome information in the six impairment categories noted previously. One measure of effectiveness in the FOTO system is the Outcomes Index, a computation of the health status change during the patient's episode of care. Another measure of effectiveness is the Patient Satisfaction Index, a computation of the overall patient satisfaction provided through a series of nine questions.[1]

A measure of efficiency in the FOTO system is the Value Index, which is the Outcomes Index divided by the average net episode cost. Another measure of efficiency is the Utilization Index, which is the Outcomes Index divided by the average number of visits. Each of the indices are provided for each of the impairment categories. The FOTO system also provides information on the mean number of visits and mean cost.[1]

IMPLEMENTATION

Two of the larger hurdles in the implementation of an outcomes measurement process are the inculcation of the long-range vision and the logistics of data collection. The rationale for this change and the vision must be carefully articulated and repeated often to both directors of facilities and their staff through multiple inservices and other extemporaneous opportunities. Shortly after beginning the new outcomes measurement process, it was apparent that few patients were entering the research. I began requiring the directors with their weekly report of new patients to list the number of enrollees into the

FOTO outcomes process. There was explanation provided for any patient who was not enrolled (e.g., neurologic patient, pediatric patient, etc.).

In the introductory stage, some of TTC's clinicians were unconvinced about the impending practice necessity for outcomes measurement, and felt unsure about the "intrusion" into patient privacy (the early FOTO outcomes measurement design involved information on the patient's socioeconomic status, and was subsequently dropped from the data set). There was also some redundancy of information collected from both the patient and clinician, such as the medical history. This implementation hurdle was helped by astute clinicians who began using the FOTO questions as part of their patient evaluation and assessment process, and alleviated by a subsequent elimination of several of the questions in the FOTO system.

Clinicians voiced a concern about the potential punitive use of outcomes information. This issue was addressed by permitting a period of time (one year) to collect a sufficient number of patient outcomes from individual clinicians, and allowing adequate time for clinicians to assume self-responsibility for improvement.

The process of outcomes measurement in our facilities began on a voluntary and experimental basis. Staff resistance to the implementation of the outcomes management process was considerable, and certainly is no different than other responses to change and unsettling of the status quo. The additional paperwork for the outcomes measurement process, albeit minimal and primarily patient-reported, was not received well. In a few months, the voluntary process was changed to mandatory. The cooperation from staff ensued with strong leadership and explanation of the long-range vision, the rationale for the change, and overcoming logistical and operational boundaries.

The enrollment of new patients into the outcomes research endeavor is not as difficult logistically as is the collection of data at the conclusion of rehabilitation. In order for an outcomes calculation to be completed with each patient, there must be either a status (interval) or discharge outcomes measurement. If discharge information is not available, or if a status measurement is utilized, there can be no calculation of outcome or the result may not reflect the full rehabilitation effect. Obtaining the discharge data was a distinct challenge, as the exact timing of each patient's final visit was very difficult to predict. Our capture rate for discharge information gradually improved with the implementation of procedures for collecting status information, providing phone interviews for the collection of patient health status data, and posting reminders throughout the facilities.

APPLICATIONS

There are three primary applications for the use of outcomes information: clinical practice; marketing to payers;

and marketing to referral sources. I would like to explore each of these applications in further detail.

Clinical Practice

The use of outcomes information has provided a means to profile the practice performance of our clinicians, and to identify areas for improvement both for our facilities collectively and for our individual staff members. Rehabilitation clinicians from a variety of professions have benefited handsomely in the past from lucrative salary and compensation benefits, and from generous merit raises, largely market-driven and bereft of performance measurement indicators. With outcomes information and clinician profiling available, there are opportunities to reward better performers. I have implemented a process that incorporates the use of outcomes information and results into compensation decisions. Although the use of outcomes information in compensation evaluation is new, it is very apparent that this trend will expand and become much more sophisticated.

The Outcomes Index provided by the FOTO system assists in the identification of specific clinical performance areas needing improvement in a *facility*. As the number of patients seen by individual clinicians and subsequently enrolled in the outcomes measurement effort grows, there is the identification of specific areas for practice improvement of *clinicians*. Continuing education can be planned more intelligently, supplementing developmental needs and areas for improvement rather than sustaining individual preferences and attendance at trendy programs.

I have avidly used outcomes information in my professional recruitment and retention campaigns, with generous allowances for continuing education. As our mission evolves to one of providing optimal and durable outcomes for the most competitive cost, I must know more about the impact of continuing education and clinical specialization on outcomes in our facilities. Do these mechanisms which purportedly make better clinicians indeed provide superior outcomes for our patients?

One of the surprises upon beginning the process of outcomes management was the discovery that in some situations the more experienced (five years plus) clinicians did *not* always provide better outcomes than the newer graduates, something that I would not have surmised. Upon my study and analysis of this situation, I discovered that some of our more experienced clinicians had become complacent and quite comfortable with the status quo. The newest clinicians were eager to prove themselves and their results. However, it became apparent that each clinician, whatever their level of experience, has an individual barometer, reaction time, and ability to change when provided a "report card" of their outcomes.

The standard FOTO outcome management report received by our organization revealed a substantial amount of comparative practice information. Although many of the measurement indicators were positive and demonstrated excellent organization performance, it was also apparent that TTC had opportunities for improvement. If the report was positive, a "marketing moment" existed. If the report was below expected levels, a management and practice betterment situation existed. In each of these cases a dimension of new information was now available: a quantification of functional change (level of effectiveness) in patients, and a comparative benchmark reference. Once this information became available and the staff became more knowledgeable, their questions became increasingly sophisticated. There were numerous requests for special reports that would enable staff to provide more definitive marketing plans or case management. I believe that an analogy exists when viewing a financial statement for the first time, and with time and experience gaining significant comprehension of the profit and loss or income statements. In some regards the outcomes management report was better, because it provided a clinical performance check. Even if our outcome results are less than optimal, we can demonstrate that we are doing something about it!

Marketing to Physicians

In a private practice the building of cogent relationships with referring physicians is absolutely essential, and a mechanism to assist in this relationship building is the creation of physician (and other referral source) specific outcomes reports. Many referring physicians are now asking for their own reports and are seeking information to provide comparisons to other physicians and specialists. For example, physicians have sought out outcomes data specifically for their patients with low back disorders, particularly in workers' compensation patients. The FOTO outcomes measurement system provides the ability to profile rehabilitation outcomes by individual physicians. With a minimum of 25 patients referred annually by a physician and enrolled in the FOTO outcomes system (which coincidentally is no small task) for the formation of a valid report, TTC has seen added marketing value through this incentive for physicians to refer additional patients.

Marketing to Payers

Health care providers are well aware that most payers continue to base contract decisions solely on price and location of facilities with little concern for quality and outcomes. However, each payer that I have presented comprehensive outcomes information (health status, satisfaction, efficiency, etc.) to has been duly impressed and excited to learn of our results and level of sophistication. I feel that as a result of our experiences in outcomes management, I have added to the information necessary for preparation of competitive capitation and other risk-sharing proposals, and have confidence in my ability to carefully "carve out" specialty services such as hand rehabilitation and industrial rehabilitation.

As rehabilitation providers, we are beginning to aptly demonstrate rehabilitation effectiveness in musculoskeletal patients, and determine the optimal expected outcomes for each patient at the initiation of service. As our experiences with outcomes management evolves we will more comfortably wear the hats of case managers, which will subsequently provide less incentive and perceived need for case review by the payer. There are clearly growing opportunities for "marketing moments," when outcomes information and prediction is available upon request.

Insights

There is a tangible learning curve in the comprehension of outcomes information, both for the clinician and change agent! The collective vision takes time to carefully assimilate and deliver to the staff. Early outcomes management reports may be laden with incomplete data and be very difficult if not impossible to interpret.

The logistics of data collection is not a task to be taken lightly. Both clinicians and staff must understand the vision for outcomes management in the organization. Patients need an explanation for the completion of health status questionnaires. Periodic meetings should be scheduled to discuss the outcomes process, and the facility and clinician results each quarter. There is continual discussion on the numbers of patients enrolled, and ensuring that adequate data are available for analysis and reporting. There must be an understanding of the need for discharge health status information, capturing the maximal impact of the outcome during the episode of care.

In new employee orientation sessions, I require staff to complete the survey forms themselves and provide an explanation of the outcomes measurement and analysis process. There must be a thorough understanding of all measure operational definitions (charges) and classification schemes (diagnoses, impairments, ICD-9-CM coding) in use with the outcomes measurement system.

The FOTO process permits the assignment of identifiers for physicians and other referral sources as well as payers. These custom fields should always be used for future outcome report purposes. There is much more powerful marketing impact in the reporting of outcomes specifically for referring physicians and identified payers.

I am and I have been convinced that TTC provides outstanding rehabilitation and was determined to show it. In order to do so, I needed a tool that would either support or disprove my conviction. I was surprised to learn early on in our outcomes management process that although we were doing well in many areas, we were not where I expected or desired to be in all areas. The FOTO data provided TTC with a baseline to determine our status, and helped set future goals for our standards of performance.

• • •

My vision for the future includes the integral use of outcomes information as an absolutely essential element in daily patient care and clinical practice management. Outcome "predictor" reports provided at intake will provide the ability to substantially determine utilization levels and resource use for the generation of optimal outcomes. I would like to base clinical compensation decisions more upon their demonstrated outcome results. In fact, already I have begun withholding or delaying scheduled merit increases when clinicians are below national outcome averages.

In this new era of health care delivery, we must seek out the best ways to rehabilitate our patients using our available resources. Factual information and data drive clinician change, not soapbox rhetoric. Clinical accountability is no longer an option but is clearly expected. The inclusion of outcomes information has made me a much better manager and has provided me with a catalyst to generate change. In the past, my extensive clinical and management experience was sufficient for responding to market situations. With the critical link between outcomes effectiveness and efficiency now a part of our business, information is now available for a variety of customer needs—clinician, payer, or physician. In order to survive and thrive in this era of managed care and changing health care paradigms, outcomes information is an essential element in patient care delivery and clinical practice decisions.

REFERENCE

1. Dobrzykowski, E., and Nance, T. "The Focus On Therapeutic Outcomes (FOTO) Outpatient Orthopedic Rehabilitation Data Base: Results of 1994–1996." *Journal of Rehabilitation Outcomes Measurement* 1, no. 1 (February 1997): 56–60.

7

Outcomes Research for Rehabilitation: Issues and Solutions

Susan C. Robertson and Anne Pas Colborn

THE DIFFICULTIES OF OUTCOMES RESEARCH

Outcomes research is essential in today's health care environment. Studies nationwide are striving to answer two key questions: (1) what strategies improve health while adhering to cost constraints; and (2) what information do practitioners need in order to improve patient health?

Yet, outcomes research is in flux. There are critics who argue that most studies have little practical application, promote overregulated practitioner behavior, and decrease clinical autonomy. Advocates take the position that outcomes research benefits patients, practitioners, and payers because it improves clinical decision and policy making by promoting a more client-centered practice.

There are two issues upon which critics and advocates agree, and both stem from the outcomes construct itself:

1. deriving accepted criteria that indicate outcomes; and
2. selecting appropriate research strategies used to understand practice processes leading to rehabilitation outcomes.

In order to determine which variables, methods, and designs are appropriate for investigating the outcomes of rehabilitation, one must first clarify what is meant by an "outcome." Measuring identified criteria is the second challenge. Each issue has serious implications for the continued recognition of rehabilitation services as critical components of health care. The purpose of this paper is to examine both of these controversial issues by offering criteria for defining rehabilitation outcomes, and suggesting research strategies suitable for today's rehabilitation outcomes needs.

J Rehabil Outcomes Meas, 1997, 1(5), 15–23

THE OUTCOMES CONSTRUCT

Defining outcomes criteria is the first key issue in outcomes research. There are two approaches to defining outcomes. The first is to contrast contemporary definitions with conventional concepts. Terms like *outcomes management, outcomes assessment, outcomes-based practice, functional outcomes, outcomes evaluation,* and *clinical outcome measures* are commonly used to describe relationships among health care practice and patient function. Outcomes management implies that there is a control over "outcomes." What is not clear is the nature of the construct under management. Functional outcomes imply that changes in patient function are the outcome measure. The problem is that function is a value-laden term with variable definitions. For example, in a patient with carpal tunnel syndrome, function may be described as 50 percent muscle strength, or the ability to fully flex and extend the wrist, or the ability to beat egg whites. Despite their widespread use, health care "outcomes" remain constructs that continue to strive for consensus definition.

There are additional variations of outcomes constructs. Managed care organizations, professional associations, health care facilities, and individual departments within a practice setting may have their own, more focused definition of outcomes. The point is that "outcomes" mean different things to different people, and the construct needs to be explicitly clear in order to study it and refine it. How outcomes are defined has great potential to challenge both the nature and form of research on rehabilitation practices.

What is the basis for current notions of outcomes? Outcomes constructs stem from two sources: (1) initiatives advanced by the health care reform movement in the United States, and (2) the World Health Organization's (WHO) conceptual frameworks. Health care reform has addressed three contemporary issues: (1) *costs* (managing increasing costs);

(2) *quality* (including measurement confirming the quality of services); and (3) *access* (all persons should have access to care).[1] Outcomes are not only about costs, quality, and access, but also about patient function.

Outcomes that include patient function have been provided by the WHO, established in 1980. Their conceptual framework for *impairment, disability,* and *handicap* considers impairments to be biological or physiological disorders, disabilities as problems performing required life activities because of impairment, and handicaps as the resulting, persistent state of needing adaptations in order to accomplish activities required by one's life roles.[2] The WHO's focus on function deemphasizes the current emphasis on costs, quality, and access.

Taken together, however, health care reform and the WHO definitions of health have effectively framed our ideas of rehabilitation outcomes. The health reform perspective leads to programmatic understandings of the outcomes of health services. On the other hand, the WHO's views on individual differences in function frame outcomes in terms of human performance. For the purposes of this paper, we have elected to distinguish *program outcomes* from *performance outcomes* because each is a complementary component of the outcomes construct. From each perspective, *optimal function* is the desired outcome of rehabilitation services.

Specific treatment processes contribute to changes in human function. Taken together, the full range of performance abilities influences overall human function and it is this overall function that measures program outcomes. This link between intervention and process outcomes as they affect program outcome has rarely been addressed in, but is essential to, current outcomes research. The next section explores the relationships among program and process outcomes.

ISSUES FOR PROGRAM OUTCOMES

Outcomes research that characterizes administrative program data, such as patient demographics, length of stay, or number of treatment sessions per diagnosis, can be called *program outcomes.* Program outcomes produce quantitative data about services provided, personnel, and resources used, overall level of independence, recidivism, and overall level of independence at the conclusion of rehabilitation. These data often infer the quality of a rehabilitation program. The inference is that rehabilitation was the sole factor for resolving impairment, minimizing handicap, or accommodating disability.

For example, a common outcome for a rehabilitation program is "increased strength." Increased strength is inferred to mean improved function, and thus, implies a positive rehabilitation outcome. The inference for practice, then, is that the rehabilitation program obtained a positive outcome by increasing a patient's strength, thus enhancing performance and overall functional health status.

For patients and practice, however, two critical questions are overlooked: *How* was increased strength obtained, and *how and why* does it contribute to a patient's health status? Program outcomes data rarely demonstrate why a particular treatment approach worked for one patient and failed with another—even though both patients had similar disease progressions, living conditions, and social supports.

Another critical issue in program outcomes research is the inference that data obtained for a group of patients has direct implications for the care of an individual patient. Grouped data might indicate that strength is best improved by a series of activities that require increasingly heavy resistance. One might assume that grading resistance is the key variable in strength development. What is missing is the view that other variables might have been causal factors. For example, perhaps the relationship with the therapist led to increased self-acceptance and motivation on the part of the patient to change strength. Or the patient was told that he could return to work and his reduced stress could have had physiological implications leading to better performance. These other possible causal factors in changing human function are rarely singled out for study. They comprise questions about the how and why of practice and may be called *process outcomes.*

ISSUES FOR PROCESS OUTCOMES

Process outcomes are changes in performance that a patient experiences during rehabilitation. They are the self views, hopes, expectations, and values that shape and are derived from the patient's involvement in therapeutic interventions. Process outcomes may be demonstrated through actions, behaviors, statements, and nonverbal communications. These ongoing outcomes guide the therapist in formulating and establishing clinical concepts of function. They are the most subtle indicators of progress in rehabilitation, but are nonetheless, extremely important. Taken together, they comprise the workings of program outcomes.

Process outcomes may be conceptualized as twofold: (1) how patients with individualized, complex needs *perform* given multiple treatment interventions, social and cultural variables, and health conditions; and, (2) why practitioners and patients *reflect* on and choose particular intervention strategies to influence performance of social, cognitive, physical, and psychological skills.

Because process outcomes are highly individualized, transient yet unfolding, and often not expressed, they require nontraditional measurement strategies. In order to produce evidence for the existence and influence of process outcomes in treatment, the research design and method must allow for recognition and incorporation of these variables into an overall study design. It is the authors' opinion that there is a need to highlight process in defining the outcomes construct.

INTEGRATING PROGRAM AND PROCESS OUTCOMES

Arguments can be made for continuing to investigate only program outcomes based on a traditional, clinical trials approach. After all, inferring positive, curative, indicators of function using a traditional clinical trials model has been the long-time standard in health care research. If *only* program outcomes are measured, practitioners assume the services they are delivering are what is making the difference in patient performance. This has the potential to be a false assumption.

While making a clear distinction between program and process outcomes has been essential in articulating these two constructs, it is also necessary to see how they relate. Process outcomes, the session-by-session changes in performance, culminate in the full functional picture of each individual. Comparing an individual from start to finish in rehabilitation yields an outcome of the rehab program, that is, the individual able to resume worker or other productive roles. A patient's time, experience, values, beliefs, and opinions about what worked *are* important because it is ultimately the responsibility of patients to carry over the positive effects (the successful session outcomes) resulting from rehabilitation interventions. The real strength of a rehabilitation program is to link program and process outcomes. If process outcomes, then, are as important as program outcomes, how can they be teased out from day-to-day practice? The next section of this paper focuses on measurement issues.

MEASURING PROGRAM AND PROCESS OUTCOMES

The second critical issue for outcomes research, the measurement of selected variables, stems from two problems. First, process outcomes have not been directly linked to program outcomes; and second, program outcomes have also been limited by available research methodologies and instrumentation.

Health care has traditionally approached outcomes using the randomized clinical trials model. The issue is whether the same method should be used to examine the outcomes of everyday practice: For example, should the designs and methods used to investigate health care products, such as new drugs, also be used to study the outcomes of noninvasive practice interventions?[3-5] The methods and designs of randomized clinical trials, considered the gold standard in medicine, are traditionally quantitative, and the resulting inferences are based on procedures that use random assignment, experimentation, and statistical techniques. While the clinical trials approach is critical for studies to determine the effectiveness and safety of new medications or invasive procedures, these same techniques yield limited information regarding the processes used by rehabilitation practitioners to obtain successful increases in function.

Using the earlier example of strength as a functional outcome, a study using a traditional clinical trials design and method would derive inferences about strength and health status by controlling, manipulating, and then testing strength with standardized instruments. Although methodologically sound, the traditional designs and methods for a clinical trials approach to outcomes can fail to account for process outcomes—the how and why of practice. It is critical for the continued success of rehabilitation to recognize, document, and demonstrate just how and why particular interventions worked for specific patients, given numerous, individualized patient and practitioner values, beliefs, and abilities, and treatment conditions.

WHY PROCESS OUTCOMES?

The need for data showing how individual patients, practices, and situational differences account for program variations has recently been approached by reexamining the quality-of-life and health status constructs. Traditional outcomes research has sought the patients' views on changes in quality of life, as a result of improved functional performance gained in rehabilitation. But this presents a number of problems.

Gill and Feinstein[6] note that each person involved in a health care intervention has a unique perspective on what constitutes quality of life, with regard to health. Different perceptions of what constitutes quality as well as outcomes are unclear and inconsistent. The search for clarifying real and perceived outcomes is leading discussions of the need for new standards for conducting research on the outcomes of practice interventions.[7] Witte notes that health care is changing from a "task" to a "process" orientation, and medical science's research philosophies and methods must follow.[8]

The next sections of this paper extend the investigation into research methods for current outcomes needs and propose that these methods are essential to the continued investigation of meaningful outcomes of rehabilitation. To begin, current changes in research paradigms will be explored.

PARADIGM SHIFT FOR OUTCOMES RESEARCH

Kuhn's now-classic work, *The Structure of Scientific Revolutions,* offers insight into how science changes its thinking. Kuhn states[(p.52)]: "As professions add new content to their fundamental bodies of knowledge [e.g., outcomes], so must they delete outdated content."[9] A new paradigm of what is considered scientific method and scientific research is fast emerging, although it may not be fully understood. A paradigm shift for outcomes research includes changes in the medical culture's ideas about the nature of questions considered relevant for patients, the instruments for collecting data, and the designs and methods used to structure a study.[7,10-13]

The ideas and opinions of practitioners, patients, and persons functioning as treatment extenders about clinical data from patient encounters are important for outcomes, as is the "everyday" data generated through practice. Methods and designs that allow systematic study and incorporation of typical practice data are much needed. Discussions of the need for multimethod approaches in outcomes research are beginning to appear in the health care literature.

NEW PARADIGM TERMINOLOGY

Simply stated, multimethod research approaches mean that different forms of data, such as words and numbers from various sources, may be used to answer the same research question. More than one data *source,* and more than one analytic *procedure,* can also be used for the same question. For rehabilitation outcomes studies, this means that formal evaluation, testing, informal clinical observations, or progress notes (data in the form of words and numbers) are regarded as sources, from which the data for systematic study may be generated.

There are some authors who use the term *methodological pluralism* to describe procedures for data consisting of words—often referred to as "qualitative" data—and numbers, "quantitative" data that may be systematically collected and processed.[13–15] Other authors use the terms *nested designs,*[16] *new generation research*[16] or *triangulation of data generation and methods*[17] to describe multimethods procedures for data management. Regardless of terminology, the strength of multimethod approaches for outcomes research is that both inductive and deductive inferences may be derived from data showing how rehabilitation practice occurs in the natural treatment environment.

NEW PARADIGM METHODS

Health care is not the first practice field to search for research methods to meet changing needs. Other practice-based fields such as business, education, and government service faced challenges similar to those of health care research during the 1970s and 1980s. Motivated to demonstrate the effectiveness of tax-supported programs, methodologists turned to then state-of-the-art scientific procedures outlined by Donald Campbell.[18] Later critiques of attempts to demonstrate program and service efficacy by Campbell himself noted how the findings of large-scaled studies were often misconstrued due to the lack of knowledge and understanding of program process.[19,20]

Methodologists in business, education, and government services fields have since been implementing applied research approaches especially useful for studying both the process and outcomes of practice. Three of the most common approaches are *case study research, evaluation research*, and *action research*. Analysis and interpretations of the data generated with case study, evaluation, and action research follow the principles of *comparative logic and inquiry*, that contain distinct procedures for either confirming or rejecting one's theory or hypothesis. Comparative logics build theories about study variables that are not suitable for experimental or traditional research procedures.[30–32]

The key to using multimethods and the logic of comparative inquiry for an outcomes study is that the techniques used to both *generate* and *interpret* data must be theoretically compatible. For example, qualitative data should not be used to "strengthen" quantitative data following a statistical procedure that produced "weak" findings.[16] It is, however, appropriate to plan at the outset to generate qualitative data via grounded theory analysis to derive text-based themes, and then conduct a quantitative content analysis in order to determine relationships among these themes. A descriptive, statistical procedure appropriate for nominal-level data is theoretically consistent for qualitative data generated through grounded theory, and then subjected to a quantitative content analysis. Thus, the interpretation of results are both theoretically consistent and compatible.

Table 1 summarizes the case study, evaluation, and action research approaches according to the type of outcome information or "product" rendered, the typical role assumed by the researcher, methodologically congruent procedures for data management, and types of inferences applied. A discussion of each approach follows.

CASE STUDY RESEARCH

Of the work by case study methodologists, Yin's[21,22] work is well-suited for both program and process outcomes. It is useful to distinguish the use of the term *case* as used in case study research from other uses familiar to health care. As an academic teaching tool, a typical or unique, single case provides learners with practice examples. In a research context, the term *case* often implies a type of design such as the one-shot case study, the single-case design, a single-system approach, or the case study mode of reporting. The case study research approach differs conceptually from these examples.

Four types of case study strategies are suggested: (1) exploratory; (2) descriptive; (3) explanatory (causal); and (4) evaluative,[21(p.38)] which has five applications:

1. to *explain* complex causal links
2. to *describe* real-life interventions
3. to *illustrate* certain topics within an evaluation
4. to further *explore* situations with no single, clear outcome
5. to perform a *meta-evaluation* of an evaluation study.[21(p.15)]

Yin notes that a researcher's choice of design depends on how the case and unit of analysis are defined.[21,22]

Vogt[23] further defines and clarifies how the terms *case* and *unit of analysis* are conceptualized for case study research design and method:

> Cases [are] subjects, whether persons or things, from which data are gathered . . . the smallest unit from which the research collects data.[23(p.30)] Units

Table 1. New Paradigm Methods for Outcomes Research

	Case Study Research	*Evaluation Research*	*Action Research*
Outcome	Program or process outcomes.	Program outcomes.	Process outcomes.
Product	Information about *how, why,* and *when* something works.	Desired end product is information about *what* works and when.	Desired end product is typically a strategy for immediate application to change the workings of practice.
Role of researcher	Researcher is often observer, recorder, and synthesizer.	Same as case study.	Same as case study, but researcher is often participant-observer.
Data management procedures (frequently used)	*Qualitative:* Grounded theory techniques. Critical Ethnography. Comparative methods including: • Pattern matching logics • Explanation-building strategies • Program logic models *Quantitative:* Time-series analysis.	*Qualitative:* Same as case study with exception of critical ethnography. *Quantitative:* Event-history analysis.	*Qualitative:* Grounded theory techniques. Critical Ethnography. Narrative analyses. Participant observation. *Quantitative:* Discourse analysis.
Typical level of data	Nominal Ordinal	Nominal Ordinal Interval Ratio	Mostly nominal
Inferences	Inductive Deductive	Mostly deductive	Mostly inductive

of analysis [are] the persons or things being studied . . . in the social or behavioral sciences [they] are often individual persons but may be groups, schools, rats, reaction times, perceptions, and so on. A particular unit of analysis from which data are gathered is called a case.[23(p.239)]

The designs and methods of the case study research approach are well-suited for the study of process outcomes, especially when specific practice variables are considered either relevant or meaningful for program outcomes. Because process outcomes often exist as practice phenomena characterizing the typical patient and practitioner rehabilitation encounter, it is useful to consider Yin's rationale when one wishes to "extract" or highlight features of practice in the natural setting:

> The major rationale for using this method is when your investigation must cover both a particular phenomenon and the context within which the phenomenon is occurring, either because; (a) the context is hypothesized to contain important explanatory variables about the phenomenon or (b) the boundaries between phenomenon and context are not clearly evident.[21(p.31)]

For example, based on informal clinical observations, a practitioner changes his or her treatment approach when working with patients in a particular stage of progressive disease. The practitioner notes that the change in treatment approach results in greater functional gains in shorter amounts of time, but he or she is not exactly sure how or why the approach facilitates these gains. Perhaps it is the treatment context in a given session. Maybe the gains occurred because the patient learned that a favorite family member could act as a treatment extender. Maybe the practitioner changed the order in which the rehabilitation modalities were introduced that day. An exploratory case study could help determine both the presence of and interactions among variables, thus setting a foundation for further study of the outcome of this specific rehabilitation process. While case study research is especially useful for the investigations of process outcomes, evaluation research is beneficial for studies of rehabilitation program outcomes.

EVALUATION RESEARCH

Evaluation research principles guide many of the current texts and procedures used for program evaluation and quality assurance in rehabilitation settings. As a form of outcomes research, both quantitative[24] and qualitative[25] evaluations may be used to test the impact or effectiveness of rehabilitation programs.[23]

Summative and formative evaluations are two types of designs frequently used in determining how a program delivers particular services. Summative evaluations describe an end product; formative evaluations are performed at specified intervals to assure the end product is obtained. Each type of evaluation targets a specific audience. Both summative and formative evaluations have an appropriate place in determining program outcomes.

Summative evaluations are often conducted for external audiences such as third-party payers, or other funding sources. The results convey program *effectiveness,* to find out what worked and what did not. Inferences through statistical procedures may show changes in a patient's length of hospital stay versus number of rehabilitation treatments, or severity of illness versus another criteria of interest to the external party. Information pertaining to treatment targets the types of interventions, the *what* kinds of questions.

Formative evaluations may obtain information pertaining to *how* a rehabilitation intervention occurred, but the study purpose is typically to target and correct potential program obstacles before they occur. For example, information on *how* something happens may show that one time of day is better for certain treatments given certain conditions. Formative evaluations may also be used to help redesign a program so that designated criteria are met. For comprehensive evaluations of program outcomes, both summative and formative evaluations are usually needed, and a variety of data sources are tapped. Typically, there is heavy reliance on in-house criteria considered relevant for collection and analysis purposes. Considering that specific criteria comprise program processes, another way of investigating outcomes is to engage both patient and practitioners in the study and search for solutions. Action research provides a framework for such investigations.

ACTION RESEARCH

The key to action research is the collaboration between subjects and researchers in order to effect change in a system. The system may be the "self," a program, or a process thought to produce an outcome. Persons other than practitioners are important in action research because they too have behaviors, roles, and actions that contribute to and affect the larger system. Often, it is the behaviors, roles, and actions of patient and practitioners that can either facilitate or interfere with the process outcomes leading to program goals or outcomes. Oquist's[26] description of action research shows its potential to target and improve practice processes: "Action research is the production of knowledge to guide practice, with the modification of a given reality occurring as part of the research process itself. Within action research, knowledge is produced and reality modified simultaneously; each occurring due to each other."[23(p.145)]

Theories of action propose that when practitioners learn about their behaviors, roles, and actions as related to a larger system, they gain information that sets into motion a "transformation" of previously held ideas, attitudes, or beliefs. These are described in studies of reasoning made popular by Argyis and Schön.[28]

There are several action research derivatives such as *collaborative research, emancipatory research,* and *participatory research.* The common link among action research and its derivatives is that they stem from the basic premise of "critical theory" as furthered by Habermas.[29] The word *critical,* according to critical theory, describes the critique of reason. A great deal of reasoning by both patients and practitioners guides the typical daily professional practice of rehabilitation. Some of this reasoning is used to guide simple task decisions in practice, but a more complex, *critical* form of reasoning may be much more important in recognizing the role of process outcomes in rehabilitation programs.

For example, a common assumption for rehabilitation practice is that when patients and practitioners recognize significant functional abilities that existed prior to a medical condition, incorporate the present, and plan for the future, positive functional changes are initiated. If the same past recognition, current status, and future functioning are then examined in light of the *reasons* behind a functional success or failure, and one "reflects" on these reasons, the process of reflection is set into motion. When this reflective process is able to bring about strategies for functional changes, it becomes *critical reflection.*

From a critical theory perspective, the ability of one to recognize, carry out, and then demonstrate increases in function from the act of critical reflection is called *transformation.* In rehabilitation, such a transformation in function is called *progress.* Data providing evidence for progress is part of the process of rehabilitation, and this is why reflection is a process outcome. These data include, but are not limited to, patient and practitioner statements or comments, both clinical and informal observations, and information from staff or caregivers. Reflection, and more specifically, critical reflection is considered both a method for generating data, and a technique for implementing change. For rehabilitation outcomes research, practice may be transformed because of new insights into the ideas, beliefs, strategies, skills, and attitudes guiding health and function.

• • •

Like traditional health care research, a decision to select case study, evaluation, or action research strategy for an outcomes study is guided by the study's purpose and research questions. Depending on how a case is defined, the case study research approach may be the most effective strategy for capturing *how* and *why* relationships among a rehabilitation program and particular processes lead to outcomes. If the purpose of an outcomes study is to investigate *what* happens and *when* during a selected course of rehabilitation, evaluation research may be the best strategy. When decisions need to be made about outcomes from selected practice problems, and it is essential that both practitioner and patient perspectives are considered, an action research approach may be best.

Case study research, evaluation research, and action research may be best described as strategies for systematically organizing and interpreting the various forms of clinical data important to the outcomes of rehabilitation practice. Assuming that outcomes stem from practitioner interventions that are part of a larger health program, the future of rehabilitation and its outcomes rests on the ability of researchers to implement designs and methods capable of capturing relationships among what the practitioner does (process outcomes) and a person's ability to improve function following rehabilitation intervention (program outcomes).

The need for meaningful health care outcomes has made it clear that both types of data, process and program, are needed in order to describe, define, and document practice so that outcomes specific to rehabilitation are clear. Case study, evaluation, and action research have great potential for guiding investigations leading to meaningful outcomes data. Each of the three approaches has a place in what may be considered a new research paradigm for health care, set forth by the need for outcomes data.

REFERENCES

1. McGlynn, E.A. "Domains of Study and Methodological Challenges." In *Outcomes Assessment in Clinical Practice,* ed. L.I. Sederer and B. Dickey. Baltimore: Williams and Wilkins, 1996.

2. Rogers, J.C., and Holm, M.B. "Accepting the Challenge of Outcome Research: Examining the Effectiveness of Occupational Therapy Practice." *American Journal of Occupational Therapy* 48, no. 10 (1994): 871–76.

3. Fuhrer, M.J. "Conference Report: An Agenda for Medical Rehabilitation Outcomes Research." *American Journal of Physical Medicine and Rehabilitation* 74 (1995): 243–48.

4. Wilson, I.B., and Kaplan, S. "Clinical Practice and Patient's Health Status: How Are the Two Related?" *Medical Care* 33, no. 1 (1995): AS209–AS214.

5. Mitchell, P.H. "The Significance of Treatment Effects: Significance to Whom?" *Medical Care* 33, no. 4 (1995): AS280–AS285.

6. Gill, T.M., and Feinstein, A.R. "A Critical Appraisal of the Quality-of-Life Measurements." *Journal of the American Medical Association* 272, no. 8 (1994): 619–26.

7. Lorig, K., et al. *Outcome Measures for Health Education and Other Health Care Interventions.* Thousand Oaks, CA: Sage, 1996.

8. Witte, D.L. "Measuring Outcomes: Why Now?" *Clinical Chemistry Forum* 41, no. 5 (1995): 775–80.

9. Kuhn, T.S. *The Structure of Scientific Revolutions.* Chicago, IL: University of Chicago Press, 1962.

10. Peters, D.J. "Quality Inquiry: Expanding Rehabilitation Medicine's Research Repertoire." *American Journal of Physical Medicine and Rehabilitation* 75 (1996): 144–48.

11. Sederer, L.I., and Dickey, B. *Outcomes Assessment in Clinical Practice.* Baltimore, MD: Williams and Wilkins, 1996.

12. Daly, J., and McDonald, I. "Covering Your Back: Strategies for Qualitative Research in Clinical Settings." *Qualitative Health Research* 2 (1992): 416–38.

13. Roth, P.A. *Meaning and Method in the Social Sciences: A Case for Methodological Pluralism.* Ithaca, NY: Cornell University Press, 1987.

14. DePoy, E., and Giltin, L.N. *Introduction to Research: Multiple Strategies for Health and Human Services.* St. Louis, MO: Mosby, 1993.

15. Miller, W.L. "Common Space: Creating a Collaborative Research Conversation." In *Exploring Collaborative Research in Primary Care,* ed. B.F. Crabtree et al. Thousand Oaks, CA: Sage, 1994.

16. Miller, W.L., and Crabtree, B.F. "Clinical Research." In *Handbook of Qualitative Research,* ed. N.K. Denzin and Y.S. Lincoln. Thousand Oaks, CA: Sage, 1994.

17. Morse, J.M. "Approaches to Qualitative-Quantitative Methodological Triangulation." *Nursing Research* 40 (1991): 120–23.

18. Campbell, D.T. "Reforms as Experiments." *American Psychologist* 24 (1969): 409–24.

19. Campbell, D.T. "Degrees of Freedom and the Case Study." *Comparative Political Studies* 8 (1975): 178–93.

20. Campbell, D.T. "Forward." In R.K. Yin, *Case Study Research: Designs and Methods.* Thousand Oaks, CA: Sage, 1994.

21. Yin, R.K. *Case Study Research: Designs and Methods.* Thousand Oaks, CA: Sage, 1994.

22. Yin, R.K. *Applications of Case Study Research.* Newbury Park, CA: Sage, 1993.

23. Vogt, W.P. *Dictionary of Statistics and Methodology.* Newbury Park, CA: Sage, 1993.

24. Mohr, L.B. *Impact Analysis for Program Evaluation.* Thousand Oaks, CA: Sage, 1995.

25. Patton, M.Q. *Qualitative Evaluation and Research Methods.* Newbury Park, CA: Sage, 1990.

26. Oquist, P. "The Epistemology of Action Research." *Acta Sociologica* 21 (1978): 143–63.

27. Tesch, R. *Qualitative Research: Analysis Types and Software Tools.* New York: Falmer, 1990.

28. Reason, P. "Three Approaches to Participative Inquiry." In *Handbook of Qualitative Research,* ed. N.K. Denzin and Y.S. Lincoln. Thousand Oaks, CA: Sage.

29. Habermas, J. *Communication and the Evolution of Society.* trans. T. McCarthy. Boston, MA: Beacon, 1979, original work published 1976.

30. Lijphart, A. "Comparative Politics and the Comparative Method." *Political Science Review* 65 (1971): 682–93.

31. Trochim, W.M.K. "Outcome Pattern Matching and Program Theory." *Evaluation and Program Planning* 12 (1989): 355–66.

32. Meckstroth, T.W. "Most Different Systems and Most Similar Systems: A Study in the Logic of Comparative Inquiry." *Comparative Political Studies* 8, no. 2 (1975): 132–56.

8

Outcome-Oriented Rehabilitation: A Response to Managed Care

Achieving cost-effective rehabilitation outcomes is a goal consumers and providers of rehabilitation have come to acknowledge and endorse. Historically, rehabilitation providers have been held accountable by their consumers (patient, family, and payer) for providing services. Today, providers are required to be accountable for the *outcome* of rehabilitation services and for ensuring patient and family satisfaction with the outcome. This shift in accountability requires rehabilitation providers to analyze closely the process by which services are conceptualized and delivered. The purpose of this article is to review a model of service delivery whereby the "outcome" from rehabilitation is agreed upon before the service is delivered. This model will be referred to as *Outcome-Oriented Rehabilitation*. It will be contrasted to a traditional "service-based" model upon which most rehabilitation organizations have been structured. Tools for delivering outcome-oriented rehabilitation will be reviewed, as will challenges inherent in providing it. The benefit of an outcome-oriented model of rehabilitation will be presented.

THE PHILOSOPHICAL BASIS OF OUTCOME-ORIENTED REHABILITATION

The philosophical basis of an outcome-oriented approach to rehabilitation focuses on aligning expectations among the payer, patient, family, and service provider regarding the outcome of care. Alignment of expectation is a process that considers

- the patient's potential for recovery and rehabilitation;
- locus of care, or the environment that is best suited for the patient's care (ie, acute rehabilitation, subacute rehabilitation, outpatient, home, or residential care);

J Head Trauma Rehabil, 1997, 12(1), 44–50
© 1997 Aspen Publishers, Inc.

- capacity of family caregiving;
- insurance/resource constraints; and
- the patient's and family's outcome expectation.

The process of "aligning expectations" is a skill that requires excellent communication and the ability to negotiate, problem solve, and resolve conflict. Often the case manager assumes this role in collaboration with the patient's physician and the rehabilitation team. Once all parties are "in alignment" regarding the anticipated outcome, the service provider is accountable to provide the services that will render the outcome. This process forms the basis for a rehabilitation outcome plan.

THE REHABILITATION OUTCOME PLAN

The rehabilitation outcome plan has four parts:

1. the agreed-upon estimated outcome for the continuum of care
2. the negotiated outcome from the designated locus of care (acute, subacute, outpatient, etc)
3. the cost for the outcome
4. the supports that must be in the patient's discharge environment in order to sustain the outcome.

Outcome goals are "front-loaded" into a rehabilitation outcome plan, which becomes the road map for the rehabilitation team, the family, and the payer. Specific services are provided for the duration needed to produce the negotiated outcome—no more and no less. For example, an agreed-upon outcome from acute inpatient rehabilitation is to return Mrs. Smith, who experienced a traumatic brain injury 3 weeks ago, to her home from acute rehabilitation with the following specific functional capabilities:

- self-feeding of solid foods
- continent of bowel and bladder
- ability to bathe and dress herself with the assistance of a checklist for cueing
- ability to climb 8 stairs to access her full bathroom with someone to stand by her for balance control
- ability to be left alone/unsupervised for up to 2 hours, with safety skills for emergencies

Intensity and frequency of services provided will take into account (1) the severity of Mrs. Smith's neurologic disability and (2) her functional strengths and limitations. All disciplines build their treatment sessions around the functional outcome goals determined by the rehabilitation experts, not by the payer. The charge, or price, of the outcome should be negotiated up front. The risk for meeting the outcome will be shared between the payer and the provider.

SERVICE-BASED VERSUS OUTCOME-ORIENTED REHABILITATION

Outcome-oriented rehabilitation stands in contrast to a traditional service-based, or cost-based, model of care in which the type and frequency of services are defined first and the outcome is often estimated and cautiously guarded. Under a service-based model, providers are paid for services or cost, regardless of the outcome result. The fee-for-service model of reimbursement, which flourished in the 1980s, created a "more is better" atmosphere in rehabilitation, with the assumption that better outcomes were proportional to service intensity. With the onset of managed care, fee-for-service was replaced with "per-diem" rates. Within a per-diem contract, the provider is paid a flat fee each day for services. Service intensity is managed by the provider.

In an outcome-oriented model of care, the provider is paid for a negotiated outcome. If the outcome is reached within the agreed-upon time frame, the provider is paid the full negotiated rate. If the outcome is not met, the provider is paid up to the agreed-upon timeframe for outcome achievement. Following that timeframe, the amount paid becomes less each day the length of stay is extended. This model reinforces outcome attainment within a specified timeframe. Providers who are best positioned to enter into an outcome reimbursement model are those who have extensive experience within rehabilitation and disability management. Tracking outcomes longitudinally is essential for the provider and the payer who enter into an outcome reimbursement model.

OUTCOMES AND SERVICE INTENSITY

In reviewing outcome literature for brain injury rehabilitation, there are no data to substantiate the "more is better"

concept. There is evidence, however, to support the fact that the timing and duration of rehabilitation services are critical to outcomes.[1-4] Hall and Wright[1] noted that better outcomes were associated with patients who received rehabilitation services earlier rather than later following their injury. Prigatano et al[2] noted that patients' outcomes in the postacute stages of recovery were affected by their "readiness" for services. They suggested that patients who displayed an awareness of their deficits were more actively engaged and motivated by the rehabilitation process and had better psychosocial and vocational outcomes than patients who had deficits of awareness. Ben-Yishay et al[3] noted that the "durability" of vocational outcomes was largely influenced by the absence of an adequate maintenance/support system. Haffey and Abrams[4] noted a significant decrease in vocational outcomes using a supported employment model when the duration of services were reduced.

These outcome studies may suggest that in a managed care environment where reimbursement is limited, or capped, rehabilitation services should be prioritized according to patient "readiness" for a particular service, and duration of service is more important than intensity. Rather than allocating all rehabilitation services into a single service location for a single length of stay, services should be streamlined over time, based on patient readiness. Access to a continuum of care is critical. Conceptualizing the long-term outcome early in the rehabilitation process and knowing when to prioritize services longitudinally is important. For example, in a managed care contract, the patient may have only 12 or fewer sessions of outpatient physical therapy, occupational therapy, and speech therapy services. Spreading these sessions over a longer period of time with a home reinforcement program would be a better resource allocation than using all sessions in succession.

PARAMETERS OF OUTCOME-ORIENTED REHABILITATION

The central organizing focus of outcome-oriented rehabilitation is the discharge environment—the environment to which the patient will return and the outcome of service will be applied. As such, a thorough assessment of the skills required by the discharge environment is essential. Family supports and resources must be identified early, as well as the family willingness and capability to assist the disabled family member. The acute rehabilitation outcome plan and treatment focus will differ significantly for a patient who will be discharged to home compared with one who will be discharged to a long-term skilled care facility.

Outcome-oriented rehabilitation seeks to reduce the level of disability and therefore must be "functional" in its approach. In the early 1980s, brain injury rehabilitation was primarily impairment focused. Rehabilitation professionals prioritized treatment of myriad underlying deficits required to effect a functional skill, anticipating that such an approach would improve the acquisition of functional skills. An example of this approach is the remediation of cognitive deficits with the use of computer-based exercises. In an era of shorter lengths of stay and reduced resource allocation, clinicians need to know whether to use compensation or remediation techniques. Knowing the approach that will most enhance the functional result in the shortest amount of time is preferable. For example, pencil-and-paper workbook activities often take up valuable treatment time that might be better spent working directly on the desired functional behavior. A patient who has significant memory impairments, and therefore cannot safely be left alone, might benefit more from learning how to use an environmental cueing device such as Neuropager[5] than from sessions spent on memory rehearsal techniques.

Teaching of family members must begin early in the rehabilitation process. In a managed care environment, the burden of care is shifted to the family almost immediately. Because patients often return home within weeks, or perhaps even days, after the brain injury, family teaching of rehabilitation is critical and may require almost as much treatment time as patient training. Families who are overwhelmed with the impact of brain injury may exhibit a reduced capacity to learn. Family teaching must be structured using written material that is user friendly rather than laden with professional jargon.

Generalization of skills must be a part of the outcome treatment plan. In addition to using a functional approach to treatment, the outcome plan must allow for, and build in, strategies for skill generalization. For outcomes to be "durable," there must be a system of support built into the discharge environment that will serve to maintain the outcome.

Outcome-oriented rehabilitation is contrasted to traditional serviced-based rehabilitation in the box, "Service-Based versus Outcome-Based Rehabilitation."

TOOLS TO FACILITATE OUTCOME-ORIENTED REHABILITATION

Tools are needed to support an outcome approach to rehabilitation and to guide the behavior of clinicians as they focus their work on outcomes. These tools include the following[6]:

- A schema for defining clinical outcomes. The schema may be program based or organized according to level of care. In either case, identified outcomes must be integrated into the program evaluation system.
- Critical pathways. Critical pathways are guidelines for mapping progression of treatment activities and anticipated outcomes within specified timeframes. Pathways should serve as guidelines rather than restrictive protocols. They should be outcome focused and goal directed. Pathways should identify the personnel accountable for accomplishing activities and may be written on the patient's chart to serve as a documentation tool.

  When outcome targets are not met, a variance report should be completed, since analysis of variance reports can be very informative. Such reports adjust the pathway to greater accuracy and identify outliers who are at risk for the planned outcomes. Such data are critical for negotiations with payers, as they substantiate and verify reimbursement and timeframes for outcome completion.
- A documentation system that is user friendly and outcome focused. Documentation focused exclusively on impairments is not useful in an outcome-oriented approach to rehabilitation. Documentation must reflect the targeted outcomes and progress or barriers toward outcome achievement.
- An outcome tracking system. A longitudinal outcome tracking system can measure effectiveness and efficiency by measuring progress toward outcome achieve-

---

Service-Based versus Outcome-Based Rehabilitation

Service-based rehabilitation	*Outcome-based rehabilitation*
• Assesses the patient's impairments	• Utilizes a patient-centered assessment
• Defines assessment parameters according to the discipline	• Defines assessment parameters according to the discharge environment; focuses on the skill requirements of the discharge environment
• Organizes treatment plan around patient limitations	• Organizes treatment plan around skill requirements of the discharge setting
• Focuses treatment on reduction of impairments that underlie skill; remediates first and compensates as last resort	• Focuses treatment on functional skill reacquisition; considers compensation first
• Sets discipline-based goals	• Sets functional goals based on the outcome result to be achieved
• Provides family teaching at the time of discharge	• Begins family teaching at admission and continues throughout duration of treatment
• Assumes skill generalization	• Builds skill generalization into treatment plan

ment. These data provide feedback about clinician effectiveness in targeting outcomes, and clinician efficiency in predicting length of time and magnitude of resources required to obtain outcomes. They assist clinicians in predicting clinical outcomes more accurately. An outcome tracking system should include at least three domains of outcomes:

1. Technical/clinical (ie, mobility, self-care, etc).
2. Cost-effectiveness.
3. Patient satisfaction: Was the patient satisfied with the program? Did the program deliver what was agreed to and expected by the patient? (*Note*: satisfaction data are based on the degree to which the patient and family were satisfied with the care they received and the outcome from those services, as opposed to being satisfied with the outcome of the injury. It is not expected that patients and their families will be satisfied with the longevity of their disability.)

CHALLENGES/BARRIERS TO OUTCOME-ORIENTED REHABILITATION

An outcome-oriented approach to rehabilitation initially appears to require only a subtle shift in the way clinicians organize and prioritize rehabilitation services. However, this system actually has a profound effect on rehabilitation organizations, because it moves them from an expert/medical driven model of care to a consumer-based model of care. Consequently, the power base of the organization is shifted. Where there was once a medical/expert orientation in which patients were the recipients of care, an outcome-oriented model gives patients, their families, and the payer equal voice in the outcome and the plan of care. Rehabilitation practitioners may feel threatened by this change. Several issues that may arise among medical and clinical staffs when moving into an outcome-oriented model are:

- "We can't predict an outcome when we don't know how the patient will respond to treatment."
- "The outcome approach forces us (the team) to work on only a few areas; we should work on all areas for total rehabilitation."
- "We went into rehabilitation to help restore the patient to the highest level of independence; now we work on only a piece of that goal."
- "If we had more time, we could complete our work" (the "more is better" concept).
- "We are forced to choose between (our ideal of) quality versus acceptable rehabilitation outcomes."

Such reactions are both predictable and reasonable. They reflect the frustration of rehabilitation professionals with a health care industry that has become increasingly restrictive with resources and demands ever-increasing accountability for results. These reactions will subside as the success of using an outcome-oriented approach to treatment becomes more evident.[6]

BENEFITS OF AN OUTCOME-ORIENTED MODEL

Employing an outcome model of rehabilitation yields the following three benefits:

1. Patients, families, and payers have clearer and more realistic expectations regarding the results of rehabilitation. This can result in assisting the patient and family with adjusting to the long-term consequences of the disability.
2. Patients, families, and payers have shared accountability for the agreed-upon outcomes with the rehabilitation provider. All consumers are stakeholders in the outcome. This promotes teamwork and momentum toward outcome achievement.
3. Outcome-oriented rehabilitation is cost-effective. Only services that support the outcome are provided. The length of stay is often reduced compared with that in a traditional service-based model because there is an alignment of the planned outcome and a focused approach to treatment.

CONCLUSION

Managed care has challenged traditional rehabilitation models, and consequently new models of care are emerging. Outcome-oriented rehabilitation is a qualitative, cost-effective method for identifying and obtaining realistic outcome results from rehabilitation, and it is an optimal way of conceptualizing, organizing, and delivering rehabilitation services. This approach acknowledges the centrality of the consumers' role in identifying and building the rehabilitation outcome plan. As we move into the future, health care and rehabilitation providers must be willing to assume responsibility and accountability for results. Outcome-oriented rehabilitation is based on shared accountability for results among the primary stakeholders.

REFERENCES

1. Hall K, Wright J. The cost versus benefit of rehabilitation in traumatic brain injury. Presented at 11th Annual Southwest Brain Injury Symposium; January 18, 1993; Santa Barbara, Calif.
2. Prigatano GP, Klonoff PS, Bailey I. Psychosocial adjustment associated with traumatic brain injury: statistics BNI neuro-rehabilitation must beat. *BNI Q.* 1987;3:10–17.

3. Ben-Yishay Y, Silver SM, Piasetsky E, et al. Relationship between employability and vocational outcome after intensive holistic cognitive rehabilitation. *J Head Trauma Rehabil.* 1978;2(1):35–48.

4. Haffey W, Abrams D. Employment outcomes for participants in a brain injury work reentry program: preliminary findings. *J Head Trauma Rehabil.* 1991; 6(3):24–34.

5. Spivack M. Neuropager. Presented at the National Brain Injury Annual Symposium; December 3–6 1995; San Diego, Calif.

6. Schmidt, N. Preparing rehabilitation teams for outcome-based rehabilitation. In: Landrum, Schmidt, McLean, eds. *Outcome-Oriented Rehabilitation: Principles, Strategies, and Tools for Effective Program Management.* Gaithersburg, Md: Aspen; 1995.

9

The Influence of Outcome Studies on Rehabilitation Policy

J. Scott Ling and Randall W. Evans

Most clinical professions are governed by ethical guidelines and a code of conduct set forth by each discipline's governing body, and most provider service organizations have set forth their own ethical guidelines, frequently as part of their mission statement.[1] Ethics are guidelines drawn from personal values, culture, and experience in the specific area of focus. The primary goal of ethical guidelines is to ensure the welfare and protection of individuals and groups affected by the service or product. Typically, a discipline's code of ethics includes statements designed to guide practitioners in their responsibility to remain up to date in their professional knowledge and awareness of confidentiality issues, obligations to protect the public and consumers, obligations to protect the welfare of research participants and others affected by the research, and a host of other specific issues and areas.

Brain injury rehabilitation, which has expanded into a highly competitive business in the marketplace of the 1990s, has been challenged by funding sources to maximize production while minimizing costs. Subsequently, service providers have increasingly attempted to develop and utilize outcomes to assess their effectiveness and economy of resources utilized, as well as to market their services. In addition, insurance providers are increasingly demanding that service providers include readily available outcome statistics as a critical negotiating point prior to approval of funding.

A standard definition of ethics would include dealing with what is favorable and unfavorable, with moral duty and obligation applied to the principles of conduct governing an individual or a group.[2] This article examines utilization of neurorehabilitation outcome data for purposes of planning and marketing treatment within the context of ethical prin-

ciples. This is a difficult process, since ethical judgments are typically defined as a standard of right behavior sanctioned by one's conscience or societal norms, with little reference to statistical models. Consequently, ethical judgments leave much room for subjective interpretation and manipulation. Furthermore, there is an inherent lack of ultimate accountability as to what constitutes an unethical act, since there is frequently misalignment between standards of ethical conduct or guidelines and enforceable legal statutes.[3]

Nevertheless, the current managed care revolution within the health care industry, combined with the ever-increasing knowledgebase regarding the effectiveness of brain injury rehabilitation, creates an opportunity in which health policy can be formed. The result of those changes will have a direct impact on determining who has access to services and who does not.

TRENDS IN NEUROREHABILITATION

Injury to the brain has been treated neuromedically and neurosurgically with increasing success in recent years, increasing the survival rate even after severe trauma. Research in neuroscience continues to provide new outlooks on brain injury. For example, our understanding of neurorecovery has led to viewing brain injury less as a static event than as a dynamic process involving plasticity of brain functions. As the survival rate after brain injury has increased, demand has also increased for more sophisticated rehabilitative services to improve an individual's functional recovery. This often leads to a more "functional" rehabilitation approach in later stages following the initial medical interventions. Consequently, recent decades have witnessed a rapid emergence of brain injury rehabilitation programs, acute and postacute, into a highly competitive industry. Accrediting bodies such as the Commission for Accreditation of Rehabilitation Fa-

J Head Trauma Rehabil, 1997, 12(1), 51–59
© 1997 Aspen Publishers, Inc.

cilities (CARF) have emerged to oversee and to ensure quality of services provided. This rapid growth of services, coupled with recent accreditation initiatives, creates an environment begging for ethical considerations.

Various research centers have responded by establishing databases to monitor types of brain injury; correlates to certain assessment procedures and treatments; and, most recently, results of interventions.[4] The National Institute on Disability and Rehabilitation Research (NIDRR) has been one of the leaders in the development, dissemination, and implementation of research that impacts on all areas of postinjury life. NIDRR directly supports research to improve the lives of persons who have sustained traumatic brain injury (TBI), as well as their families, friends, and employers. This is accomplished through the TBI Model System Projects, including research and training centers, engineering centers, and specific research and knowledge dissemination projects.[5] In addition to this publicly funded project, there have been numerous outcome studies conducted in various clinical settings.[4]

TBI, the leading cause of death and disability to children and young adults,[6] with an overall incidence rate of nearly 2 million cases each year, results in medical intervention costing billions of dollars.[7,8] The longer term consequences and ramifications of TBI continue to become more apparent and multidimensional over time. There frequently are disruptive consequences to the lives of the patient's family, friends, and employers. Legal matters often ensue. In addition, there are ever-increasing financial expenditures, frequently as a result of employment disability.

Attempting to ascertain the effectiveness of various clinical interventions has catalyzed researchers to examine the recovery process and corresponding treatment techniques and other factors. For example, recent advances made in understanding the functional anatomy of the brain have led to an understanding of differences between injury to white matter and injury to gray matter, and also to the influence of location and severity of injury, although point-to-point correlations are still lacking. Through many therapeutic strategies, billions of dollars have been spent rehabilitating individuals with TBI. Although most of those patients respond positively to treatment, it is still unclear whether this response is due to therapeutic strategies, the natural healing process (spontaneous recovery of the brain), or the interrelationship of the two. Lack of standardized procedures to monitor the stages of recovery, interventions, and ultimate outcomes has led to a growing confusion among consumers and financial providers alike in their search for the most clinically appropriate and economically appropriate paths. In an effort to clarify this central issue, the American Congress of Rehabilitation Medicine has expended substantial effort in attempting to standardize various definitions, treatment approaches, and outcome measures of neurorehabilitation.

OUTCOME STUDIES: ACQUIRED BRAIN INJURY

As researchers collect outcome data following TBI, many engage in independent projects but communicate little with other researchers. This has resulted in a great discrepancy among the variables utilized across most studies, including everything from classification of subjects (independent variables) to definitions of outcome measures (dependent variables). This leads to the classic dilemma of comparing "apples and oranges" when plotting the merits of one study versus another.[4]

Control groups have often not been included in outcome studies, since it has not seemed "ethical" to withhold treatment. Although some outcome studies have examined survival rates, acute care progress, and other neuroanatomic or neurophysiologic factors, the preponderance of outcome studies fall in the quasi-experimental (ie, retrospective analysis or absence of a control group) category. While it is a valid and respectable means of examination, such a design calls for more cautious interpretation and generalization of results.[9]

For example, Keith[10] argues against making causal inferences from many rehabilitation outcome studies, because clinical outcomes may not reflect the effects of clinical interventions, in large measure due to the presence of uncontrolled variables such as spontaneous recovery. In his review of the complex factors that can be included in analysis of treatment outcomes, Keith suggests concentrating on more global outcome measures such as discharge destination, need for assistance, level of productive activity, and costs. A growing literature supports this utilitarian approach.[11–13] A global approach to outcome measurement allows nonclinical and laypersons to participate knowledgeably in outcome discussions.

MARKETING REHABILITATION SERVICES

In 1990 the National Head Injury Foundation (now known as the Brain Injury Association) reported that there were over 500 programs specializing in brain injury rehabilitation.[14] A more recent estimate suggests the number of programs may have grown to over 700.[15] Ulicny,[16] in reference to such growth, describes the risk of marketing practices of a less than ethical nature, referring to errors of commission and omission. While some of the potentially misleading advertising may even be intentional by design, other concerns raised when interpreting outcome data may be influenced by a lack of understanding and sophisticated appreciation for research design and application of statistical analysis by the consumer of such data. Ulicny argues that outcome data used for marketing purposes should be viewed with the same scrutiny and held to the basic standards of any scientifically valid statistical model. Therefore, conditions that need to be carefully addressed include selection criteria for patients included in the study; classification of characteristics such as age, severity of injury, or time intervals since onset of injury; and use of operational definitions for various measures.

Consumers who may not be educated or "savvy" in interpreting information are commonly targeted for marketing and advertising outcome data. Such data presented may seem legitimate on the surface, despite containing serious methodologic flaws. Certain factors that may influence outcome such as severity of injury, medical complications, family situations, preinjury history, and funding source may not be reported in the marketing material. An advertisement is potentially misleading if it contains an unqualified claim that cannot be evaluated properly with further inquiry.[3,17] Marketing should balance presentation of information in a manner that can be understood by the consumer and ensure validity. Failing either criterion may discredit the information.

Emphasis on outcomes management, customer satisfaction, and quality management requires that consumers of services have access to information about the effects (ie, outcomes) of services rendered. This would allow informed decisions to be made by consumers of services. On the other hand, it also creates a scenario of possible abuse in the marketing and selling of patient outcomes. It would seem ethical that as outcome data are reported, the potential *limitations* of treatment are mentioned in addition to the positive effects of services rendered. In summary, the rehabilitation industry must report outcome data in an ethically responsible and scientifically valid manner, treating consumers and practitioners as *simultaneous* users of the information.

APPLICATION TO MANAGED CARE

The benefits of providing rehabilitation services for persons with acquired neurologic injury has been adequately addressed from the standpoint of improving patient/client overall levels of functioning.[4] Furthermore, those studies that have investigated the "investment" aspect of rehabilitating the injured person show clear and convincing financial rewards[18] of treatment. However, *access* to various levels of rehabilitation (eg, acute or postacute) may be curtailed and/ or eliminated in today's marketplace.[19] Several theories account for the potential lack of accessibility to care:

- high initial expense
- few long-term follow-up effectiveness studies
- few published standards of performance among similar providers
- industry tainted by negative press
- few prescriptive models of care/service delivery

Neurologic recovery demonstrates that the brain indeed has "spontaneous" anatomic recovery features, given an adequate medical or social support environment.[20] It is generally accepted that barring secondary complications, patients with

mild injury achieve optimal spontaneous recovery within 3 months, and patients with severe injury do so within 18 to 24 months of injury.[20] Unfortunately, there is little discussion in the rehabilitation *treatment* literature regarding methods to maximize optimal outcome status within these recovery periods. To complicate matters, many rehabilitation services are time limited and funded by health maintenance organizations (HMOs) to the acute phase of recovery, allowing limited access to rehabilitation beyond the initial hospitalization period.

Many would argue that while rehabilitation of persons with acquired neurologic injury, particularly severe TBI, usually reaps clinical and financial (long-term) "return on investment," predicting the eventual long-term outcome within the restrictive guidelines of many of today's funding policies becomes a dangerous guessing game—that is, clinical outcome research and current payment models have yet to coalesce into a rational system to drive allocation outcome data and the dollars available for it, from a health policy standpoint, with specific attention to the efficiencies of managed care strategies. Managed care includes a variety of plans of payment and service delivery. These include the following:

- *Capitation.* This is a payment system in which physicians or physician groups are paid a negotiated monthly amount based on the number of members enrolled in a plan. Capitation rates are based on the number of services required in an average month for that membership.
- *Fee-for-service.* This is the traditional arrangement by which physicians receive payment for the services they provide. Patients usually have considerable choice within this model.
- *Group model HMO.* A group (ie, employer) contracts with an entity to manage and deliver medical care to the entity's members. Physicians are all employees or contractees of the group and share in the profits of the group.
- *HMO.* This is an entity that provides managed health care services to members for a prepaid payment.
- *Managed competition.* This is an economic process in which managed health care delivery systems compete with each other, allowing market forces to contain the cost of services.
- *Point-of-service (POS) plan.* This is an HMO-style plan in which members may choose to receive health care services from a primary care physician in the HMO network (in-network) or from a provider outside of the network (out-of-network).
- *Preferred provider organization (PPO).* A list of participating physicians provide discounted rates to health plan members. There is no organization structure or quality review for this type of organization.
- *Prepaid health plan (PHP).* Employers or individual members pay a monthly premium to a health care entity,

compensating it for all covered services rather than submitting claims for each visit. Members contribute a flat co-payment at the time of service rather than a percentage of charges.

- *Staff model HMO.* Physicians are salaried employees of an HMO and treat solely the members of the HMO. There is no option for partnership, but physicians may receive bonuses based on performance.
- *Traditional indemnity insurance.* This is the traditional system in which insured individuals submit claim forms to be reimbursed for covered services. This system has recently been considered too patient friendly and less attentive to efficient models of care.

The ability to predict and therefore potentially reduce the cost of providing services (the marching cry of managed care practices) is a feature desired in each of these plans. Unfortunately, the existing rehabilitation literature does not address which may be in the best interest, particularly the long-term interest, of the person receiving rehabilitation services. Therefore, lacking clear and convincing clinical data to support more costly options, the payer of services is tempted to choose the least expensive, usually short-term, option. In other words, without a clinical compass, financial issues will predominate.

Within the last few years, a few studies have attempted to promote models of care that consumers and payers of services can utilize as reliable and valid.[13,21–23] Unfortunately, these models of care usually focus on clinical issues alone, with little or no guidance to provide fiscal management or control.[24] Current managed care strategies do not seem to be based upon neurologic theories of recovery or published outcome research; therefore, neurorehabilitation health care policy, either in the public or private sector, is listless or ambiguous at best.

We contend, however, that current rehabilitation outcome research does allow for preliminary discussions about integrating reliable clinical/neurologic information, quantifiable outcome data, and existing financial options in order to form a preliminary framework for rehabilitation health care policy.

POLICY FRAMEWORK ASSUMPTIONS

The following assumptions, although not exhaustive, provide a framework to apply rehabilitation theory and outcomes to reimbursement models.

Clinical/Neurologic Assumptions

- Severe, diffuse injuries usually require involvement of multiple clinical disciplines for maximum recovery.
- Spontaneous recovery rates tend to predictably decelerate over time.

- Early rehabilitation efforts improve long-term outcomes.
- Chronic (greater than 2 years) acquired neurologic deficits are more difficult to remediate than acute, transient deficits.

Outcome Data Assumptions

- Acute rehabilitation generally improves long-term functional capacities (medical stability, independence in activities of daily living [ADLs]).
- Postacute rehabilitation generally improves long-term functional capacities (independence in ADLs, return to work).
- Early predictor variables (such as severity of injury, posttraumatic amnesia, preexisting health) account for some of the statistical variance regarding long-term outcome.
- Intact psychosocial and medical supports (family, employer, community) improve overall outcome.

Financial Data Assumptions

- Rehabilitation and medical costs for severe, catastrophic injury can easily exceed $500,000 per case.
- "Unmanaged" rehabilitation does not adequately address cost-benefit issues.
- Predictability of cost and outcome should occur as soon after the injury as possible.
- The law of diminishing returns applies to neurologic rehabilitation.

Examples

In 1991, Learning Services Corporation, a private, for-profit, nationally accredited postacute neurorehabilitation company, published a pilot study regarding its Outcome Validation System (OVS).[11,25] The OVS, designed with significant consumer input, captures functional outcome data following postacute rehabilitation from TBI. The system contains a follow-up component whereby *durability of outcome* is measured as well as initial outcome. This pilot study showed that the OVS was a reliable and valid indicator of change following postacute rehabilitation.

In 1992, a more extensive version of the OVS was published.[26] In this study, it was suggested that "managed care" practices (specifically HMOs) may have both positive and negative impacts on overall outcome. On the positive side, it was obvious that managed care practices allowed patients more rapid access to appropriate rehabilitation services. On the other hand, patients were being discharged from rehabilitation services after shorter lengths of stay than previously recorded in published studies. In addition, rehabilitation was often concluded prior to completion of spontaneous recovery. A rapid "step-down" to little or no rehabilitation was found to have a negative impact on the durability of the rehabilitation outcome following discharge from programs.[11,26]

From another angle, Metropolitan Life Insurance Company created "Centers of Excellence" for levels of rehabilitation, whereby a national spectrum or approved network would promote efficient entry and transfer among "approved" providers. In addition, shared databases were established to link providers from various regions, thereby producing efficiencies in communication and evaluation services. Preliminary outcome data from these networks are very encouraging.

Another strategy to combine clinical outcome statistics with financial data is a case management model with a "shared risk" strategy. In this strategy, payers and providers negotiate agreed-upon outcomes and costs prior to implementation of a rehabilitation plan. Providers are encouraged to manage cases efficiently so as to meet or undercut the cost to deliver an agreed-upon outcome. In circumstances in which the outcome is not reached, the provider may be obligated to continue to provide services until the agreed-upon outcome is obtained (shared risk component), without further reimbursement. The practice is relatively new and is encouraged with one national company.[27] This practice is in alignment with the ethical code and standards that direct clinical providers to provide therapy with an end in mind, rather than to be occupied with means.

DISCUSSION

Application of outcome results to funding allocations, service delivery models, and marketing practices highlights significant conceptual and ethical issues. Biases and flaws in decision making may limit or influence access to funding for those individuals in need of treatment. In light of the apparent "insensitivity" to some payment practices, many outcome studies may be misinterpreted due to variability of outcome definitions, variability of comparable groups, and the marketing temptation to present skewed, favorable data. For example, failure to identify subjects according to age, gender, ethnicity, and cultural diversity lines[28] may impact functional outcome following TBI.[29] The effect of establishing a policy on the length of rehabilitation, or financial limits to rehabilitation, may be to reduce access to and quality of services, and to create a risk of underserving patients with high needs.

Society currently has no mechanism whereby medical and rehabilitation needs may be prioritized in certain ways, and guidelines are not available for how to proceed in an ethical manner in an environment of curtailing excessive costs, although the state of Oregon has tried with their "ration" process. Cervelli and Banja[2] provide five suggestions on ways to improve ethical conditions surrounding the financing of rehabilitation of persons with catastrophic brain injuries. These suggestions rely on (1) the development of more socially responsible ways to reimburse care necessitated by the onset of catastrophic disability and (2) education of health insurance purchasers regarding the economic realities assumed upon purchase of a health care insurance policy. They encourage ongoing dialogue between insurers and rehabilitation providers regarding several dimensions of the provisions of services. They also encourage providers and insurers to commit to improved data collection and analysis to facilitate improved decision making by all parties. They claim that doing so will improve the ethical performance of the industry through implementation of meaningful measures of accountability.

CONCLUSION

The struggle between health care providers, consumers of service, and health care insurers is unlikely to simplify or achieve equilibrium in the near future. Each player in this competitive engagement has qualitatively different expectations and definitions of successful outcome. This inherent "misalignment" will continue to challenge the ethical position of all parties involved. The overall access to health care by the general public is of growing concern among employees, politicians, and the employers that are burdened with much of the financial responsibility to ensure this.

Relevant to the access issue, one study reported that survivors, TBI unable to pay for health care had less improvement in functional independence at 12 to 24 months after injury and a poorer quality of life.[30] Other variables contributed or subtracted to both functional independence and quality of life. One could speculate from some of the current results in the literature that individuals suffering catastrophic TBI, or even mild TBI with significant impairment, who are denied optimal resources for rehabilitation, will consistently demonstrate decreased performance both vocationally and socially. The cost to the marketplace and to society, although difficult to quantify, suggests that short-term perspectives that protect the cash reserves of the payer will result in long-term, unnecessary cash payouts.

The Brain Injury Association, along with many other organizations and individuals, continues to press for research and implementation of public policy and legislation to improve provision of and access to services and also to decrease the occurrence of disabling brain injuries. If the suggestions concerning "data collection, funding decision, access to services, and accountability" made by Cervelli and Banja,[2] Papastrat,[24] the Brain Injury Association,[31] and others[12,16,32] were addressed in earnest by providers and payers alike, those participating in the rehabilitation effort would more than likely meet their own business and clinical objectives.

REFERENCES

1. American Psychological Association. *Ethical Principles of Psychologists and Code of Conduct.* Washington, DC: American Psychological Association; 1992.

2. Cervelli L, Banja JD. Ethical dilemmas resulting from insurance coverage for catastrophic rehabilitative care. *J Head Trauma Rehabil.* 1995;10(1):90–93.

3. Ford G, Calfee J. Recent developments in FTC policy on deception. *J Marketing.* 1986;50:82–103.

4. Cope N. The effectiveness of traumatic brain injury rehabilitation: a review. *Brain Injury.* 1995;9(7): 649–670.

5. Melia RP. Research, consumer involvement, and models of care. Presented at Traumatic Brain Injury: Models and Systems of Care Conference; April 11–13, 1996; Washington, DC.

6. Kraus JF, Fife D, Cox P, et al. Incidence, severity, and external causes of pediatric brain injury. *Am J Dis Child.* 1986;140:687–693.

7. Bush G. Calculating the cost of long term living: a four step process. *Journal of Head Trauma Rehabilitation.* 1990;5(1):47–56.

8. Brooks CA, Lindstrom J, McCray J, Whiteneck G. Cost of medical care for a population-based sample of persons surviving traumatic brain injury. *J Head Trauma Rehabil.* 1995;10(4):1–13.

9. Rappaport M, Herrero-Bake C, Rappaport MC, Winterfield KM. Head injury outcome up to ten years later. *Arch Phys Med Rehabil.* 1989;70:885–892.

10. Keith RA. Conceptual basis of outcome measures. *Am J Phys Med Rehabil.* 1995;74(1):73–80.

11. Evans RW, Jones ML. Integrating outcomes, value, and quality: an outcome validation system for post-acute rehabilitation programs. *J Insurance Med.* 1991;23(3):192–196.

12. Evans RW, Ruff RM. Outcome and value: a perspective on rehabilitation outcomes achieved in acquired brain injury. *J Head Trauma Rehabil.* 1992;7(4):24–36.

13. Malec JF, Basford JS. Post-acute brain injury rehabilitation. *Arch Phys Med Rehabil.* 1996;77:198–207.

14. Head Injury Foundation. *National Directory of Head Injury Rehabilitation Services.* Southborough, Mass: Head Injury Foundation; 1992.

15. *National Head Injury Foundation Resource Guide.* Washington, DC: National Head Injury Foundation; 1996.

16. Ulicny G. Marketing brain injury rehabilitation services: toward a more ethical approach. *J Head Trauma Rehabil.* 1994;9(4):73–76.

17. Gardner DM. Deception in advertising: a conceptual approach. *J Marketing.* 1975;39:40–46.

18. Ninomiya J, Ashley MJ, Raney ML, Krych DK. Vocational rehabilitation. In: *Traumatic Brain Injury Rehabilitation.* Ashley MJ, Krych DK (eds.). New York, NY: CRC Press; 1995.

19. Banja J, Johnston MV. Outcomes evaluation in TBI rehabilitation, part III: ethical perspectives and social policy. *Arch Phys Med Rehabil.* 1994;75:19–26.

20. Levin HS, Grafman J, Eisenberg HM. *Neurobehavioral Recovery from Head Injury.* New York, NY: Oxford University Press; 1987.

21. Johnston MV, Hall KM. Outcomes & evaluations in TBI rehabilitation, part I: overview and system principles. *Arch Phys Med Rehabil.* 1994;75:2–9.

22. Hall KM, Johnston MV. Outcome evaluation in TBI rehabilitation, part II: measurement tools for a nationwide data system. *Arch Phys Med Rehabil.* 1994; 75:10–18.

23. Hall KM, Cope N. The benefit of rehabilitation in traumatic brain injury: a literature review. *J Head Trauma Rehabil.* 1995;10(1):1–13.

24. Papastrat LA. Outcome and value following brain injury: a financial provider's perspective. *J Head Trauma Rehabil.* 1992;7(4):11–23.

25. Outcome Validation System. Durham, NC: Learning Services; 1989.

26. Jones ML, Evans RW. Outcome validation in post-acute rehabilitation: trends and correlates in treatment and outcome. *J Insurance Med.* 1992;24:186–192.

27. Cope DN, Olear J. A clinical and economic perspective on head injury rehabilitation. *Journal of Head Trauma Rehabilitation.* 1993;8(4):1–14.

28. Gervasio AH. Gender, ethnicity, and cultural diversity. Presented at Traumatic Brain Injury: Models and Systems of Care Conference; April 11–13, 1996; Washington, DC.

29. Reeder K, Rosenthal M, Licktenberg P, Wood D. Impact of age on functional outcome following traumatic brain injury. Presented at Traumatic Brain Injury: Models and Systems of Care Conference; April 11–13; 1996. Washington, DC.

30. Webb CR, Wrigley M, Yoels W, Fine PR. Explaining quality of life for persons with traumatic brain injuries 2 years after injury. *Arch Phys Med Rehabil.* 1995;76(12):1,113–1,119.

31. National Head Injury Foundation. *Ethical Marketing and Service Delivery Practices for Health Care Providers Engaged in Head Injury Management.* Southborough, Mass: National Head Injury Foundation; 1992.

32. Ashley MJ, Persel CS, Krych DK. Changes in reimbursement climate: relationship among outcome, cost and payor type in the post acute rehabilitation environment. *J Head Trauma Rehabil.* 1993;8(4): 30–47.

10

Values and Outcomes: The Ethical Implications of Multiple Meanings

John D. Banja

The term "outcome" is a marvelously descriptive term, denoting a phenomenon or reality that literally "comes out of" something else. While this coming-out-of obviously involves a process of cause and effect, people normally desist from using the word *outcome* for simple cause and effect occurrences wherein brute matter interacts with brute matter. For example, the release of energy as heat following an explosion of gasoline would not ordinarily be called *outcome*. However, without hesitation, health care professionals would call a stroke patient's Functional Independence Measure (FIM) score of 85 at discharge—in contrast to his or her FIM score of 50 on admission—an *outcome* (Oczkowski & Barreca, 1993). What, then, accounts for this reserved, specialized usage of *outcome* even though the stroke patient's outcome may be as much a causally induced phenomenon as heat following an explosion of combusted gas?

Perhaps the answer lies in how an outcome reflects the value-laden intentions, estimations, and goals of those who launch a causal process aimed at—but not guaranteeing—the restoration of function. True, the rehabilitation patient's outcome is as factually and measurably apparent as any other phenomenon occurring in nature. However, a rehabilitation outcome not only reflects scientific causality vis à vis physicians, nurses, and therapists trying to alter the nature or course of pathophysiological events. It also reflects a process that witnesses countless decisions over what is desirable or undesirable, acceptable or unacceptable, reasonable or unreasonable, and appropriate or inappropriate. Most importantly, it witnesses how all of these decisions eventuate in an outcome to which subjective assessments of worth or value will be attached. Professional accountability requires an evaluation of health care outcomes along with the processes

that presumably account for them. Just as *evaluate* implies, there is no way that ascriptions of worth, significance, and importance—which are the sum and substance of valuing—can be excluded from accountability determinations.

Because health care is ultimately a valuative enterprise insofar as the restoration of health and function represents an important social good, health care outcomes become the realities that a society will seize upon in deciding whether that social good has been achieved. However, values, especially in a democracy, tend to be notoriously heterogeneous and divisive. The United States was founded on the notion of individual rights and freedoms that grant citizens as much latitude as possible in evolving personal value systems that direct their lives (Rorty, 1990). It is not surprising, then, that an industry like health care, which admits numerous stakeholders, each with a specific, value-driven agenda, will provide a fertile ground for valuative disputes and conflicts. Certain of these problems will be discussed below, beginning with a discussion of the ethical requirement to perform outcome studies.

PROFESSIONAL INTEGRITY AND ATTRIBUTIONS OF CAUSALITY

An issue that might strike many as purely scientific and without valuative or ethical import is the act of attributing an outcome to a particular process or chain of causation. Ever since David Hume pointed out in the 18th century that we never actually observe or perceive causation but only the conjunction of two phenomena wherein one seems consistently to succeed or follow from another (Hume, 1967), scientists have evolved an acute appreciation of the need to secure data-gathering methods and evidence that rationally compel ascriptions of causality.

Rehabilitation researchers, of course, insist on the scientific dimensions of outcome studies, such as validity, reli-

Top Stroke Rehabil, 1997, 4(2), 59–70
© 1997 Aspen Publishers, Inc.

ability, errors of measurement, norms and scaling, measures development, and general standards (often articulated in technical manuals and guides) for the use of those measures (Johnston, Keith, & Hinderer, 1992). However, the basis of these concerns goes deeper than a professional demand for methodological rigor. On a fundamental level, these concerns reflect attitudes about the moral integrity of science and its fiduciary responsibility to the society expecting to benefit from science's discoveries.

Outcomes research is the most visible and obvious expression of rehabilitation accountability, prompted largely by demands that rehabilitation justify its frequently considerable cost by demonstrating its effectiveness. However, rehabilitation has entered the outcomes era only recently and reluctantly. In 1994, Marcus Fuhrer, Director of the National Center for Medical Rehabilitation Research of the National Institutes of Health, remarked that "There's no secret to what credible, well designed outcomes studies look like—we're just not yet doing them" (Novack, 1994, p. 7).

Indeed, like virtually every other health care discipline, rehabilitation has subjected relatively few of its treatment modalities and interventions to rigorous outcomes research and analysis. In a fairly recent essay notable for its criticism of the state of stroke rehabilitation research, Matyas and Ottenbacher (1993) went so far as to declare that "the cumulative evidence has not produced a general consensus on the effectiveness of stroke rehabilitation" (p. 559). They lament the "methodological heterogeneity" of 30 years of stroke research and "the confusion and conflict that appears to exist in the stroke rehabilitation literature" (p. 559).

Consider, then, the moral implications of a rehabilitationist's touting a particular intervention, perhaps one that he or she has mastered over the years, enjoys practicing, and for which he or she can summon some clinical justification, if not in the research literature, at least from other practicing colleagues. The therapist "feels" that the treatment "works." From the start, the therapist has made two distinctly valuative decisions: (1) that the endpoint of his or her therapeutic efforts has a "reasonable," "acceptable," or "adequate" probability of occurring and (2) that the "quality" of the outcome is "worth" the clinical effort.

The valuative parameters of probability and quality determinations will be discussed later. For now, just consider that without an empirically validated knowledgebase, this therapist is relying on a "best guess" to justify his or her therapeutic plan. Ethical considerations enter this picture when it is recognized that although the therapist's best guess might be the optimal therapeutic approach, it may just as well have seriously missed the mark. For all the therapist "knows"—which, in the absence of a methodologically adequate, rigorously controlled outcome study, must be deemed problematic—another treatment approach might secure a superior or similar functional result with less clinical effort and financial expense. However, if that is so, this therapist, his or her employing organization, and, by extension, the profession the therapist represents are minimally guilty of professional lassitude that can easily evolve into suspicions of fraud and patient rights violations: fraud because a third party payer is being billed for a treatment that might admit a less expensive option and violating patient rights in that the patient is denied an opportunity to consent to a therapeutic alternative that might be at least as good as the therapist's preference.

Although these observations might sound harsh, ample evidence attests to ways health providers will—sometimes unconsciously, sometimes because it is all they know, but virtually always without sufficient critical scrutiny—inject their notions of "appropriateness" into treatment decisions. Examples from acute, invasive treatments are numerous, such as a 1989 study of 4,500 hospital records of Medicare patients, which reported that one sixth of those undergoing coronary angiography and upper gastrointestinal endoscopy and one third of those undergoing carotid endarterectomy had procedures that a consensus panel considered "inappropriate" (Epstein, 1990). A 1995 study of acute low back pain among patients seen by primary care practitioners, chiropractors, and orthopaedic surgeons showed that the times to functional recovery, return to work, and complete recovery from low back pain were similar among patients seen by all the practitioners, although the treatment costs were highest among the orthopaedic surgeons and chiropractors (Carey et al., 1995). A rehabilitation example might be the outcome study recently reported by Keith, Wilson, and Gutierrez (1995) that indicated virtually no difference in discharge-to-community rates among stroke patients seen in acute rehabilitation centers versus those seen in subacute care. Like the low back pain study, however, the care costs were substantially different, with acute inpatient rehabilitative care considerably more expensive.

The ethical point of all this is that in the absence of outcome studies to guide clinical practice, payers and consumers of care are at the whim of their providers as to what counts as the "appropriate" thing to do. However, if there is little data-driven consensus among those very providers about appropriateness, ample room exists for them to inject their own preferences into the care plan, especially as those preferences are driven (or, indeed, conflicted) by incentives that are specific to the provider rather than to the patient.

Ethics require better. The present state of affairs invites suspicions about the degree to which the rights and values of at least consumers and payers may be compromised, given the absence of a sufficient, outcome-driven knowledgebase. Related moral considerations are discussed in the next section.

"PEOPLE MAKE VALUE JUDGMENTS DIFFERENTLY"

An important analytical contribution to discussions about withholding or discontinuing life-prolonging treatment was recently made by pointing out that estimations about treatment "futility" invariably admit both a quantitative as well as qualitative dimension: quantitative in that mathematical estimates about how a "low" success probability intertwines with qualitative estimations about a "poor result" bearing on the meaning of *success* (Schneiderman, Jecker, & Jonsen, 1990). These quantitative and qualitative dimensions of futility speak as much to clinical anticipations of "worthwhile" success that urge treatment. Presumably, the decision to provide care occurs because the professional believes the treatment has "enough" chance of realizing a "valued" outcome. How much is "enough," and how "valuable" ought the outcome be?

Consider cardiopulmonary resuscitation (CPR). If probabilistic estimates about the likelihood of a code's success never occurred, then the code ought, theoretically, never be stopped since one could not say with *absolute* certainty that continuing for another 5 min, 50 min, or 5 hr would not eventuate in "success." Providers must be allowed to reach a point of "reasonable" rather than "absolute" certainty that the code has physiologically failed. On the other hand, definitions of a successful outcome from CPR vary considerably, as some references translate successful CPR as sheer biologic survival immediately following the intervention; others use survival at 24 hr; and still others examine survival at 30 days or at discharge (Murphy & Matcher, 1990). Other commentators object to these definitions because they ignore quality of life issues (Podrid, 1989). At least one other viewpoint, sounding its admittedly vested interest in rehabilitating patients who might receive CPR, has suggested that "successful" CPR connote survival with *rehabilitation potential* (Bilsky & Banja, 1992).

Success probability coupled with quality of life—or, perhaps, quality of function—estimations are inevitable in stroke rehabilitation. The very notion of rehabilitation *potential* implies the value-laden, clinical belief that rehabilitation interventions will not provide "sufficient" benefits to all individuals who have sustained serious musculoskeletal or neurological impairments. If that is true, then what criteria are customarily used in rehabilitation to make such prognoses? Are these criteria mutually understood and agreed upon by all rehabilitation providers (i.e., is there good reliability in their implementation)? How probable ought a treatment's success be before it is deployed? How ought health care professionals qualitatively define *success*?

There are at least four reasons values cannot be prescinded from these determinations about outcomes, regardless of which outcome measures are used and which statistical measures are implemented to process the data. The first is that most outcomes, especially in stroke rehabilitation, cannot be guaranteed. Because an element of probability exists as to whether or not a projected outcome will materialize, questions inevitably revolve around how probable that outcome need be—and how certain clinicians need be about that prob-

ability—so as to justify the allocation of that treatment. Bohannon, for example, declared in 1993 that stroke patients whose flaccid upper extremity remains so after 3 weeks of physical therapy ought not continue receiving it (cited in Colan, 1993). This relatively straightforward, seemingly innocuous declaration is, in fact, morally provocative. If physical therapy were stopped at 2 weeks rather than 3, would a morally unconscionable degree of uncertainty have been allowed to compromise the stroke patient's right to a "reasonable" degree of rehabilitative treatment? On the other hand, suppose a rigorously controlled study was performed that showed 8% of patients who were without functional return in a flaccid upper extremity after 3 weeks began, during a 4th week of therapy, to evince certain movements that suggested some hope of meaningful functional use. Ought that finding compel additional therapy? Again, how are we to understand "some hope" and "meaningful"—both of which recall the observations made above about the inevitability of quantitative and qualitative conjecturing in making treatment decisions about outcomes?

As amply demonstrated by the last half-century of philosophical reflection, there appear to be no objective ethical standards to which individuals can refer to calculate the *moral point* at which "success probability" and its appropriate confidence interval justify the deployment of rehabilitation or any kind of care (Engelhardt, 1996). Even if an outcome study found a particular treatment to be "successful" 33% of the time, it would still be an entirely speculative matter as to whether or not a 33% rate of success was "acceptable." A treatment success rate of 33% might be marvelous if it could save a life, but considerably less marvelous if the person's quality of life would only be barely improved.

A second reason values are inevitable in outcome determinations is that an "outcome" is not a solitary phenomenon but the one dimension of which means different things to different people. As Haas (1988) observed, "People make value judgments differently" (p. 330). "Quality of life," for example, may seem a strikingly obvious rehabilitation outcome the value of which no one, in good moral conscience, could repudiate. Nevertheless, consider the following:

> Clearly, quality of life varies according to its judge—practitioner, patient, or family. Some may equate it with independence in activities in daily living; others with economic productivity, working regularly, or living independently; still others, with functioning satisfactorily in social and interpersonal relationships. Although criteria are not generally agreed on, the concept of quality of life is rarely challenged in the rehabilitation setting. Thus, practitioners who base decisions upon it may not recognize the subjective nature of such decisions. (Haas, 1988, p. 330)

The fundamental reason determinations of quality outcomes are inevitably subjective is that outcomes either satisfy or frustrate personal desires. Rehabilitation is delivered in order to satisfy the desire of a patient and family for functional recovery and the desire of rehabilitation providers to advance their patients' welfare and sell their services. However, desires are by nature subjective and can become decidedly problematic in rehabilitation scenarios when their satisfaction is viewed as nonmeritorious, unrealistic, or unfair to others.

As the brief but extremely provocative literature on the psychodynamics of transference and countertransference in rehabilitation has pointed out, rehabilitation providers have well-defined professional objectives that they seek to realize in treatment sessions. Gans (1987) has noted that rehabilitation team members are often "young, healthy, in control. . . . Rehabilitation staff members are extremely goal-oriented and often experience patients' achievements of these goals as evidence of their own competence. In the process they unwittingly assign to patients the task of preserving their self-esteem" (pp. 186–187). Indeed, an unbridgeable, phenomenological gulf separates the patient and therapist, in that the former subjectively experiences his of her functional impairment and all the (frequently intensely negative) feelings, emotions, and attitudinal formations that attach to it. The therapist, of course, cannot experience this but only his or her concentration on and gratification (or disappointment) in the degree to which the patient's progress approaches those functional goals. Both the therapist and patient are constrained by the pathophysiology of the patient's impairments, and both have a decidedly narcissistic involvement with the therapeutic outcome. However, for one, that narcissism attaches to his or her interest in reclaiming a life worth living. The other's narcissism is attached to the degree to which the patient's success derives from applying the treatment plan and achieving or surpassing the outcomes that were initially projected (Gunther, 1994).

It is perfectly understandable, then, how patient and provider can differ on the meaning of rehabilitation "success." One might measure success in terms of FIM points gained, while the other, in terms of increased feelings of happiness. One might target ability in activities of daily living; the other might target returning to employment or playing golf. The only way to resolve whatever valuative disputes might exist between them would be for one to surrender or for both to negotiate the outcome in which they are invested or deem "reasonable" or "good." On the other hand, to the extent that other parties in the patient's rehabilitation, such as his or her family, employer, or insurer also maintain vested interests in an outcome he or she deems desirable, this negotiation might have to be repeated over and over.

This leads to a third reason rehabilitation outcomes are inherently value-laden, which is that, very frequently, an individual's functional status at discharge may impose burdens on other persons to which they, in turn, will attach values of acceptability or unacceptibility, desirability or undesirability (Callahan, 1988). Thus, a stroke patient's discharge to home without home health benefits might mean a halt to the insurer's financial responsibility for care and thus satisfy the insurer's desire to terminate reimbursement. To the patient's family members, however, that same discharge home might require their having to manage certain challenges and lifestyle disruptions that they find distinctly undesirable. This problem returns to the same valuative disputes discussed above. To what extent might a caregiver's at-home burden be "unreasonable?" To what extent ought a humane society seek to relieve these burdens?

These questions point to a fourth reason values are inevitable in these types of conversations: namely, the degree to which the body politic is economically disposed to invest in the value of health care outcomes. On the one hand, if sufficient reservoirs of money existed whereby cost would not be a factor in allocating rehabilitative care, concerns about the success probability of a treatment justifying its allocation would seem beside the point. One would simply adopt a thoroughgoing, patient-centered ethic that says that as long as even the most modest evidence exists for a treatment's success—say, a 1 in 10,000 chance—the patient deserves that chance. (This is not terribly different from the allocation attitude that existed in the fee-for-service reimbursement era of the late 1960s and 1970s, which witnessed little concern about reimbursement and, not surprisingly, little concern over deploying treatments whose chance of success might be remote at best.) Furthermore, where enough money exists so that one person's benefit does not become another's burdens, valuative disputes over inequity or injustice—as represented by a caregiver's having to assume unreasonable or excessive responsibilities—would not be an issue. By subsidizing the costs of those burdens, their oppressiveness and undesirability, and, hence, the burdens presenting to others, would disappear.

However, the degree to which a society is disposed to allocating these kinds of economic resources for health care involves a valuative balancing of the worth of health care with other social goods, such as education, welfare, national defense, and so forth. How much society is willing to spend on health care—whether in insurance premiums or taxes—entails valuative choices of the first order (Daniels, 1994).

All of these issues pose significant moral questions as to how rehabilitation providers as well as their employing organizations should understand outcomes, especially if outcome data are used to make allocational decisions. What any professional owes to a consumer of services encompasses a host of ethical considerations about rights, duties, promises, and fidelity. The point to be appreciated is that values are inherent and inevitable in not only rehabilitative but any kind of health care decision that sets its sight on some "outcome." What is inevitable in all of this, however, is the way that values elicited by rehabilitation outcomes will reflect back upon the rehabilitation process as the engine that produces that outcome. As clinicians value certain outcomes but not others, and as they simultaneously consider whether certain outcomes are "reasonably" attainable, clinicians will operationalize valuative decisions by modifying the rehabilitation process. A discussion of some of these possibilities follows.

THE IMPACT OF VALUES ON REHABILITATION PROCESS

If outcomes are as imbued with values as the above suggests, then as outcome studies become more definitive, their findings will elicit reactions that cause the rehabilitation process to change in accordance with whose values are asserted most compellingly and powerfully. Although it presently seems that the rehabilitation process functions as an independent variable with outcome the dependent variable, these identities will be reversed as outcomes studies progress. Put simply, outcomes will drive process. The following will speculate on the ways values will affect that phenomenon.

Economics

Some individuals may assert that the economic aspects of care are not an outcome per se but rather a measure of resource utilization. They want to reserve "outcome" for only those functional dimensions of patient-centered care. Third party payers as well as hospital administrators, however, will almost certainly regard costs as an outcome, which perhaps illustrates the point that what one identifies as an outcome is, at least partially, valuatively driven.

Whether considered an outcome or not, as costs continue to be carefully studied and linked as efficiency measures to functional outcomes achieved, valuative questions are sure to arise. A brute variable affecting rehabilitation process involves how the patient's degree of functional restoration may be profoundly associated with the economic resources upon which he or she can call. The question as to how aggressive or prolonged the rehabilitation process can be—and, presumably, what kinds of functional attainments can therefore be expected—may largely be answered by another question: "How much functional restoration can the patient buy?" In short, if length of stay and the therapies an individual receives constitute the formal and substantive aspects of the rehabilitation process respectively, then they will wax and wane according to ability to pay. However, that ability to pay (and the point is exquisitely illustrated by Medicare tax revenues that reimburse so much of stroke rehabilitation) is largely a function of social values that express a willingness or reluctance to set aside "sufficient" revenues for stroke rehabilitation (Daniels, 1994).

Valuing Clinical Contributions

In addition to the economic impact on the rehabilitation process, sophisticated outcome studies will also want to track the clinical contribution of each member of the rehabilitation team to the outcome achieved (Banja & Johnston, 1994). To the extent this is demonstrable, rehabilitation process will predictably be orchestrated with greater precision that, in turn, might ultimately have profound implications for the rehabilitation team approach that has evolved over the last half-century.

While the analogy might provoke anger, it nevertheless seems fair to say that many rehabilitation teams frequently function like assembly lines (whose members admittedly exercise more creativity and cross communication than their industrial counterparts) wherein the "product" (patient) is nevertheless shuttled back and forth from therapy to therapy. Very little is known, however, about how much each individual therapist contributes to the patient's ultimate outcome. As Keith (1991) and others have wondered, is a team effort required for any given patient, or might the patient's impairments "sufficiently" respond only to physical and recreational therapy but not, say, occupational or speech-language therapy?

The ramifications of these outcomes studies on rehabilitation process are immense: Not only might outcomes studies demonstrate that certain rehabilitation impairments are not worth the therapeutic effort traditionally expended in treating them, but these studies might have significant bearing for the professional preparation of rehabilitationists themselves. That is, in treating certain types of impairments, ought therapists be more trained or can more therapies be safely and effectively delivered by assistants and aides? Bella May (1996) has wondered the following:

> Does it require a physical therapist to teach gait training to an individual who is medically stable? Can a physical therapist assistant effectively teach exercises to an individual following transtibial amputation? Is it even physical therapy to walk behind an elderly individual who needs only supervision but no instruction? Do we delegate tasks appropriately? We are and should continue to be a client-centered, hands-on profession, but we need to clearly define what is and is not physical therapy and who is appropriately educated to provide what services. (p. 1,237)

Inevitably, how values determine a "reasonable" or "good" outcome will predictably influence the development of standards as to the degree of professional skill and knowledge therapists ought to demonstrate.

Quality of Life

In addition to questions about how "good" clinicians want an outcome to be, the questions raised above will elicit basic valuative responses about how much clinicians believe they "owe" to rehabilitation consumers—especially by way of how much reimbursement they are willing to allot in the process—and, not unimportantly, how deeply they value the historical precedent of the rehabilitation team and are politically intent on keeping it. Suppose, for example, outcome studies show that although certain patients do not respond well to certain therapies, patients who nevertheless experienced a team effort did better overall than those who had a disparate or fragmented array of treatments. For example, suppose clinicians begin finding that quality of life outcome measures in rehabilitation are consistently higher among patients treated by a rehabilitation team than by a more piecemeal rehabilitation effort that absents, say, a rehabilitation psychologist, recreational therapist, and chaplain. Suppose they further find that individuals who experience a team effort maintain their functional gains longer after rehabilitation discharge than those patients who are not exposed to a team approach. Outcome findings such as these will only spur valuative questions about "how long" rehabilitation gains ought to endure after discharge in order to justify a team or, in fact, any rehabilitation effort. Again, though, the question will be settled on valuative, not empirical, grounds.

Caregiver Burden and Family Support

An extremely important outcome measure is the effect of the rehabilitation process on relieving caregiver burdens (Callahan, 1988). Presumably, the primary means of relieving caregiver burden will be through securing greater functional restoration for the patient, but this will only reiterate the question as to "how much" benefit—now understood as directed to families—should accrue in order to justify deploying rehabilitation services. Will payers be willing to reimburse increased lengths of stay if outcome studies show that significant diminution on caregiver burden will result? Might the rehabilitation process significantly shift to the home, where families can receive more direct instruction on how to manage their loved one's recovery?

Indeed, a family's declared interest in caring for their loved one after rehabilitation discharge—which tends to vary and, in the absence of a legal mandate that requires their doing so, represents a valuatively driven choice—may exert enormous impact on the rehabilitation process. The family who is intent on providing care at home might desire as much professional support and education as monies will allow in contrast to not-so-eager counterparts. However, suppose that as outcome studies become more sophisticated, clinicians find that the *absence* of a supportive family means that a par-

ticular type of rehabilitation patient's functional gains will not be maintained after discharge. In cases where a nursing home placement is extremely probable and recognized early, how far can one even begin to justify an aggressive and vigorous rehabilitation?

What is most troubling about this entire crop of questions is that because there is no overarching set of "correct" values to which all the persons making or influencing rehabilitation decisions can refer to settle valuative disputes, clinicians are left with their disagreements and the realization that resolution can only occur through consensus, not through the discovery of an absolute, unconditionally, and eternally right set of values. It is worth asking, then, whether the heterogeneity of values prompted by the above questions renders outcome assessments hopelessly relativistic and prey to whomever might have the most "political" power to compel his or her agenda into prominence or whether there might be some moral signposts that can guide disputes over valuative dimensions of outcomes. The next section will consider certain directions these signposts might offer.

CONSIDERATIONS FOR THE FUTURE OF OUTCOMES ACCOUNTABILITY

No matter how disputatious the intersection of values with outcomes becomes, a patient-centered or patient-focused ethic must prevail. This minimally means that the patient's values must be accorded a *prima facie* priority. Admittedly, the patient's values or functional aspirations may be constrained by economics or the gravity of the patient's impairments. However, where the patient's values and aspirations are reasonable, health care ethics will insist that their status "trumps" the values of others.

There are many reasons for a patient-centered ethic but none better than the history of moral reflection's demanding the centrality of the consumer's wishes in a health care—or, indeed, any professional—arrangement (Bayles, 1989). That history flatly repudiates self-regarding actions or behaviors as "moral." On the one hand, to say that actions that ultimately preserve one's own interests at the cost of everyone else's are moral, virtuous, or right seems a gross contradiction to the intuitive understanding of those terms laid down since the ancient Greeks. On the other hand, in the moral understandings relevant to that special class of *professional* relationships, it is explicitly understood by both the provider and consumer of the service that the uppermost objective of the relationship is to advance the consumer's welfare. This is precisely what the consumer expects and to which the professional is socially and legally expected to respond (Bayles, 1989). The implication of all this for outcomes is clear. Unless there are compelling moral reasons to think otherwise—such as cognitive impairments affecting the patient's decision making—the patient's notion of what constitutes a "desirable" outcome must be accorded priority.

The primacy of a patient-centered ethic nicely returns this discussion to the elevated status persons hold in all of creation by way of their extraordinarily broad ability to value. The great German philosopher Immanuel Kant (1964) observed that it was precisely the valuing ability of human beings that gave them infinite and unconditional worth. Things and events around individuals take on worth or value, Kant noted, because people intend those objects with value. However, that means that values originate in the individual as the valuer. Because the individual can reflect on and choose certain values while rejecting others—in contrast to the rest of creation, which cannot—the individual is especially precious as an originator of value. In social terms, one's significance as an originator or creator of value means that others must respect one's preciousness as a valuer of unconditional worth and that the individual similarly respects theirs.

As a final word on value, then, perhaps the rehabilitation community should remind themselves of the special dignity that attaches to human beings as valuers and the compromise of that dignity by the onset of disability. Not only is disability an outrageous narcissistic injury, as Gunther (1994) has observed, but it interferes precisely with people living their lives according to the valuative choices they make. Where function has been compromised because of a neurological or musculoskeletal impairment, moral intuitions about human dignity seem, if not to demand, at least to encourage that such impairments be remediated. Unfortunately, though, moral rhetoric or exhortations that rest on intuitions are extremely vulnerable, not only because they are rebuttable by the intuitions of others but because without more compelling rationales or arguments to support them, a simple recitation of one's personal intuitions about what is right or wrong might well sound inordinately subjective, narcissistic, uninformed, self-serving, or wearisome to those with differing intuitions.

Still, the choices people make and the values they call upon in making them ultimately determine the artifacts, services, and relations that typify society and through which they will be known to future generations. Human beings are, as the existentialists like to observe, their choices. One might observe, then, that society seems on the verge of a valuative crisis in health care as the morality of the marketplace threatens to submerge the moral attitudes that have been traditionally identified and associated with respecting human dignity (Yarmolinsky, 1995). Note that two parties stand to lose here: not just persons with disability, who, without care, might be forced to accept a lower functional status than they could attain with therapy, but the rehabilitation provider as well, who is prohibited from deploying his or her skills in an optimally therapeutic way.

• • •

Those of us in rehabilitation would be well advised to consider articulating a vision of human functioning that speaks directly to the dignity of being human. The outcomes of rehabilitation interventions will obviously hold center stage in this conversation. While it is impossible to predict how this conversation will play out, one can be sure that if the traditional values of rehabilitation, centering on independence and functional restoration, are not powerfully put forward, the values of some other ideological group will be.

REFERENCES

Banja, J. & Johnston, M.V. (1994). Outcomes evaluation in TBI rehabilitation part III: Ethical perspectives and social policy. *Archives of Physical Medicine and Rehabilitation, 75,* SC19–SC26.

Bayles, M.D. (1989). *Professional ethics* (2nd ed.). Belmont, CA: Wadsworth.

Bilsky, G.S., & Banja, J.D. (1992). Outcomes following cardiopulmonary resuscitation in an acute rehabilitation hospital: Clinical and ethical implications. *American Journal of Physical Medicine and Rehabilitation, 71*(4), 232–235.

Callahan, D. (1988). Families as caregivers: The limits of morality. *Archives of Physical Medicine and Rehabilitation, 69*(5), 323–328.

Carey, T.S., Garrett, J., Jackmann, A., McLaughlin, C., Fryer, J., Smucker, D.R., & North Carolina Back Pain Project. (1995). The outcomes and costs of care for acute low back pain among patients seen by primary care practitioners, chiropractors, and orthopedic surgeons. *New England Journal of Medicine, 333*(14), 913–917.

Colan, B.J. (1993, September 20). Making judgments in evaluating patients with stroke. *ADVANCE for Physical Therapists,* p. 19.

Daniels, N. (1994). Four unsolved rationing problems: A challenge. *Hastings Center Report, 42*(4), 27–29.

Engelhardt, H.T. (1996). *The foundations of bioethics* (2nd ed.). New York: Oxford University Press.

Epstein, A.M. (1990). The outcomes movement—will it get us where we want to go? *New England Journal of Medicine, 323*(4), 266–270.

Gans, J.S. (1987). Facilitating staff/patient interaction in rehabilitation. In B. Caplan (Ed.). *Rehabilitation psychology desk reference* (pp. 185–217). Rockville, MD: Aspen Publishers.

Gunther, M.S. (1994). Countertransference issues in staff caregivers who work to rehabilitate catastrophic injury survivors. *American Journal of Psychotherapy, 48*(2), 208–220.

Haas, J.F. (1988). Admission to rehabilitation centers: Selection of patients. *Archives of Physical Medicine and Rehabilitation, 69*(5), 329–332.

Hume, D. (1967). *A treatise of human nature.* Oxford, England: Clarendon Press.

Johnston, M.V., Keith, R.A., & Hinderer, S.R. (1992). Measurement standards for interdisciplinary medical rehabilitation. *Archives of Physical Medicine and Rehabilitation, 73*(12–S), S3–S12.

Kant, I. (1964). *Groundwork of the metaphysic of morals* (H.J. Paton, Trans.). New York: Harper Torchbooks.

Keith, R. (1991). The comprehensive rehabilitation team. *Archives of Physical Medicine and Rehabilitation, 72*(5), 269–275.

Keith, R.A., Wilson, D.B., & Gutierrez, P. (1995). Acute and subacute rehabilitation for stroke: A comparison. *Archives of Physical Medicine and Rehabilitation, 76*(6), 495–500.

Matyas, T.A., & Ottenbacher, K.J. (1993). Confounds of insensitivity and blind luck: Statistical conclusion validity in stroke rehabilitation clinical trials. *Archives of Physical Medicine and Rehabilitation, 74*(6), 559–565.

May, B. (1996). The twenty-eighth Mary McMillan lecture: On decision making. *Physical Therapy, 76*(11), 1,232–1,241.

Murphy, D.J., & Matcher, D.B. (1990). Life-sustaining therapy: A model for appropriate use. *JAMA, 264,* 2,103–2,108.

Novack, J. (1994). Joseph N. Schaeffer lectureship. *Excellence, 4*(1), 7.

Oczkowski, W.J. & Barreca, S. (1993). The functional independence measure: Its use to identify rehabilitation needs in stroke survivors. *Archives of Physical Medicine and Rehabilitation, 74,* 1291–1294.

Podrid, P.J. (1989). Resuscitation in the elderly: A blessing or a curse? *Annals of Internal Medicine, 111,* 193–195.

Rorty, R. (1990). The priority of democracy to philosophy. In A. Malachowski (Ed.), *Reading Rorty* (pp. 279–302). Oxford: Basil Blackwell.

Schneiderman, L.J., Jecker, N.S., & Jonsen, A.R. (1990). Medical futility: Its meaning and ethical implications. *Annals of Internal Medicine, 112,* 949–954.

Yarmolinsky, A. (1995). Supporting the patient. *New England Journal of Medicine, 332*(9), 602–603.

11

Linking Treatment to Outcomes through Teams: Building a Conceptual Model of Rehabilitation Effectiveness

Dale C. Strasser and Judith A. Falconer

THE PARADOX OF TEAM CARE IN REHABILITATION

A curious paradox permeates the provision of rehabilitation services for individuals who have suffered a stroke or another disabling condition. From the professional organizations and residency training guidelines to the medical corporate boardrooms and marketing brochures, the primacy of a team approach is extolled. Nevertheless, little agreement exists on how teams should function and the process in which the team approach actually makes a difference in patient outcomes. Rehabilitation literature reflects this paradox in the extensive opinion-based articles and few scientific studies on teams (Halsted, 1976; Keith, 1991). The team approach is more an act of faith than a proven strategy in inpatient medical rehabilitation.

Team care remains the dominant paradigm in rehabilitation (Keith, 1996). Its legitimacy is codified in regulatory guidelines such as Health Care Financing Administration (HCFA) requirements for Medicare diagnosis related group (DRG) exempt designation (*Federal Register,* 1985) and the Committee on Accreditation of Rehabilitation Facilities Guidelines. Nevertheless, financial concerns increasingly challenge the practice of team treatment. Economic considerations have resulted in markedly diminished lengths of hospitalization and a reliance on alternative models of care delivery such as home care, outpatient services, day hospitals, and subacute facilities. In addition, pressures exist to provide specific services less expensively, such as the use of more technicians instead of certified therapists and the provision of group therapy instead of individual therapy. These forces challenge the current structure of rehabilitation services and even question the viability of the team approach. In the words of the Board of Governors of the American Congress of Rehabilitation Medicine (1996), "The classic team of the 1970s . . . has largely passed into history" (p. 319).

Even before the contemporary financial challenges, many professionals were frustrated with the team approach. In particular, rehabilitation specialists bemoan the discrepancy of the avowed worth and the actual practice of team care. The inability to achieve significant levels of interprofessional collaboration is cited as a shortcoming of the current practice of teams (Fordyce, 1981; Melvin, 1980). Though some rehabilitation professionals bristle when their activities are compared to toddlers, others share the sentiments of Dr. Jerome Siller (1969) when he compared team activity to "two-year-olds where despite physical proximity everyone is busy with his independent play" (p. 292). In more measured tones, a consensus does exist on the lack of theoretical foundations and empirical proof of the value of team care (Diller, 1990; Keith, 1996). The paradox of rehabilitation teams suggests an ambivalence among rehabilitation specialists. On the one hand, we believe teams are important, but on the other, we appear to have limited insight on how to use them effectively.

Historical developments can provide perspectives on contemporary issues. Origins of the team approach trace back to the beginnings of rehabilitation medicine in the United States and geriatrics in the United Kingdom (Strasser, 1992). Rusk championed the importance of functional assessment and intervention with his pioneering work with disabled soldiers during World War II (Gritzer & Arluke, 1985; Rusk, 1977). In London in the 1930s, Warren spearheaded a new

Special thanks to Robert Allen Keith, PhD, Research and Planning Center, Casa Colina Hospital, Pomona, California, for insightful comments and encouragement and to Barbara Steele-Trower for her assistance with manuscript preparation.

Top Stroke Rehabil, 1997, 4(1), 15–27
© 1997 Aspen Publishers, Inc.

approach in the management of the chronically disabled and frail, older patients. Similar to Rusk, she emphasized functional assessment and practical interventions. In the process, she laid the foundation of modern geriatric medicine (Matthews & Warren, 1984) much like Rusk did in rehabilitation. In each of these examples, a team approach evolved from an emphasis using comprehensive functional assessments to guide therapeutic interventions. Rusk and Warren independently concluded that treatment teams were essential to the management of functional disabilities. Both became vocal advocates for the team approach. This legacy of the intrinsic worth of the team approach is still evident in the practice of rehabilitation professionals. Building on this tradition, contemporary theorists highlight the importance of linking team treatment to patient outcomes (Diller, 1990; Keith, 1996).

THE WHOLE IS GREATER THAN THE SUM OF ITS PARTS

A foundation for team treatment and for problem solving in general is the gestalt notion that the whole is greater than the sum of its parts. Whether in health care, manufacturing, or education, many examples of the superiority of group versus individual effort in solving complex problems exist. One of the dramatic changes in industry in the last 20 years is precisely the rise and perceived value of the work group. Prominent examples in industry include the Japanese automotive and American computer software companies. Likewise, teachers have embraced the value of group activity and collaborative learning. The issue is not whether teams work but, rather, how they work and when it is most effective to use them.

In rehabilitation medicine, this team notion may be framed as multidisciplinary versus interdisciplinary teams (Fordyce, 1981; Melvin, 1980). *Multidisciplinary teams* refer to groups of multiple professionals working in parallel, and *interdisciplinary teams* emphasize concerted integration and collaboration of staff activity in addition to the involvement of multiple professionals. Some professionals have even suggested that transdisciplinary teams would be an even more desirable stage of team development (Diller, 1990; Melvin, 1989). Transdisciplinary team members transcend their particular disciplines in the provision of optimal team treatment. In the descriptive literature on teams, the interdisciplinary and transdisciplinary teams are the overwhelming preference over the multidisciplinary teams.

In general, teams exist because they are felt to be more productive than individuals acting in isolation. Extrapolating from this belief, one could argue that the success of a team depends on the ability to evaluate and intervene in effective ways across disciplines. Teams coordinate and integrate the evaluations and interventions of a diverse group of rehabilitation professionals. The tools of team activity are the tools of this coordination and integration, namely, communication, problem solving, goal setting, and consensus building.

PERSPECTIVES FROM OTHER HEALTH FIELDS

Tantalizing evidence exists from other fields that organizational practices in general and the team approach in particular directly affect patient outcomes. For example, in geriatrics, changes in organizational structure of service delivery involving elements of a team approach have been associated with improvements in functional outcome (Applegate et al., 1990), survival (Applegate et al., 1990; Rubenstein et al., 1984), and resource utilization (Rubenstein et al., 1984). In the intensive care unit (ICU) setting, caregiver interaction was associated with a lower risk-adjusted length of stay and with higher perceived quality of care (Shortell et al., 1992, 1994). In emergency departments, organizational structure and social psychological factors are associated with clinical and economic effectiveness (Georgopoulos, 1986).

In each of these examples, researchers found evidence that organizational structures and processes with elements of teams were associated with improved outcomes. Rubenstein et al. (1984) evaluated the effectiveness of a geriatric assessment unit in a Veterans Administration (VA) setting, while Applegate et al. (1990) looked specifically at the outcomes of older adults in a rehabilitation setting. In both studies, the interventions studied emphasized comprehensive functional evaluations with targeted interventions to optimize outcomes. In ICU settings, Shortell et al. (1992, 1994) examined the physician–nurse interaction. The quality of communication, leadership, and conflict resolution correlated with desirable patient outcomes. Georgopoulos' (1986) landmark study on effectiveness in emergency departments highlighted the importance of organizational structure and problem solving as determinants of clinical and economic effectiveness. These studies present compelling evidence for the potential to improve outcome by improving team care.

RESEARCH ON HEALTH CARE TEAMS AND INTERPROFESSIONAL RELATIONS

Some evidence does exist on the variability of rehabilitation team characteristics and their possible relationship to outcomes. Strasser, Falconer, and Martino-Saltzmann (1994) studied the perceptions of rehabilitation team members on a variety of social psychological and sociological variables. They found interteam differences on group measurements of involvement, practical orientation, and program clarity and interprofessional differences on questions related to professional boundaries. Halstead and colleagues (1986) conducted an experiment in team building designed to improve patient participation on treatment rounds. Patients treated by the experimental team showed increased participation in rounds, and the team itself improved on measures of team environment.

In geriatric medicine, Farrell, Schmitt, and Heinemann (1987, 1988; Heinemann, Schmitt, & Farrell, 1994) found differences in team processes, as reflected in team development. This group of researchers related health care team development to patient outcome. In a small but elegant study, they examined four health care teams in a diabetic clinic. Team membership was identical for the master's-level nurse, the bachelor's-level nurse, and the dietitian. Only the physician differed on each of the four teams. The primary outcome, control of blood glucose, was directly correlated to the measures of team development. These studies suggest that team process, as assessed by stages of team development, appears to affect major patient outcomes.

Interprofessional relations have been extensively described and examined as important, if poorly appreciated, factors on rehabilitation and other health teams (Kane, 1975; Melvin, 1980; Rothberg, 1985; Schmitt, Farrell, & Heinemann, 1988). Professional roles typically exert a stronger influence on staff behavior than treatment team membership (Horwitz, 1970). In customary organizational practice, decisions regarding hiring, firing, raises, assignments of work responsibilities, and reporting mechanisms provide much of the glue to hold organizations together. In contrast, rehabilitation teams typically have few of these cohesive forces. Individual team members identify primarily with their affiliated department or organizational hierarchy while the team affiliation is secondary.

The team also operates within and is influenced by factors extrinsic to the team process such as the professions and the overall hospital's culture and treatment process. A clinical trial designed to improve efficiency in inpatient stroke rehabilitation may offer insights into the importance of extrinsic factors on team process and outcome (Falconer, Naughton, Dunlop, Roth, Strasser, & Sinacore, 1994). In this experiment, enhanced team communication and problem solving, without alteration in the larger culture and organization within which the team functioned, could not sustain improvements in clinical or economic outcomes.

ASSESSING OUTCOMES IN STROKE REHABILITATION

Despite our limited knowledge of team care per se, extensive evidence exists that supports the superiority of specialized rehabilitation units over the delivery of similar services on general medical wards. As reviewed by Dombovy, Sandok, and Basford (1986) and Ottenbacher and Jannell (1993), rehabilitation services dedicated to particular diagnostic entities, such as stroke, usually have superior patient outcomes compared to comparable therapy services delivered in nonspecialized units. Given the consensus on the value of the team treatment approach, a reasonable case can be made in favor of team care versus no team care. However, as an alternative explanation, these improved outcomes could simply reflect increased intensity of service or improved professional skills of individual therapists instead of an indication of the superiority of the team approach.

The alternative explanation of increased therapy intensity has not been supported by the empirical studies. Heinemann, Hamilton, Linacre, Wright, and Granger (1995) looked at traumatic brain injury (TBI) and spinal cord injury patients ($n = 246$) and failed to reveal any association with the intensities of physical, occupational, or speech therapies and functional outcomes measured by the Functional Independence Measure (FIM; Stineman & Granger, 1994). Taking advantage of the natural experiment with the implementation of the Medicare 3-hr regulation, Johnston and Miller (1986) studied patient outcomes before and after the implementation of this regulation. While the amount of physical and occupational therapy increased on the average of 0.55 hr per patient, no detectable differences in outcomes as assessed by improved functional status or living arrangement were revealed.

The recent growth in subacute rehabilitation services offers another test of the relationship of service intensity to patient outcomes. Advocates for these services contend that similar outcomes to those in hospital-based inpatient rehabilitation can be achieved at reduced costs in subacute settings. Cost reductions are achieved primarily by reductions in service, including nursing, physician, and therapy. A retrospective study comparing acute and subacute rehabilitation services for stroke patients found that the outcomes for those treated in the acute setting demonstrated greater functional gains as measured by the FIM, but these gains were not necessarily associated with higher rates of discharge to the community (Keith, Wilson, & Gutierrez, 1995). Likewise, stroke patients treated on acute inpatient rehabilitation services demonstrated greater functional gains than those treated in either regular nursing homes or rehabilitative nursing homes (Kane, Chen, Blewett, & Sangl, 1996). No difference in outcomes was found between those treated in regular nursing homes and rehabilitative nursing homes.

Taken together, these studies on the intensity of service and outcomes suggest the involvement of other factors, perhaps akin to the relationship of the student-to-teacher ratio and the amount learned in school. More intense inpatient services have not been shown to improve outcomes, while some evidence has been presented that suggests that less intense services in nursing homes may have poorer outcomes. A critical factor in explaining this relationship of treatment to outcome could be the service delivery itself and not simply the amount of service provided. The medical, social, and psychological issues associated with disabled stroke patients challenge rehabilitation professionals to "put it all together."

Since no one professional orientation can provide comprehensive care to the multifaceted stroke patient, the way the services are delivered probably has a great deal of an impact on the outcomes.

A MODEL OF TREATMENT EFFECTIVENESS IN INPATIENT STROKE REHABILITATION

In the remaining section of this article, a model of treatment effectiveness is proposed (Figure 1). The model places the team approach at the center of treatment effectiveness and hypothesizes relationships that can be studied and used as bases for interventions. While this model may have generalizability beyond stroke rehabilitation, the biopsychosocial complexity of stroke patients represents a disabling condition likely to benefit from the team approach.

Based on critical analyses of diverse perspectives and extensive clinical experience, a model of team effectiveness is presented in the following section. With particular attention to the dynamics of treatment, the model relates characteristics of the organization, treatment, and participants to each other and, more importantly, to patient outcomes. While the importance of patient characteristics in predicting functional status and resource utilization is acknowledged, this model focuses on dimensions of team process that are believed to influence patient outcomes. The model proposes that team process (interprofessional relations, social climate, leadership, and team practices) affects patient outcomes through

the dynamics of effective coordination of diverse staff activities in the context of functional evaluation and intervention. Such a model may prove useful to rehabilitation specialists in understanding how inpatient rehabilitation works and in devising strategies to improve treatment effectiveness.

Patient Outcome

The primary focus of this model is the patient. Other potential outcomes not directly addressed by this model include those of the organization, treatment, and staff. Organizational outcomes that could also be of interest are financial, relations with referring sources, and the mission of the organization. Therapy and treatment outcomes could emphasize efficiency and efficacy. Staff outcomes of rehabilitation commonly involve salary, satisfaction, stability, and professional advancement. The outcomes of interest in this model relate broadly to patient-centered issues, such as discharge destination, functional status gain, and functional status at discharge.

Health Care Organization and Behavior

Health care organizations, including hospitals, consist of a structure, a culture, organizational processes, and patterns of operations. Each element is potentially a determinant of team behavior. Components of hospital structure that could reasonably relate to team effectiveness include size, staff composi-

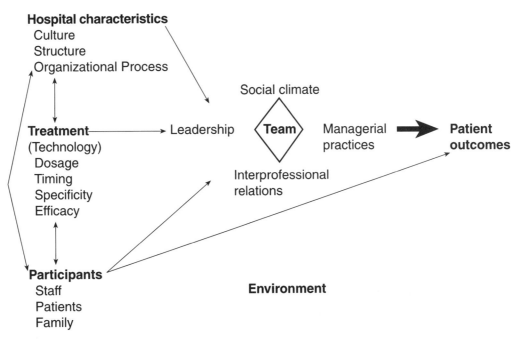

Figure 1. Model of treatment effectiveness in inpatient stroke rehabilitation.

tion, and formal structure (e.g., as represented in the organizational chart). Organizational culture consists of the values of an organization as demonstrated in the normative beliefs and shared behavioral expectations of its members (Cooke & Szumal, 1993). Organizational processes are, in brief, the way things get done in the organization and are related to structure and culture. Included in organizational processes are communication, conflict resolution, goal setting, and evaluations.

Hospital characteristics of structure, culture, and process have been related to staff performances and patient outcomes. Hospital size is associated with variations in resource utilization in rehabilitation (Keith & Breckenridge, 1985) and with staff attitudes toward continuous quality improvement/total quality management principles (Shortell et al., 1995). Organizational culture is a useful construct in explaining patient outcomes in ICU settings (Shortell, Rousseau, Gillies, Devers, & Simons, 1991), in characterizing nursing services (Thomas, Ward, Chorba, & Kumiega, 1990), and in understanding innovation and turnover in health care (O'Reilly, 1989). In rehabilitation, specific organizational processes, such as admissions procedures, directly influence case mix and relations with referral sources.

Hospital (Osberg, Haley, McGinnis, & DeJong, 1990) and regional (Keith & Breckenridge, 1985) variations have been associated with resource utilization in inpatient rehabilitation along with a host of patient characteristics (McGinnis, Osberg, DeJong, Seward, & Branch, 1987; Granger, Hamilton, & Fiedler, 1992; Stineman, 1995). While DRGs have been useful in predicting resource utilization in acute-care hospitals, DRGs alone only explained 12% of the variation in charges in inpatient rehabilitation (McGinnis, et al., 1987). Case mix is highly correlated with patient lengths of stay and functional outcomes (Stineman, Hamilton, Goin, Granger, & Fiedler, 1996). The determinants of case mix in a particular setting are influenced by the evaluation and admission processes which, in turn, reflect the organization's mission and value. Hence, the health care organization including the rehabilitation hospital or unit must profoundly influence rehabilitation treatment and outcomes.

Treatment

Four components of treatment postulated to influence team effectiveness are (1) dosage, (2) timing, (3) specificity, and (4) efficacy. Dimensions of treatment *dosage* include intensity, frequency, and duration. *Timing* refers to the time of treatment relative to a precipitating event or stage of recovery. *Specificity* relates to the precision of the treatment relative to the nature of the problem. *Efficacy*, as opposed to effectiveness, is the laboratory in vitro effect of the treatment technique or strategy.

The treatment component of our model deals with efficacy, while the overall patient outcomes relate to effective-

ness. A number of rehabilitation interventions have been efficacious in controlled trials (Agency for Health Care Policy and Research, 1993). However, an efficacious treatment may not effectively transfer into good clinical outcomes for a variety of real-world reasons. Efficacy studies typically involve highly selected populations and strict adherence to treatment protocols under controlled conditions. Compared to efficacy studies, clinic work involves a more diverse population, treatment protocols are more often adapted or modified, and control over the treatment conditions is more variable. For example, mobility outcomes may be compromised by patient-specific factors, such as cognitive capabilities or problems related to the method of instruction (i.e., type and amount of feedback or follow up), dose (i.e., inadequate opportunities to practice developing skills), or the environment (i.e., limited access to appropriately challenging and varied practice settings).

Participants: Staff, Patients, and Family

For rehabilitation to achieve the goal of functional well-being, the participants in the rehabilitation treatment process—staff, patients, and family—must come together productively in an environment that promotes the acquisition and maintenance of behavioral and functional skills. Characteristics of these participants, much like the importance of particular students, parents, and teachers in a classroom, have a major influence on the success of the rehabilitation effort.

Patient-level characteristics that have been associated with functional outcome after stroke include clinical features related to premorbid health and function, comorbid conditions, type and severity of impairments (i.e., incontinence, visuospatial deficits) and disabilities (activities of daily living [ADL] status), and onset to admission interval (Jongbloed, 1986; Stineman, & Granger, 1994). Less studied, but acknowledged for their role in enabling the individual to benefit from treatment, are behavioral factors such as personal goals, beliefs, motivation, expectations, and preference for treatment.

Using patient-specific characteristics, the ability to predict resource utilization, functional gains, and other patient outcomes for patients suffering a stroke who receive inpatient rehabilitation has been enhanced by the work of Stineman, Escarce, Hamilton, Granger, & Williams (1994) and Harada, Kominski, and Sofaer (1993). Patient-level variables combined with Functional Related Groups (FRGs) and the (FIM) can account for up to 30% of the variances in rehabilitation lengths of stay. The FIM/FRGs and other approaches provide a tool to control for patient and institutional characteristics, including case mix, in an analysis for interinstitutional effectiveness.

Compared with patient-level characteristics, fewer staff-level characteristics have been examined for their effect on stroke rehabilitation effectiveness. It is reasonable to assume, however, that a variety of staff characteristics may directly and indirectly influence patient outcomes. Staff knowledge, skills, attitude, training, and experience are potential determinants of the effectiveness of patient treatment. Appreciation and understanding of sociocultural concerns for patients influence medical care generally and likely play a similar role in determining patient outcomes in stroke rehabilitation.

The family and other psychosocial supports contribute significantly to patient outcomes. As reviewed by Bishop and Evans (1995), family issues have profound influences on patient outcome. The presence of a caregiver was a significant predictor of discharge destination for stroke patients undergoing inpatient rehabilitation (Davidoff, 1992). Furthermore, family variables are associated with long-term adjustment to a stroke (Evans, Bishop, Matlock, & Noonan, 1987). Given that much of inpatient rehabilitation strives for the optimal balance between the patient and his or her environment following discharge, the family plays a critical role in the establishment of this homeostasis.

Treatment Team

At the core of this model of treatment effectiveness is the team itself. Four major dimensions of the team are offered to explain the translation of the organization, treatment, and participants into desirable patient outcomes. Two of these dimensions—interprofessional relations and social climate—are the foundation of team work, while the other two—leadership and managerial practices—provide insight into team activity. Team process—a function of these four dimensions—transforms the inputs (hospital, treatment, and participants) into patient outcomes.

A foundation of team activity is manifested in the interprofessional relations among the team members. Interprofessional relations among team members constitute a forum for team activity. However, professional roles typically exert a stronger influence on staff behavior than treatment team membership (Horwitz, 1970). This influence is evident when tensions between an individual's role as a member of a professional group and as a member of a treatment team occur. In these circumstances, most team members identify primarily with their professional discipline. Nevertheless and somewhat paradoxically, it is precisely the professional diversity that distinguishes the team approach.

The social climate of the team modulates this tendency for primary identification with one's discipline over treatment team. *Social climate* refers to the distinctive "personality" of a treatment team and is a cause and consequence of team activity. Just like individuals, teams differ on friendliness, task orientation, and rigidity. Teams have distinctive social climates that influence the behavior of individuals in that environment (Moos, 1994a, 1994b). Staff form global ideas

of the team from specific perceptions of the social climate. The resulting perceptions of the social climate influence how a team member acts.

Empirical evidence exists in support of the utility of these constructs of interprofessional relations and social climate. With respect to interprofessional relations, rehabilitation staff report the most discord in areas of professional boundaries (Strasser et al., 1994). An inverse relationship between an individual's professional identification and identification with a health care team has been found on VA health care teams (Farrell, Schmitt, & Heinemann, 1994). Measurements of social climate on health treatment teams have been useful in characterizing rehabilitation teams (Strasser et al., 1994) in revealing discipline-specific differences among VA health care teams (Schmitt, Heinemann, & Farrell, 1994) and in measuring change after a successful intervention to improve patient participation on rehabilitation team rounds (Halstead, et al., 1986).

While the foundation of team activity resides in the interprofessional relations and social climate, the realization of team activity comes through the dimensions of team leadership and managerial practices. The team is "dealt" a particular hand from the health care organization, treatment parameters, and the rehabilitation participants in the context of a particular environment. The team "plays" this hand through its leadership and managerial practices. Hence, leadership and managerial practices represent the actions by which the team conducts its work.

The dimension of team leadership encompasses attributes of leaders and managers. Managers take charge of activities for task accomplishment, and leaders influence, guide, and set directions (Bennis & Nanus, 1985). Managers are needed to understand the specifics of rehabilitation and to integrate the activities of a diverse group of professionals. Leaders communicate a vision and establish a shared purpose for the context of rehabilitation team activities. Team leaders may be called upon to negotiate with nonteam professionals and with the hospital administration. Successful team leadership requires both good leaders and good managers (Strasser, 1988).

While leaders and managers usually refer to individuals, leadership has more of a functional connotation. Multiple roles crucial to team activities are performed by different team members, and the relative importance of an individual team member in a leadership function will vary according to the situation. For example, the multifactorial roles inherent in team activity have been classified as case management, team management, primary patient relationship, charismatic leader, and medical decision (adapted from Parker, 1972). These leadership functions significantly affect the team as a cohesive and effective group.

The managerial practices of the team are the operations of team process. These practices represent the "nuts and bolts" of team activity. Core elements of managerial practices consist of communication, coordination, and problem solving (adapted from Shortell et al., 1991). Hence, this model proposes that rehabilitation treatment effectiveness is modulated by team process, which is a function of the team's interprofessional relations, social climate, leadership, and managerial practices.

•   •   •

Based on the belief that even a primitive tool is better than no tool at all, a theoretical model of team effectiveness was proposed. While couched in reference to empirical studies and reasonableness of constructs, this model places the team in a unique position to the work of others, precisely at the center of meaningful inpatient rehabilitation activity. The selected constructs and associated measures have been employed by researchers in other settings and are measurable. Hence, interested individuals may find this model beneficial in devising clinical interventions and studies of rehabilitation effectiveness. The team orchestrates three interrelated themes (hospital, treatment, and participants) to produce a composition of outcomes. In the best of scores, the student responds harmoniously providing music to the ears of a satisfied staff.

REFERENCES

Agency for Health Care Policy and Research, Public Health Service, U.S. Department of Health and Human Services. (1993). *Critical literature review: Clinical effectiveness in allied health practices,* (AHCPR Publication No. 94-0029). Rockville, MD: Author.

Applegate, W.B., Miller, S.T., Graney, M.J., Elam, J.T., Burns, R., & Akins, D.E. (1990). A randomized, controlled trial of a geriatric assessment unit in a community rehabilitation hospital. *New England Journal of Medicine, 322,* 1,572–1,578.

Bennis, W., & Nanus, B. (1985). *Leaders: The strategies for taking charge.* New York: Harper Perennial.

Bishop, D.S., & Evans, R.L. (1995). Families and stroke: The clinical implications of research findings. *Topics in Stroke Rehabilitation, 2*(2), 20–31.

Board of Governors, American Congress of Rehabilitation Medicine. (1996). Editorial: Evolution and vision. *Archives of Physical Medicine and Rehabilitation, 77*(4), 319.

Cooke, R.A., & Szumal, J. (1993). Measuring normative beliefs and shared behavioral expectations in organizations: The reliability and validity of the organizational culture inventory. *Psychology Reports, 72,* 1,299–1,330.

Davidoff, G.N. (1992). Who goes home after stroke: A case control study. *NeuroRehabilitation, 2*(2), 53–62.

Diller, R. (1990). Fostering the interdisciplinary team, fostering research in a society in transition. *Archives of Physical Medicine and Rehabilitation, 71,* 275–278.

Dombovy, M.L., Sandok, B.A., & Basford, J.R. (1986). Rehabilitation for stroke: A review. *Stroke, 17,* 363–369.

Evans, R.L., Bishop, D.S., Matlock, A.L., & Noonan, W.C. (1987). Prestroke family interaction as a predictor of stroke outcome. *Archives of Physical Medicine and Rehabilitation, 68,* 508–512.

Falconer, J.A., Naughton, B.J., Dunlop, D.D., Roth, E.J., Strasser, D.C., & Sinacore, J.M. (1994). Predicting stroke inpatient rehabilitation outcome using a classification tree approach. *Archives of Physical Medicine and Rehabilitation, 75,* 619–625.

Falconer, J.A., Roth, E.J., Sutin, J.A., Strasser, D.C., & Chang, R.W. (1993). The critical path method in stroke rehabilitation: Lessons from an experiment in cost containment and outcome improvement. *Quality Review Bulletin,* 8–16.

Farrell, M.P., Schmitt, M.H., & Heinemann, G.D. (1987). Assessing the validity of an index of team development. Paper presented at the Ninth Annual Interdisciplinary Health Care Team Conference, State University of New York-Stoney Brook, NY.

Farrell, M.P., Schmitt, M.H., & Heinemann, G.D. (1988). Organizational environments of health care teams: Impact on team development and implications for consultation. *International Journal of Small Group Research,* 31–53.

Farrell, M.P., Schmitt, M.H., & Heinemann, G.D. (1994). Social networks, team development, and the quality of team functioning in geriatric care. Paper presented at the 16th Annual Interdisciplinary Team Conference, Chicago, IL.

Federal Register (1985, July 31), *50*(147), 31041.

Fordyce, W. (1981). On interdisciplinary peers. *Archives of Physical Medicine and Rehabilitation, 62,* 51–53.

Georgopoulos, B.S. (1986). Conclusions and implications. In *Organizational structure, problem solving and effectiveness,* (pp. 283–303). San Francisco: Jossey-Bass, Publishers.

Granger, C.V., Hamilton, B.B., & Fiedler, R.C. (1992). Discharge outcome after stroke rehabilitation. *Stroke, 23,* 978–982.

Gritzer, G., & Arluke, A. (1985). *The making of rehabilitation.* Berkeley, CA: University of California Press.

Halstead, L.S. (1976). Team care in chronic illness: A critical review of the literature of the past 25 years. *Archives of Physical Medicine and Rehabilitation, 58,* 507–511.

Halstead, L.S., Rintala, D.H., Kancellos, M., Griffin, B., Higgins, L., Rheinecker, S., Whiteside, W., & Healy, J.E. (1986). The innovative rehabilitation team: An experiment in team building. *Archives of Physical Medicine and Rehabilitation, 67,* 357–361.

Harada, N., Kominski, G., & Sofaer, S. (1993, Spring). Development of a resource-based patient classification scheme for rehabilitation. *Inquiry, 30,* 54–63.

Harada, N., Sofaer, S., & Kominski, G. (1993). Functional status outcomes in rehabilitation: Implications for prospective payment. *Medical Care, 31,* 345–357.

Heinemann, A., Hamilton, B.B., Linacre, J.M., Wright, B.D., & Granger, C.V. (1995). Functional status and therapeutic intensity during inpatient rehabilitation. *American Journal of Physical Medicine and Rehabilitation, 74*(4), 315–326.

Heinemann, G.D., Schmitt, M.H., & Farrell, M.P. (1994). The quality of geriatric team functioning: Model and methodology. Paper presented at the 16th Annual Interdisciplinary Team Conference, Chicago, IL.

Horwitz, J.J. (1970). Professionalism, professionalization, and the interdisciplinary team. In *Team practice and the specialists: An introduction to interdisciplinary teamwork* (pp. 111–146). Springfield, IL: Charles C Thomas.

Johnston, M.V., & Miller, L.S. (1986). Cost-effectiveness of the Medicare three-hour regulation. *Archives of Physical Medicine and Rehabilitation, 67,* 581–585.

Jongbloed, L. (1986). Prediction of function after stroke: A critical review. *Stroke, 17,* 765–776.

Kane, R.L. (1975). Interprofessional teamwork. In *Manpower Monograph Number Eight,* Syracuse, NY: Syracuse University School of Social Work.

Kane, R.L., Chen, Q., Blewett, L.A., & Sangl, J. (1996). Do rehabilitative nursing homes improve the outcomes of care? *Journal of the American Geriatrics Society, 44*(6), 545–554.

Keith, R.A. (1991). The comprehensive treatment team in rehabilitation. *Archives of Physical Medicine and Rehabilitation, 72,* 269–274.

Keith, R.A. (1996). Treatment theory in the design and conduct of medical rehabilitation outcomes research. In M.J. Fuhrer (Ed.), *Medical rehabilitation outcomes research.* Baltimore: Paul H. Brookes Publishing.

Keith, R.A., & Breckenridge, K. (1985). Characteristics of patients from the hospital utilization project data system: 1980–1982. *Archives of Physical Medicine and Rehabilitation, 66,* 768–772.

Keith, R.A., Wilson, D.B., & Gutierrez, P. (1995). Acute and subacute rehabilitation for stroke: A comparison. *Archives of Physical Medicine and Rehabilitation, 76*(6), 495–500.

Matthews, D.A., & Warren, M. (1984). The origins of British geriatrics. *Journal of the American Geriatric Society, 32,* 253–258.

McGinnis, G.E., Osberg, J.S., DeJong, G., Seward, M.L., & Branch, L.G. (1987). Predicting charges for inpatient medical rehabilitation using severity, DRG, age, and function. *American Journal of Public Health, 77,* 826–829.

Melvin, J. (1980). Interdisciplinary and multidisciplinary activities and the ACRM. *Archives of Physical Medicine and Rehabilitation, 62,* 51–53.

Melvin, J. (1989). Status report on interdisciplinary medical rehab. *Archives of Physical Medicine and Rehabilitation, 70,* 273.

Moos, R.H. (1994a). *Group environment scale manual* (3rd ed.). Palo Alto, CA: Consulting Psychologist Press.

Moos, R.H. (1994b). *The social climate scales: A user's guide.* Palo Alto, CA: Consulting Psychologist Press.

O'Reilly, C. (1989). Corporations, culture, and commitment: Motivation and social control in organizations. *California Management Review, 31,* 9–25.

Osberg, J.S., Haley, S.M., McGinnis, G.E., & DeJong, G. (1990). Characteristics of cost outliers who did not benefit from stroke rehabilitation. *American Journal of Physical Medicine and Rehabilitation, 69,* 117–125.

Ottenbacher, K.J., & Jannell, S. (1993). The results of clinical trials in stroke rehabilitation research. *Archives of Neurology, 50,* 37–44.

Parker, A.W. (1972). The team approach to primary health care. In *Neighborhood health center seminar program* (Monograph Series, No. 3, pp. 31–33. Berkeley, CA: School of Public Health, University of California.

Rothberg, J.S. (1985). Rehabilitation team practice. In J. Lecca & J.S. McNeil (Eds.), *Interdisciplinary team practice: Issues and trends.* (pp. 19–41). New York: Praeger Publishing.

Rubenstein, L.Z., Josephson, K.R., Wieland, D., English, P.A., Sayer, J.A., & Kane, R.L. (1984). Effectiveness of a geriatric evaluation unit. *New England Journal of Medicine, 311,* 1,664–1,670.

Rusk, H.A. (1977). *A world to care for: The autobiography of Howard A. Rusk, M.D.* New York: A Reader's Digest Press Book, Random House.

Schmitt, M.H., Farrell, M.P., & Heinemann, G.D. (1988). Conceptual and methodological problems in studying the effects of interdisciplinary geriatric teams. *Gerontologist, 28*(6), 753–764.

Schmitt, M.H., Heinemann, G.D., & Farrell, M.P. (1994). Discipline differences in attitudes towards interdisciplinary teams, perceptions of the process of team work, and stress levels in geriatric health care teams. Paper presented at the 16th Annual Interdisciplinary Team Conference, Chicago, IL.

Shortell, S.M., O'Brien, J.L., Carman, J.M., Foster, R.W., Hughes, E.F.X., Boerstler, H., & O'Connor, E.J. (1995). Assessing the impact of continuous quality improvement/total quality management: Concept versus implementation. *Health Services Research, 30*(2), 377–401.

Shortell, S.M., Rousseau, D.M., Gillies, R.R., Devers, K.J., & Simons, T.L. (1991). Organizational assessment in intensive care units: Construct development, reliability, and validity of the ICU nurse-physician questionnaire. *Medical Care, 29*(8), 709–726.

Shortell, S.M., Zimmerman, J.E., Gillies, R.R., Duffy, J., Devers, K.J., Rousseau, D.M., & Knaus, W.A. (1992). Continuously improving patient care: Practical lessons and an assessment tool from the national ICU study. *Quality Review Bulletin, 18,* 150–155.

Shortell, S.M., Zimmerman, J.E., Rousseau, D.M., Gillies, R.R., Wagner, D.P., Draper, E.A., Knaus, W.A., & Duffy, J. (1994). The performance of intensive care units: Does good management make a difference? *Medical Care, 32*(5), 508–525.

Siller, J. (1969). Psychological situation of the disabled with spinal cord injuries. *Rehabilitation Literature, 30*(10), 292–296.

Stineman, M.G. (1995). Case-mix measurement in medical rehabilitation. *Archives of Physical Medicine and Rehabilitation, 76,* 1,163–1,170.

Stineman, M.G., Escarce, J.J., Hamilton, B.B., Granger, C.V., & Williams, S.V. (1994). A case-mix classification system for medical rehabilitation. *Medical Care, 32,* 366–379.

Stineman, M.G., & Granger, C.V. (1994). Outcome studies and analysis: Principles of rehabilitation that influence outcome analysis. In G. Felsenthal, S.J. Garrison, & F.V. Steinberg (Eds.), *Rehabilitation of the aging and elderly patient* (pp. 511–522). Baltimore: Williams & Wilkins.

Stineman, M.G., Hamilton, B.B., Goin, J.E., Granger, C.V., & Fiedler, R.C. (1996). Functional gain and length of stay for major rehabilitation impairment categories: Patterns revealed by function related groups. *American Journal of Physical Medicine & Rehabilitation, 75*(1), 68–78.

Strasser, D.C. (1988). Team leadership—who, what and how. *Archives of Physical Medicine and Rehabilitation, 69*(9), 717.

Strasser, D.C. (1992). Geriatric rehabilitation: Perspectives from the United Kingdom. *Archives of Physical Medicine and Rehabilitation, 73,* 582–585.

Strasser, D.C., Falconer, J.A., & Martino-Saltzmann, D. (1994). The rehabilitation team: Staff perceptions of the hospital environment, the interdisciplinary team environment, and interprofessional relations. *Archives of Physical Medicine and Rehabilitation, 75,* 177–182.

Thomas, C., Ward, M., Chorba, C., & Kumiega, A. (1990). Measuring and interpreting. *Journal of Nursing Administration, 20*(6), 17–24.

PART II

Patient Satisfaction

12

Measuring Patient Satisfaction in an Outpatient Orthopedic Setting, Part 1: Key Drivers and Results

Teresa L. Elliott-Burke and Lori Pothast

SCOPE OF THE STUDY

This four-year study of 19,834 patients offers an in-depth look at patient satisfaction in the outpatient orthopedic rehabilitation setting. It provides insight into the following inquiries: Why measure patient satisfaction? How is patient satisfaction actually measured? How does patient satisfaction relate to an outcomes management process? What can it reveal about the management, service, and care in an outpatient orthopedic setting?

MEASURING PATIENT SATISFACTION

Patient satisfaction measurement has grown in response to increasing involvement and awareness of the patient and family in health care, the use of capitated payment plans, the application of total quality management (TQM) in the health care setting, and the growing competition among health care providers for clients.[1] The standardized patient satisfaction survey issued in 1995 by the National Committee for Quality Assurance (NCQA) promoted satisfaction as one of the performance measures for health plans and increased the emphasis on patient satisfaction in a variety of health care settings.[2] Measurement of patients' perceptions by a standard satisfaction survey is increasingly important to the success of a health care organization.

Clinicians are cautious of measuring patient satisfaction. They are concerned about bias of the negative responses from "difficult" patients or those with personal motivation to report a negative result. As Roush points out, physical thera-

pists (PTs) and occupational therapists (OTs) have generally ignored standardized evaluation of patient satisfaction.[3]

Standardized and reliable patient satisfaction studies can assist clinicians in six crucial ways.

1. Educating clinicians to better understand the patient's paradigm

It is important to consider the patient's expectations and perceptions of the service and care he or she receives. Clinicians often think of delivering care only from their point of view. As DiMatteo, Prince, and Taranta concluded, physicians and other health care professionals who hope to provide effective continuous care to their patients need to learn to communicate caring and concern. They must listen, amply explain, and educate. It has been shown that patients are responsive to these efforts.[4]

2. Providing an important component of outcomes measurement

Outcome is a complex issue with minimal agreed-upon standardization within rehabilitation. Patient satisfaction is one element of an overall process of outcomes management. In addition to satisfaction with health care, outcomes can include changes in health status, changes in knowledge or behavior pertinent to future health status, and satisfaction with health care.[5] The growing attention given to customers' views about quality make satisfaction an increasingly important element in evaluating the end results of care. The expressions of satisfaction (or lack of it) with certain elements of care might be considered a nonintrusive indicator of the art of medical practice. Patient reports can be regarded as valid measures of one aspect of the care received.[6]

J Rehabil Outcomes Meas, 1997, 1(1), 18–25
© 1997 Aspen Publishers, Inc.

3. Predicting health-related behaviors and health care utilization

Satisfaction may predict the likelihood a patient will return to care. One study concluded that successful physicians were ones who were able to overall satisfy patients enough so that they would return for treatment.[7] Marquis et al. agreed that patient satisfaction is predictive of how patients will behave in the future and that patient dissatisfaction may cause provider change.[8]

4. Determining a patient's compliance to his or her treatment program

Ongoing patient satisfaction contributes to increased compliance of care and eventually leads to successful therapy outcomes. Donabedian identified patient satisfaction as a factor directly influencing compliance with medical regimens.[9]

5. Offering data to be used in a continuous process improvement program

There is a growing consensus that satisfaction with care may be one of our most important measurements of quality health care.[10–12] The improvement of quality requires knowledge of discrete factors pertinent to health care delivery. An ongoing, standardized patient satisfaction survey provides a mechanism to evaluate quality in a rehabilitation program on a regular basis.

6. Creating a service-oriented culture

The provision of quality service and service training of employees have been common in successful businesses and in industries for years. Health care has had a tendency to sponsor clinically oriented training programs, with less attention to service delivery training. Nelson and Larson stated that health care providers who are serious about improving quality may want to do their own customer research. This would offer insight into what the providers might do to delight and avoid disappointing their patients and what they should do consistently, efficiently, and compassionately to meet basic expectations of their patients.[13]

THE STUDY

This patient satisfaction project involved measurement of over 120 outpatient orthopedic rehabilitation centers, the majority providing physical therapy services, with approximately 15 centers also providing occupational therapy. These centers were owned by a publicly traded health care corporation. The typical center averaged 40 patients per day and was staffed with 3–4 clinicians.

In 1992 patient satisfaction measurement was initiated for two reasons. The first was to support a service initiative. The goal was to train all personnel on service standards and concepts with the expectation that these principles be put to use. The patient satisfaction surveys helped to measure the results of this training. The second reason this process was initiated was to support an outcomes management initiative. This initiative measured four components: patient satisfaction, clinical effectiveness, cost, and utilization. Clinical effectiveness was measured by improvement in functional status, return to work, and goal achievement. Utilization was defined as the number of treatments a specific patient with a specific diagnosis received. Cost was included to ensure the best outcome for the least cost. Measuring patient satisfaction showed commitment to the service and outcomes initiatives.

Building the Instrument

Zastowny et al. suggested that focus groups provide essential help in individualizing the assessment measure to the nature of health care being delivered and to the unique context-based set of patient experiences and expectations.[14] Five patient focus groups were convened to identify the range of aspects of care and service that was to be measured. Groups were held in locations that reflected company geographical concentrations of centers: two in Chicago, one in Phoenix, and two in Austin, Texas. The groups consisted of 10–12 former or current physical therapy patients from our centers and local competitors. Participants were randomly selected by an outside agency. Each session lasted two hours and was led by a contracted facilitator. As a result of these focus groups, 26 points of service were identified. These 26 points represented 5 service dimensions: overall satisfaction, therapist interaction, center operations, facility, and billing (see Table 1).

The Gallup Organization was then employed to help create and administer the standardized patient satisfaction survey. An outside agency was chosen to eliminate internal bias and provide greater credibility with all our customers (payers, physicians, and patients). As reported by NCQA, greater confidence is given to information collected and reported by a credible entity with experience in conducting survey research and one that is independent of the health care being provided.[15]

Surveying Patients

A total of 19,834 patients was interviewed between April 1992 and December 1995. Each year the number of interviews increased as the result of new center acquisitions. We began in 1992 with 3,340 interviews and completed in 1995 with 6,705. Patients were selected randomly by the surveyors from a monthly computer list of all discharged patients in

Table 1. The five service dimensions: a description of the points of service

Dimension	Points of service
Overall satisfaction	• The experience, considering all aspects of the service you received at your local center • Willingness to refer a family member or friend to the center
Therapist interaction	• Explanation of your treatment program • Amount of personal attention from therapists • Number of different treating clinicians • How knowledgeable the clinicians were about case • Amount of personal input into setting treatment goals • Frequency therapists made you aware of progress • Amount of empathy or concern expressed by therapists for your level of discomfort/pain
Center operations	• How quickly patients were able to schedule first appointment • The convenience of the center's hours of operation • Orientation to the center • Amount of waiting time • The helpfulness and courteousness of office staff
Facility	• Appearance of center was neat, clean, and organized
Billing	• Explanation of billing procedures • Monthly billing statements were accurate • Resolution of billing problems

each location. A discharged patient was classified as one who had been discharged from care or had no attendance for 30 days. This patient population was chosen over the active patient population because they had completed the total physical therapy experience.

On average 25 patients were surveyed quarterly for each orthopedic rehabilitation center in 1992, 1993, and 1994. Industrial rehabilitation centers were excluded. In 1995, due to the cost of the surveys and increased number of centers, 20 patients per center were surveyed quarterly. Newly acquired centers were initially surveyed following their second full quarter of operation in the new parent company. By the end of 1995 more than 120 centers had been surveyed, representing 12 states (Arizona, Maryland, New Jersey, Ohio, Illinois, Indiana, Texas, California, Washington, Missouri, South Carolina, and North Carolina).

All interviews were conducted via the phone and lasted 4–5 minutes. Phone interviews were chosen over mailed-back surveys with the intent to obtain higher response rates in the available time and a greater representation of the sample. A telephone interview may also decrease responder bias. (A patient may be motivated to respond more positively when the survey is given at the same location the care is provided.) Also the quantity of information gathered during a phone interview may be greater than other survey formats. One study showed that, when presented with written questionnaires, patients were reluctant to write any meaningful comments and even when patients did write important comments they were too few in number to provide useful information.[16]

Refining the Instrument

The original survey consisted of 32 questions encompassing the 26 points of service that were determined in the focus groups, plus population demographic and screening questions. The satisfaction questions required a response on a Likert-type (five point) scale. The five responses were:

5 Very satisfied
4 Somewhat satisfied
3 Neither satisfied nor dissatisfied
2 Somewhat dissatisfied
1 Very dissatisfied

After an initial use of the survey, the instrument was refined by (1) soliciting feedback from clinicians and other center staff, (2) determining the drivers of overall satisfaction via regression analysis, and (3) interviewer feedback.

Following nine months of survey use, several changes were made to increase the focus on satisfaction. Low satisfaction impact questions were removed, such as several billing questions, parking convenience, and working status of center equipment. Also removed were questions requesting factual responses instead of satisfaction levels, such as waiting time, number of treating therapists, types of billing problems, and how the patient dealt with billing problems.

In 1995 a total of 17 questions requiring a response on a five-point scale and one open-ended question remained. The open-ended question regarding service improvement was the same as the original version: "What one thing could the center have done to better satisfy you?" This question was in response to the understanding that each care setting is likely to generate its own set of unique expectations and potential problems when patient expectations are unfulfilled.[17] Patients were provided with the opportunity to address these situations. Also in 1995 a question was added to enhance the overall satisfaction dimension. This question assessed a patient's willingness to refer a family member or friend to the center in which he or she was treated.

The responses were tabulated by the Gallup Organization and reported each quarter by center, for each region cluster, and totaled nationally. This comparative reporting mechanism allowed us to internally compare the results between centers, and begin to identify and benchmark superior performers. Each quarter the center could compare its results to the national and regional scores as well as the top performers. This method of reporting provided a quarterly trending of results for the past four quarters.

The time delay for processing the results of a phone survey is less than a written survey method with a reduced time for data collections management. Reports were published 3–4 weeks following the end of each quarter sampled. A quarterly reporting schedule was effective in maintaining ongoing center quality improvement plans. The downside to the quarterly reporting was the inability to respond immediately to a problem. As a result, many centers continued to use a nonstandardized written survey or a suggestion box.

ASSESSING SURVEY RESULTS

Patient Characteristics and Reported Satisfaction Rates

Patient characteristics were collected during each survey. The demographic data were recorded as financial class, ICD-9 diagnosis code, gender, age, and number of visits. The report of these demographics allowed the organization to identify the key patient customer groups and provide appropriate clinical programs. The individual center could compare the current patient population and scores demographically with other quarters' populations to determine the influence of the type of patients sampled.

Patient-specific demographics were collected from our existing financial database and from questions asked by Gallup. Additional descriptive data collected were (1) who would you say had the most influence as to when your treatment program ended, (2) how did your injury or condition occur, and (3) what is the current status of your injury?

Overall Satisfaction

The overall satisfaction dimension includes two questionnaire items. They were (1) "Overall, considering all aspects of the services you received at the center, how satisfied were you with your experience?" and (2) "If a friend or family member asked your opinion about the center, would you recommend it?" Question one was initially asked in the beginning of the survey and repeated at the end of the survey. The responses remained consistent regardless of the placement of the question. Because of this consistency during the first nine months of survey use, the question was placed at the end of the survey to allow for a natural summary and ending to the telephone interview.

An overall satisfaction rate of 93–96 percent satisfied and 78–80 percent very satisfied was maintained over the four years of this survey (Table 2). This is similar to other health

Table 2. Percent very satisfied (5.0 response) per dimension for 1992–1995

Year	1995	1994	1993*	1992**
Sample size	6,705	5,796	3,993	3,340
Dimension	%	%	%	%
Overall satisfaction	78	80	78	79
Clinician/patient relationship	77	79	79	78
Center operations	85	87	86	86
Billing	71	68	70	72
Center	89	80	80	80

*1993—sampled 3 quarters only as computer system conversion in Quarter 1 left patient sampling information unavailable.
**1992—sampled 3 quarters only as measurement initiated in Quarter 2 of 1992.

care surveys[18–20] where most people reported they were satisfied with their health care. However, it is difficult to compare results across studies due to methodological and measurement variations.[21]

The overall satisfaction dimension was correlated with all questions to determine the impact on patients' overall satisfaction. Although all questionnaire items impacted overall satisfaction, the top five items were the focus of our quality assurance initiative. Nationally the top five service areas that most drive overall satisfaction were found to be:

1. *Explanation of treatment.* The patient's perception of the clinician's ability to thoroughly communicate the treatment plan.
2. *Personal attention.* The perceived quality time the clinician spent with the patient.
3. *Number of different treating clinicians.* The satisfaction with receiving consistent service regardless of the number of treating clinicians.
4. *How informed clinician is of the patient's case.* Patients have a need to feel the clinician understands their medical history, diagnosis, and treatment plan. For some patients this question also covered the clinician's ability to understand the patient's financial situation, for example, payer limitation, personal financial situation, or an understanding of workers' compensation or Medicare.
5. *Amount of patient input in treatment goal setting.* Clinicians must be patient focused. The patient and clinician must be in agreement regarding appropriate functional goals.

The Pearson correlation coefficient analysis indicates the impact that the perceived service on each of the questions had on overall satisfaction. The actual correlation coefficients are listed in Table 3. These correlation coefficients have remained fairly consistent over the life of the project.

Table 3. Correlation coefficient of survey question to overall satisfaction, August 1995 (based on 2,269 patients)

Question	Correlation coefficient (r^2)
1. Explanation of treatment	.6659
2. Amount of personal attention	.6471
3. Number of different treating clinicians	.6237
4. How knowledgeable clinician was about care	.6218
5. Amount of personal input in setting goals	.5976
6. Frequency clinicians made aware of progress	.5953
7. Amount of empathy or concern expressed by clinicians for your level of discomfort/pain	.5895
8. Orientation to the center	.4519
9. Helpfulness and courteousness of office staff	.4183
10. Billing procedures were clearly explained to you	.3511
11. Monthly billing statements were accurate	.3990
12. Amount of waiting time during treatment	.3390
13. Appearance of center was neat, clean, organized	.3072
14. How quickly first appointment scheduled	.2366
15. Hours of operation were convenient to you	.2255

Improving Satisfaction

Each patient surveyed was asked one open-ended question: "What one thing could the center have done to better satisfy you?" The responses provided additional insight into the service component of patient satisfaction. In our most recent survey of fourth quarter 1995, 51 percent of the patients said nothing could be done even though 12 percent of that group were less than satisfied with their overall experience. Another 14 percent of the total patients said they didn't know what could be done. Thirty-five percent of those surveyed responded to the open-ended question (Table 4).

The responses to this open-ended question were most helpful at the individual center level. At the center level the staff could take these suggestions and comments and create specific action plans. Responses were reported and placed in categories according to similarities in issues (Table 5).

DRAWING CONCLUSIONS FROM SURVEY RESULTS

A Closer Look at the Top Drivers of Satisfaction

The importance of the top five drivers of patient satisfaction, those items with the highest correlation to overall satis-

Table 4. Improve satisfaction: responses to "What one thing could the center have done better to satisfy you?" Quarter 4, 1995 (1,676 patients)

Response	Percent of respondents
Nothing	51
Don't know	14
Suggestion given*	35

*See Table 5 for description of suggestions.

faction, must be explored if maximal patient satisfaction is to be achieved. These top drivers provide insight into how daily practice by rehabilitation professionals should be conducted.

In the daily treatment of patients, therapists must remember that the technical skills they possess and share with the patients are only a small portion of the treatment they impart. Taking time to explain a treatment to a patient is a necessity. This study found explanation of treatment is the patient's number one priority. The majority of therapists would agree with this statement and yet many treatments are performed without consent or explanation to the patient. As more demands are placed on the clinician's time, it is imperative that this explaining continue to occur and not be neglected or excluded.

Therapists need to be especially aware of the fact that patients may not have enough information to formulate questions regarding their treatment program. A clinician should not assume that because patients are not asking questions that they have a solid understanding of evaluation and treatment issues.[22] A basic rule of communication could be applied here as the clinician may want to ask the patient to describe the procedure in his or her own words versus just asking if he or she understands. How the explanation takes place is also important. Many explanations are given in medical terms that the patient cannot understand. Developing a simple language to explain all treatments is necessary.

The second key driver, personal attention, can be exhibited in many ways: listening to a patient, taking enough time to let him or her relate how he or she responded to the previous treatment, not being distracted by a multitude of other things during the patient's treatment. This does not mean that more than one patient cannot be treated simultaneously; it does mean that a clinician's full attention should be given to the patient when speaking, listening, or working hands-on with him or her. This will give the required personal attention to the patient and assist therapists in formulating a more accurate clinical assessment. Kovacek also noted that therapists considered to be high producers (those seeing more patients or doing more treatments than peers) exhibit good listening skills and intense eye contact, and that the patient's perception of contact time is skewed high.[23]

Table 5. Improvement suggestions: a summary of all patients offering specific comment, Quarter 4, 1995 (567 patients)

Suggestion category*	Specific comments	Percent responding
Conditions pertaining to the clinician	• Provide better skilled or trained clinicians • Discontinue use of nonlicensed personnel (for example, aides) • Better communication and/or explanation of therapy • More personalized attention	34.2
Billing	• Improve billing process • Eliminate errors	22.9
Operational issues	• Extend hours to more evenings and weekends • Improve consistency in scheduling clinicians • Improve service from office staff • Decrease waiting time	20
Center	• Larger therapy rooms • More privacy • More personal amenities	11.4
Other	• Eliminate my need to be there • Increase contact with the primary physician • Control the temperature in the center	11.4

* Responses were placed in categories according to similarities in issues.

The third driver is how informed the clinician is of the case. We were not able to differentiate between therapists who were not informed adequately of the case history and therapists who failed to communicate this knowledge to the patient. It is most probably some mixture of both that results in a dissatisfied experience. It is often difficult to obtain complete information from the physician; still, an attempt must be made to ease this transition to the treating clinician. All parties will benefit from the exchange of information. It is a clinician's obligation to define the best way to communicate with a physician (fax, written mail, through the nursing or front office staff) and to put that information to use.

The fourth driver that deals with interpersonal skills is the amount of patient input in treatment goal-setting. Again, most therapists would agree that this is a practice that should be instituted with all patients, yet in reality it often gets overlooked. Goal-setting may become even more confusing when considering all parties involved. This may include the utilization goals of the payer, the physician's postsurgical goals, the patient's return to work or activity goals, and the clinician's goals. Therapists are in the unique position of being able to bring together the patient, the payer, and the physician expectations to address the appropriateness of care and set attainable goals.

The fifth driver of satisfaction, having the same clinician treating the same patients each time, is increasingly difficult in today's mobile environment. Because of the emphasis on decreased visits and lowest cost delivery of care, once the initial evaluation is complete the patients are often moved from therapist to therapist assistant or an aide. As this trend is a reality in today's health care environment, care needs to be taken to make these transitions as seamless as possible. This continues to challenge a clinician to practice excellent communication and interpersonal interactions.

Support for the Top Five Drivers

The importance of the top drivers is substantiated by the following:

First, when improvements are made to correct service problems identified as having high correlation coefficients, we find an increase in overall satisfaction. Instead of focusing only on the frequency of a problem, our focus is on the problem with the highest correlation or the greatest influence on patient overall satisfaction. A problem may occur more frequently but because of its low coefficient has less impact on overall satisfaction than a higher correlator that occurred only once.[24]

Secondly, the responses to the open-ended question also support the positive correlation between strong interpersonal skills and patient satisfaction. Responses such as improve communication, provide explanation of therapy, offer personalized attention, demonstrate better understanding of the patient's condition, improve courtesy, increase patient input, explain billing and charges, improve the service from the office staff, and increase contact with the primary physician, all reflect the same needs as the top five drivers.

Finally, four of the key drivers (explanation of treatment, personal attention, how informed the clinician is of the case, and the amount of patient input into treatment goal-setting) deal with communication and interpersonal skills. Consistent with our findings, multiple sclerosis patients in Roush's satisfaction study cited specific interpersonal characteristics as positive aspects of their relationships with their therapists more frequently than they cited the physical effects of treatment.[25]

• • •

Patient satisfaction is an invaluable aspect of outcome measurement and care delivery. This study of satisfaction in outpatient orthopedic rehabilitation should be expanded to evaluate other settings and other patient populations. Although similarities can occur between settings, further research is needed to determine potential, unique patient expectations in each setting.

Keeping this in mind, the five drivers of overall satisfaction have implication for how physical therapists deliver care in an outpatient setting. In the changing health care environment, this information can assist therapists in providing the type of care our patients desire. The five drivers could become part of a center's quality initiative. This information should also be used in academic curricula to assist in the nontechnical education of therapists.

Measuring patient satisfaction from an organizational point of view provides an internal benchmarking mechanism to assist in evaluating multiple sites. Without benchmarking measurement is incomplete. Measuring without having anything to compare it with does not allow one to understand if the measurement is high, low, or average. The ideal would be to benchmark to an external database. In the absence of this, internal benchmarking allowed us to compare peers. As health care organizations become more geographically widespread, satisfaction measurement is a consideration in maintaining a consistent level of service and care delivery across all centers. It must be stressed that patient satisfaction is only one element of quality assessment to consider.

Finally, the uses for the patient satisfaction data are numerous. In part two, the internal and external applications for the data will be discussed. Included will be detailed information on how to:

1. select the correct person(s) to manage the patient satisfaction process,
2. initiate continuous process improvement with the data,
3. utilize the data for sales and marketing, and
4. incorporate patient satisfaction data into a clinician's incentive compensation.

REFERENCES

1. Zastowny, T.R., et al. "Patient Satisfaction and Experience with Health Services and Quality of Care." *Quality Management in Health Care* 3, no. 3 (1995): 50–61.
2. National Committee for Quality Assurance. "The Enrollee Satisfaction Survey." 1994 NCQA Report Card Pilot Project/Technical Report. Washington, D.C.: NCQA, 1994.
3. Roush, S.E. "The Satisfaction of Patients with Multiple Sclerosis Regarding Services Received from Physical and Occupational Therapists." *International Journal of Rehabilitation and Health* 1, no. 3 (1995): 155–66.
4. DiMatteo, M.R., Prince, L.M., and Taranta, A. "Patients' Perceptions of Physicians' Behavior." *Journal of Community Health* 4, no. 4 (1979): 280–90.
5. Donabedian, A. "The Role of Outcomes in Quality Assessment and Assurance." *Quality Review Bulletin* 18, no. 11 (1992): 356–60.
6. Lohr, K. "Outcome Measurement: Concepts and Questions." *Inquiry* 25 (Spring 1988): 37–50.
7. DiMatteo, Prince, and Taranta, "Patient's Perceptions of Physicians' Behavior."
8. Marquis, M.S., Davies, A.R., and Ware, J.E. "Patient Satisfaction and Change in Medical Care Provider: A Longitudinal Study." *Medical Care* 21, no. 8 (1983): 821–29.
9. Donabedian, "Role of Outcomes."
10. Zastowny et al., "Patient Satisfaction."
11. Lohr, "Outcome Measurement."
12. Marquis, Davies, and Ware, "Patient Satisfaction and Change in Medical Care Provider."
13. Nelson, E.C., and Larson, C. "Patients' Good and Bad Surprises: How Do They Relate to Overall Patient Satisfaction?" *Quality Review Bulletin* 19, no. 3 (1993): 89–94.
14. Zastowny et al., "Patient Satisfaction."
15. NCQA, "The Enrollee Satisfaction Survey."
16. Zimney, L., et al. "Patient Telephone Interviews: Valuable Technique for Finding Problems and Assessing Quality in Ambulatory Medical Care." *Journal of Community Health* 6, no. 1 (1980): 35–42.
17. Zastowny et al., "Patient Satisfaction."
18. Ibid.
19. Roush, "The Satisfaction of Patients with Multiple Sclerosis."
20. Health Services Research Group. "A Guide to Direct Measures of Patient Satisfaction in Clinical Practice." *Canadian Medical Association Journal* 146, no. 10 (1992): 1727–30.
21. Ibid.
22. Roush, "The Satisfaction of Patients with Multiple Sclerosis."
23. Kovacek, P.R. *The Productive Clinician.* Harper Woods, Mich.: Kovacek Management Services, Inc., 1996.
24. Zastowny et al., "Patient Satisfaction."
25. Roush, "The Satisfaction of Patients with Multiple Sclerosis."

13

Measuring Patient Satisfaction in an Outpatient Orthopedic Setting, Part 2: Utilizing Data To Improve Quality and Market Services

Teresa L. Elliott-Burke and Lori Pothast

THE IMPORTANCE OF PATIENT SATISFACTION DATA

Patient satisfaction is an invaluable component of outcomes management and care delivery.[1,2] The measurement and implementation of a patient satisfaction process is an arduous task.[3] The value of patient satisfaction data is gained by communication of the results to the organization and its customers.

In Part 1, "Key Drivers and Results," we discussed the importance of measuring patient satisfaction. A methodology for designing and implementing a patient satisfaction survey in an outpatient rehabilitation setting was presented along with the results of a four-year study. From 1992 to 1995, patient satisfaction data were collected quarterly in 120 outpatient rehabilitation facilities in 12 states. A total of 19,834 patient surveys were completed. The Gallup Organization was employed to assist in the creation, administration, and analysis of the standardized patient survey. The five primary service areas impacting overall satisfaction were found to be: (1) explanation of treatment, (2) personalized attention, (3) number of different treating clinicians, (4) how informed the clinician is of the patient's case, and (5) the amount of patient input in treatment goal setting.[3] We continue with the topic of patient satisfaction and explore the applications of the data obtained.

The determination of how the patient satisfaction data will be applied prior to initiating the process allows an organization to obtain optimal results. Understanding uses for the data also aids in the design of the questionnaire and data collection process. The data provide value by being an integral part of the facility marketing program, thus enhancing the

number of referrals. Patient satisfaction information should be available to improve care delivery and enhance results. The positive benefits of a successful patient satisfaction strategy include patient retention, customer loyalty, and demonstration of facility effectiveness.

The broad utility of patient satisfaction information encompasses both internal and external applications. The data are used within a facility as part of a process of continuous quality improvement, and externally in support of a marketing plan for a facility. The identical data are formatted differently for both of these applications. The internal reports require more in-depth review of specific areas that require improvement, that is, explanation of the patient's treatment program. The external reports provide more general information to confirm the organization's commitment to its patients over an extended period of time, that is, the overall satisfaction score over the past four quarters.

The internal and external applications of patient satisfaction information overlap. External customers are often interested in how the data are used internally. Successful internal use of the data is determined by the extent to which the staff endorses the patient satisfaction process, supports the collection and use of the data, makes the recommended changes, and shares an ability to explain the information to all customers.

INTERNAL USE

Each facility received a quarterly report of its results. The survey questions were grouped into five dimensions: overall satisfaction, therapist interaction, center operations, facility, and billing. The facility's report contained a satisfaction score for each dimension, and comparisons to regional and national results within the organization. The report included dimension scores, patient demographic statistics, results of each survey question, *Best In Class* facilities, an *Action Plan*

J Rehabil Outcomes Meas, 1997, 1(2), 16–22
© 1997 Aspen Publishers, Inc.

Worksheet, and the listing of the correlation coefficients of each survey question to overall satisfaction.

Patient satisfaction measurement was used in several continuous quality improvement projects. The quarterly satisfaction report maintained focus on customer requirements by periodic assessment of the clinical improvement activities and results. The internal uses of the satisfaction results were:

- *Best In Class* Facilities
- *Action Plan Worksheet*
- Patient Service Award
- Organizational Quality Plan
- *Field Incentive Program*
- Service Training

Within our organization the patient satisfaction data and reports were issued by facility, region, and for the entire network. Oliver Goldsmith, an English author, stated people "seldom improve when they have no other model but themselves." The survey report encouraged comparison and initiated the ability to benchmark facilities through a program entitled *Best In Class.* For example, a Chicago area facility could benchmark its overall satisfaction performance to other facilities within its geographic region, with other regions, and to the entire organization. The comparison of scores and the sharing of program improvement was encouraged within our diverse national system of 120 facilities.

Within each quarterly patient satisfaction report was a list of the ten *Best In Class* facilities for each of the five primary survey questions that correlated to overall satisfaction. For example, a facility desiring to improve in "explanations of treatment programs" was encouraged to contact a *Best In Class* facility to become familiar with the methods and processes that contributed to their success. The five survey questions, in order of importance, that presented the highest correlation to overall satisfaction were:

1. satisfaction with explanation of treatment program
2. satisfaction with number of treating clinicians
3. satisfaction with amount of personal attention from clinician
4. satisfaction with clinicians' knowledge of the patient's case
5. satisfaction with amount of patient input in setting treatment goals.[3]

The amount of data collected each quarter was sizable. The use of an action plan was encouraged as a mechanism for identifying and prioritizing areas of improvement and implementing change. An *Action Plan Worksheet* was provided to monitor quality improvement activities in the facility. All staff members within a facility were involved in the action planning process. The written plan encouraged goal setting on aspects of service delivery that most negatively affected the overall satisfaction score. A designated staff member made contact with a *Best In Class* facility and through their assistance developed a written action plan. Staff meetings with the clinicians, operations staff, and management encouraged collaboration and total team accountability for the facility's success. An action plan template is noted in Figure 1.

The organization made several global process changes as a result of patient satisfaction measurement. These changes included: increased hours of operation, increased emphasis on mutual goal setting (patient and clinician), improved explanation of the patients' insurance benefits, and awareness of scheduling patients with the same clinician or team of clinicians.

In addition to local improvement efforts in each facility, several projects developed in the administrative offices. A business operations regional management team developed an ongoing record of patient satisfaction issues regarding billing and orientation of new patients. These processes were discussed at local management meetings. The clinical programs department included the patient satisfaction data in their creation of the annual quality plan for the organization. An overall patient satisfaction goal of 95 percent was established and progress was reported internally to management on a quarterly basis. Patient satisfaction performance and process improvement was often requested by managed care organizations.

A brief description of the Gallup process was included within each quarterly facility report. The information helped inform the staff on patient satisfaction improvement objectives, the schedule of data collection, and the current patient population demographics. This was especially useful to new employees and new facility acquisitions. The frequency of quarterly patient satisfaction kept employees focused on the items patients perceived as adding value to their service. The organization's mission mirrored the philosophy that the only way companies in service industries like health care stay in business is by keeping customers happy.[4]

In the initial year of patient satisfaction measurement, a *Field Incentive Program* (FIP) was developed to encourage facility staff, both clinicians and operations, to excel in service provision to patients. The incentive compensated a facility's team for exceptional service and encouraged employees to meet and exceed the customers' requirements. The incentive calculation was based in part on achievement of a facility overall patient satisfaction performance of at least 80 percent "very satisfied" and at least 90 percent "satisfied" (a combination of very satisfied and satisfied responses). Incentive compensation was payable to the staff with achievement of these ratings, with concomitant achievement of each facility's gross profit plan.

The *Patient Service Award* was another method developed to provide incentive for exceeding customer expectations. Recognition of exceptional achievement in overall patient satisfaction was given at the annual national management

Action Plan Worksheet

As your center analyzes this quarter's data, use this worksheet to prioritize the dimension weaknesses and keep written notes outlining your action plan. Next quarter, refer back to the plan and compare the improved strength of the dimension!

Quarter

Dimension	Best dem. center	Strongest question	Weakest question	Action plan	Who's responsible?
Overall sat.					
Pt-therapist					
Operations					
Billing					
Facility					

KEY: DIMENSION—The dimensions are listed in the order of the importance to overall satisfaction. Remember this as you prioritize dimensions.

BEST DEMONSTRATED CENTER—Record the center with the strongest scores within the dimension your center is directing your plan and contact them for assistance.

STRONGEST QUESTION—List the number of the question within this dimension that received the highest score.

WEAKEST QUESTION—List the number of the question within this dimension that received the lowest score.

ACTION PLAN/WHO'S RESPONSIBLE—Briefly describe your center's response to the weakest question or other priority within the dimension chosen.

Figure 1. Sample Action Plan Worksheet.

---

meeting. The award was given to the facility in each region that attained the highest score on a combination of overall patient satisfaction and a quality audit. The audit was based on facility compliance to divisional policy and procedures. The award included a banner, which the facility proudly displayed in their location to publicize their success, and a gift certificate to provide for a team activity. The *Patient Service Award* was a catalyst for inculcating patient satisfaction ideals and the organization's commitment to the process. Public recognition at a national forum was a powerful motive for teams to improve their patient satisfaction results.

All facility staff received training on service delivery and responding effectively to customers. A module on customer service was included in orientation of all new employees. The emphasis in the training was on how to deal with a variety of customer personalities, problem solving, identifying customer needs, and appropriate responses to difficult situations.

EXTERNAL USE

The primary emphasis for the external use of the patient satisfaction data was for marketing, such as sales and relationship management, initiation of contact with referral sources, and

maintenance of customer relationships. The data were used to enhance and develop relationships with our major customer groups and to facilitate business development. A format for presentation of the information required development before the data could be used for marketing purposes.

DEVELOPING THE EXTERNAL REPORT

In developing the reporting mechanism for external uses, the four major considerations were (1) the length of the report, (2) the clarity of the report, (3) ease of understanding the report, and (4) the use of the report. The report needed to encompass the requirements of all customers. As a result the *Report Card* (Figure 2) was developed. The report card format remained consistent from one reporting period to the next. This consistency in reporting assisted with a customer's ability to immediately recognize the type and source of information and increased recognition for the organization. The one-page format provided a precise illustration of patient satisfaction results and at the same time an explanation of the methodology. The results were presented as percentages and in pie graph formats. This provided visual impact and assisted in clarifying the data for the customer.

The Report Card

Patient Satisfaction

1995 SECOND QUARTER RESULTS

COMPANY:

Caremark Centers for Physical Therapy

PATIENTS CONTACTED TO DATE:

16,087 Nationally

REGION

East Region

NOTE: THIS SURVEY PROGRAM HAS BEEN ONGOING FOR 12 CONSECUTIVE QUARTERS

PROGRAM OVERVIEW

Since April 1992, Caremark Centers for Physical Therapy have contracted The Gallup Organization, one of the premiere research and polling companies in the U.S., to contact patients and monitor their satisfaction levels with various aspects of their rehabilitation experience. Reports come out quarterly, with results as follows:

PERCENT OF RESPONDENTS:

■ **VERY SATISFIED**
▨ **SATISFIED**
☐ **ALL OTHER RESPONSES**

OVERALL SATISFACTION
The key measure of customer satisfaction, this question is phrased as follows: "Overall, considering all aspects of the services you received at your local center, how satisfied were you with your experience?"

91%*

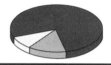

THERAPIST INTERACTION
This area explores the important topic of the patient/therapist relationship. Communication, attention, empathy, and willingness to listen are some of the specific topics covered.

95%*

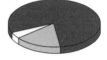

BILLING
Satisfaction with the explanation of billing procedures, interaction with insurance providers, resolution of problems, and billing statement accuracy are monitored in this area.

90%*

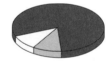

CENTER OPERATIONS
This area covers satisfaction with operational issues such as how quickly patients were able to schedule first appointments, the convenience of the center's hours, and the helpfulness of the orientation process and office staff.

97%*

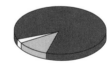

FACILITY
Questions asked in this area probe for patient satisfaction with the amount of privacy they had as well as with the neatness and cleanliness of the physical therapy facility.

97%*

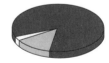

*Percent of patients surveyed this quarter indicating they were either satisfied or very satisfied with Caremark in this area.

Figure 2. A sample report card on patient satisfaction.

USES OF THE REPORT WITH CUSTOMERS

The four major customer groups that the report card targeted were payers, referral sources, employers, and patients. The report was used as an introductory topic to gain access to decision makers in managed care organizations and physician practices. The use of a reputable firm such as The Gallup Organization was beneficial in gaining credibility for the process and results. The report card was instrumental in initiating conversation and interest in our organization.

Many customers were impressed by the well-planned methodology of this study and subsequent action planning to improve patient satisfaction.

As several studies indicate, patients who are satisfied with their care or care experience are less likely to change providers.[5,6] This was of great interest to payers who were increasing their focus on maintaining contracts with a wide variety of employers and to referral sources who were keenly interested in patient retention. Satisfied patients expressed their support for the current health plan to their employers.

It is more likely that dissatisfaction rather than satisfaction is reported by patients. Payers and referral sources are negatively impacted by reports made to them by patients of health care provider dissatisfaction. Addressing these concerns also takes valuable administrative time on the part of the payer and referral source staffs. All attempts on the part of the provider to direct attention to the resolution of these complaints is seen as positive by the external customers.

Payers were most responsive to the content of the patient satisfaction survey, the analysis process, and in the results attained. Patient satisfaction was used by the payers as an indicator of the level of the quality being provided. The payers were the first customer group to shift the emphasis from the survey, data collection, and results to the methodology of how the data were utilized within the organization.

Referral sources were interested in the quality of services delivered by rehabilitation providers. Our organization made this information readily available, thus substantiating our commitment to quality and our patients. Physicians, particularly orthopedic surgeons, view physical therapy as an extension of their practice. Therefore satisfaction with the rehabilitation provider is indicative of the patient's satisfaction with the physician. Thus, patient satisfaction was mutually important to our organization and our referral sources. Most referral sources were interested in the demonstrated results versus the methodology or use of the data within the organization.

Many patients were curious about the process. A report card was displayed in each facility to provide an awareness of the process, results, and our commitment to meeting patient needs. The display also acted as a reminder of a potential future call from The Gallup Organization.

Patient satisfaction information was also used during the process of our organization's acquisition of privately owned rehabilitation facilities. The *Report Card* was evidence of our company's commitment to patients. Potential prospects found attractive the organization's sharing of patient satisfaction information and the process of internal benchmarking.

DISCUSSION

The successful implementation and overall effectiveness of a patient satisfaction measurement process is highly dependent upon management support, deliberate selection of the leaders and change catalysts responsible for the process, and the attitude of the staff receiving the results.

Management must consistently support the patient satisfaction process and hold the facility staff accountable for results. Management support is required to keep the emphasis on the process. It is also essential that management advocate the use of the information to continuously improve the service and care of the patient.

The careful selection of the person(s) that have the responsibility of analyzing and interpreting the data is also critical. Data analysis goes beyond statistical methods to applying and managing the information. The questions include, "What do the data signify for the organization?" and "What should be done with this knowledge?" A team approach or an individual with multiple skill sets (clinician/administrator) is ideal. There are clinical, financial, strategic, and marketing implications of patient satisfaction data. Whether it is a team approach or an individual, it is recommended that authority and accountability for the entire patient satisfaction process be theirs. This method minimizes conflict and places equal importance on the collection, analysis, and management of the information.

The staff attitude and receptiveness for change upon review of the data was important. Some clinicians became defensive and rationalized the results of the patient satisfaction survey. The more constructive and positive attitude was to use the data as an improvement opportunity. The clinician's acceptance of the facility's performance was critical in facilitating an ongoing improvement process. If the clinicians did not feel accountable for the facility's success in the survey and reporting process, the information was not often utilized. Leaders within the organization advanced the process and encouraged use of the data in a nonpunitive manner.

• • •

Measuring patient satisfaction is a process (Figure 3). Patient satisfaction performance measurement provides valuable information for improvement of clinical practice. The design of the process should carefully consider both internal and external applications of the data.

Patients are only one of the customers served by outpatient rehabilitation. Understanding the drivers of satisfaction for our other customers is an important consideration as outpatient rehabilitation ensures its place in the health care of the future. Therefore, consideration should be given to additionally measuring the satisfaction of referral sources, payers, and employers.

The use of patient satisfaction information is highly recommended to organizations competing in the changing

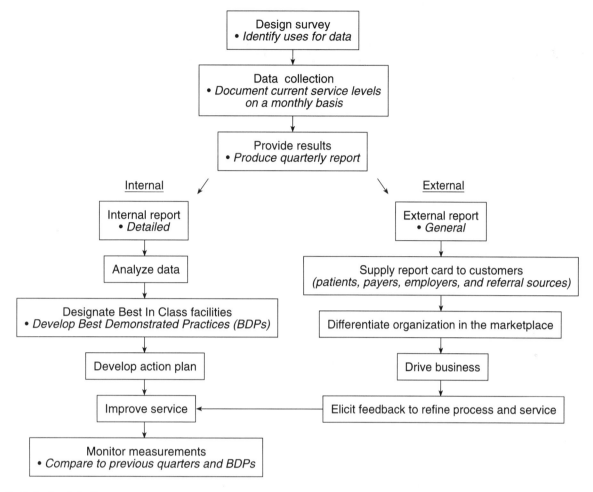

Figure 3. Patient satisfaction process.

health care environment. Patient satisfaction measurement benefited our organization by assisting with the following:

- setting and measuring service expectation
- providing value through multiple uses of the data with a variety of internal and external customers
- quantifying the quality of service provided.

We advocate the use of patient satisfaction within all rehabilitation facilities. Patient satisfaction is an invaluable aspect of outcomes management and care delivery. Rehabilitation clinicians need to become more sophisticated in measurement and use of patient satisfaction data. Ongoing patient satisfaction contributes to increased compliance of care and eventually leads to successful therapy outcomes.[2]

REFERENCES

1. Lohr, K. "Outcomes Measurement: Concepts and Questions." *Inquiry* 25 (1988): 37–50.
2. Donabedian, A. "The Role of Outcomes in Quality Assessment and Assurance." *Quality Review Bulletin* 18, no. 11 (1992): 356–60.
3. Elliott-Burke, T., and Pothast, L. "Measuring Patient Satisfaction in an Outpatient Orthopedic Setting—Part 1: Key Drivers and Results." *Journal of Rehabilitation Outcomes Measurement* 1, no. 1 (1997): 18–25.
4. Montague, J. "Making Hospitals More Hospitable." *Hospitals & Health Networks* 69 (September 1995): 64.
5. DiMatteo, M.R., Prince, L.M., and Taranta, A. "Patients' Perceptions of Physicians' Behavior." *Journal of Community Health* 4, no. 4 (1979): 280–90.
6. Marquis, M.S., Davies, A.R., and Ware, J.E. "Patient Satisfaction and Change in Medical Care Provider: A Longitudinal Study." *Medical Care* 21, no. 8 (1983): 821–29.

14

Validation of a Measure of Family Members' Perceptions of Service Quality in Nursing Homes

Teresa M. Steffen and Paul C. Nystrom

Increasingly, directors of nursing, nursing home administrators, governmental regulators, and payers are interested in the degree to which residents and their families are satisfied with the quality of service being provided within long-term care facilities. Residents' satisfaction with service quality is frequently reported as an outcome measure. Such measures attempt to assess the effect of nursing intervention on clients' perceptions of quality in health care settings where nursing is the primary service provider.

The researchers sought to assess whether nursing homes could utilize the questionnaire SERVQUAL[1] to determine service quality. SERVQUAL had demonstrated its usefulness in a variety of industries,[2] including accounting services,[3] financial services,[4] and hospitals.[5–7] Davies[8] suggested using SERVQUAL to obtain feedback from nursing home residents' families. Our study follows through on this suggestion by examining the reliability and validity of adapting SERVQUAL for family members of residents in nursing homes.

LITERATURE REVIEW

SERVQUAL

The questionnaire assesses five dimensions of customer perceptions of service quality (see Appendix for the SERVQUAL items). *Responsiveness* refers to having prompt service, *Reliability* refers to having the service provided correctly the first time, *Assurance* refers to the employees' ability to convey trust and confidence, *Empathy* refers to the caring nature of the service provided, and *Tangibles* refers to the appearance of the facilities and staff.

Parasuraman, Zeithaml, and Berry[1] reported high interitem reliability (.90) and convergent validity when they studied services in four industries (banking, credit, repair and maintenance, and phone services). They found customers' perception scores were high on each SERVQUAL dimension, with average scores of 5 on a 7-point Likert scale. The original version of SERVQUAL (1986)[1] had 26 items. SERVQUAL published by the same authors in 1988 had 22 items.[9] The goal of their research was to help service organizations seek profitable ways to differentiate themselves. In the absence of objective measures, they sought to define a quantitative yardstick against which to gauge perceptions.

The original 1986 26-item version of the SERVQUAL instrument was used in a hospital setting to collect data using phone interviews (performed by the marketing departments of two hospitals) with 575 discharged patients.[6] Four of the five SERVQUAL dimensions demonstrated adequate reliability. Tangibles dimension was the one dimension found unreliable. Babakus and Mangold[5] modified SERVQUAL into a 15-item questionnaire when they studied 443 discharged patients from one hospital. Their perception subscales yielded acceptable coefficient-alpha reliabilities: Responsiveness (.90), Reliability (.76), Assurance (.89), Empathy (.87), and Tangibles (.78). Finally, SERVQUAL was used with 300 phone respondents in one hospital setting.[10] In this study the authors changed the rating scales and items from previous research on SERVQUAL, so meaningful comparisons cannot be drawn. Each of these three studies was conducted in one or two organizations, which restricts one's ability to generalize to other organizations.

Reasonableness of Measuring Customer Satisfaction

Customers can derive satisfaction from the conditions under which care is provided, and from the manner in which

J Rehabil Outcomes Meas, 1997, 1(4), 1–9

they are treated. "One must never forget that, as far as these nontechnical matters are concerned, the clients are the ultimate authority on the criteria of good care."[11] When assessing customer satisfaction, one asks whether customer opinion truly reflects quality of care given? The literature indicates that most researchers have found that customers can provide valid information about the quality of their medical care.[12] Studies indicate that customers' ratings of interpersonal or technical quality of their care in outpatient settings are not substantially affected by purported sources of bias.[13] Additional studies have shown that customers can rate technical quality of care and that their ratings agree with those of physicians.[14,15]

Problems of Measuring Satisfaction in Nursing Homes

The health care field lacks a well-developed theoretical framework concerning customer satisfaction.[16–18] Nevertheless, a few research projects have tried to measure satisfaction with nursing care in nursing homes. Bennett[19] asked residents 12 open-ended questions, such as "What do you think of the nurses?" But the test–retest reliability was totally inadequate (.27). McCaffree and Harkins[20] used structured interviews to ask people to rate the importance, along 4-point scales, of 15 aspects of being in a nursing home, such as "have a place to be alone." They found an adequate interitem reliability of .78. Kane et al.[21] revised this scale to include 17 items measuring residents' satisfaction with issues directly related to the environment and caregivers. They converted scaling into a yes, no, and unsure format, and found a coefficient–alpha reliability of .88. Subsequently, Kruzich, Clinton, and Kelber[22] reported a coefficient alpha of .80 for that same measure.

Kleinsorge and Koening[23] developed a survey instrument consisting of 32 statements regarding nursing home quality. Areas covered include food, nursing administration, environment, housekeeping, empathy, and home issues. The survey required both residents and family members to express their opinions, using 5-point scales. Coefficient–alpha reliabilities ranged from .51 to .73, based on data from 50 residents. They only received nine responses from residents' family members, and those coefficient–alpha reliabilities ranged from .63 to .94. The authors alluded to the higher reliability levels of the family sample over those of the residents, and suggested screening residents to identify individuals who are able to complete a survey.

Gustafson, Sainfort, Van Konigsveld, and Zimmerman[24] developed the Quality Assessment Index (QAI) for measuring total nursing home quality by the state surveyors. QAI addresses seven components: direct resident care outcomes (grooming, mood, awareness, and physical condition), resident care process (plan of care, medical records, staff issues), recreation activities, staff qualifications and number, facil-

ity, dietary, and resident/community ties. The reliabilities for the components ranged from .71 to .96.

The problems with the measurement of customer satisfaction in nursing homes thus far include how to deal with the cognitive impairments of residents,[23] the inadequate reliabilities of some of the instruments,[19] and the lack of validity testing of the questionnaires.[19–22] Collecting primary data for comparative field studies in nursing homes is difficult,[25] which may be a reason for the prevalence of studies focusing on one or two facilities.[5,23,26,27] More recently, external funding has assisted some researchers in gaining access to larger numbers of nursing homes, although none of these studies utilized random sampling.[22,28–32] Our research project builds on the existing literature and utilizes suggestions of previous authors on how to surmount past limitations of nursing home research on satisfaction.

METHODOLOGY

Our study contains 41 skilled nursing home facilities reported in the *Wisconsin Nursing Home Directory & Factbook,*[33] and each home has 50 or more beds. All administrators or directors of nursing in these 41 homes signed an organizational consent form approved by the University's Institutional Review Board for the Protection of Human Subjects.

The first author randomly selected one unit within each home. Then, 25 residents were randomly selected from each selected unit, and a SERVQUAL questionnaire was mailed to the person listed as the resident's health care representative, closest relative, or friend. The Omnibus Reconciliation Act of 1987 requires that a resident's health care representative be informed of all changes in that resident's status. The term *health care representative* refers to that person who makes health care decisions on behalf of a nursing home resident. Every nursing home must identify a health care representative for each resident who cannot make independent informed decisions. In nursing homes, the majority of residents tend to be sufficiently cognitively impaired or unaware to prevent their giving informed consent. The *Wisconsin Nursing Home Utilization 1990*[34] data reported 65 percent of residents have impaired memory. In our study, pilot work examined 10 residents whom the RN recommended as being cognitively able to answer questions on the survey. All but 1 of the 10 clients rated everything as perfect, had difficulty understanding the reversed-scored items, and required significant coaching. Formal cognitive testing of clients had not been conducted in any of the homes on a regular basis. For these reasons, the family members or health care representatives were surveyed about their level of satisfaction. These representatives make the decisions about transferring the resident to another institution, and they often provide financial support as well as social support, so their opinions matter.

A total of 416 customers of the 1,025 included in the mailing actually completed the questionnaires (40 percent response rate); their distribution ranged from 5 to 20 respondents per nursing unit, with a mean and median of 10 respondents per nursing unit and a mode of 9. The staff on the unit were not informed of the survey, in order to avoid potential biased results due to behaving in an uncharacteristically responsive manner. Following suggestions by previous authors,[6,35-37] SERVQUAL perception items were used.

DATA ANALYSIS AND RESULTS

Customer Demographics

Past studies reveal few significant correlations between customer demographics and customers' perceptions of service quality.[5,6,12,14] Nonetheless, researchers should routinely examine such potential relationships in order to determine whether demographic factors account for observed differences in perceptions of service quality. Four demographic questions were asked: length of residents' stay, relationship to the resident, amount of visitation, and age. Length of stay was measured with categories of less than one month (2.4 percent), 1–6 months (10.8 percent), 6–12 months (12.7 percent), 1–2 years (14.9 percent), greater than 2 years (57 percent), missing (2.2 percent). Future research should differentiate more categories over 2 years. Length of stay does not correlate significantly with any of the SERVQUAL measures.

Daughters of the nursing-home residents were the most frequent respondents (34 percent), followed by sons (20 percent), nieces (7 percent), wives (5 percent), husbands (5 percent), nephews, sisters, friends (4 percent each), brothers (2 percent), others or missing data (16 percent). This question enabled us to identify 207 respondents as female and 128 as male. A set of t tests show no significant difference between the genders with respect to any of the SERVQUAL measures. When visiting spouses ($N = 30$) are compared with visiting children ($N = 179$), t tests show no significant differences on any of the SERVQUAL measures.

Representatives visited a median of one to two times per week. Responsiveness ($r = -.16, p < .01$) and Empathy ($r = -.14, p < .01$) correlate significantly with frequency of visitation. Administrators of nursing homes that seek to improve customer satisfaction may want to begin by focusing on the most frequent visitors because these customers tend to be more critical of current conditions.

Ages of the respondents were distributed as follows: younger than 41 years old (4 percent), 41–50 (18 percent), 51–60 (28 percent), 61–70 (30 percent), and older than 70 years (20 percent). Only two of the six correlations between customer age and service quality are significant: Reliability ($r = .19, p < .001$) and Assurance ($r = .17, p < .01$). These

results suggest that older people tend to rate service quality higher than do middle-aged people.

In summary, this study found low or no significant correlations between sociodemographic factors and family member satisfaction with care. This is a desirable finding, because it means that observed differences in perceptions of service quality are not likely to be due to demographic factors.

Descriptive Statistics as Norms

This section provides descriptive statistics so that other researchers can use them as norms to compare findings from their own particular nursing home with ours for 41 nursing homes. Mean scores of the dimensions demonstrate a similar order of relative importance whether analyses refer to individual customers or to their aggregations by nursing home. Table 1 lists the means of the service–quality dimensions for both individuals and organizations. The scale ranges from 1 = "strongly disagree" to 7 = "strongly agree."

The means on SERVQUAL are lower and show greater variance than they have done in previous studies within the health care field.[5,6] In other words, we did not encounter a range-restriction problem that would have thwarted statistical analyses.

Factor Structure

Factor analysis of SERVQUAL used oblique rotation in order to be consistent with previous researchers. It converged in 10 iterations upon three factors, instead of the five factors suggested by its developers (see Table 2). Reliability and Assurance dimensions factored together here, as they had in Shewchuck, O'Connor, and White's[38] study conducted in a health care setting. The high correlation between Reliability and Assurance may be unique to health care organizations. Table 2 also shows that Responsiveness and Em-

Table 1. Mean Scores of Customers and Nursing Homes on SERVQUAL Dimensions

Service quality dimension	Aggregated by nursing home[†]		Customers[*]	
	Mean	SD	Mean	SD
Responsiveness	5.03	1.63	4.99	.88
Reliability	6.16	.94	6.13	.47
Assurance	6.12	.95	6.11	.44
Empathy	5.92	1.37	5.89	.60
Tangibles	6.16	.87	6.12	.44

[*]$N = 363–393$ customers.
[†]$N = 41$ nursing homes.

Table 2. Factor Analysis of SERVQUAL

Item	Factor 1	Factor 2	Factor 3
1			.84
2			.79 TANGIBLES
3			.64
5	.71		
6	.77		
7	.82 RELIABILITY		
8	.73		
9	.70		
10		−.66	
11		−.83	
12		−.81 RESPONSIVENESS	
13		−.73	
14	.81		
15	.77		
16	.76 ASSURANCE		
17	.62		
18		−.84	
19		−.86	
20		−.81 EMPATHY	
21		−.76	
Eigenvalues	9.18	1.92	1.43
Variance	45.9%	9.6%	7.2%

pathy factored together, and they both contained the negatively worded items. Overall, the factor structure here resembles the original authors' dimensions. However, one item (item 4) in the dimension about Tangibles did not load on any factor. We noted problems when coding this item, and its wording clearly allows a respondent to interpret it in two different manners, so we eliminated item 4 from further analyses. Parasuraman, Berry, and Zeithaml[39] had a panel of experts review SERVQUAL and they, too, suggested that item 4 be revised.

Reliability

The Cronbach coefficient alpha for SERVQUAL overall is very high (.93). Coefficient alphas for the separate dimensions range from very high to moderate yet acceptable levels: Responsiveness (.85), Reliability (.89), Assurance (.79), Empathy (.90), and Tangibles (.74).

Validity

Construct validity links psychometric notions and practices to theoretical notions. Basically, the question involves the extent to which an operationalization really measures the concept it was intended to measure.[40] Construct validity typically becomes established by an ongoing process of assess-

ing other types of validity, particularly convergent validity and criterion-related validity.

Convergent Validity

Convergent validity refers to the extent that multiple attempts to measure one concept do agree with each other. Representatives answered two questions about overall satisfaction with nursing service, using 7-point Likert scales. Each representative's responses to these two items were averaged to form an index of service quality. This overall index of satisfaction correlated significantly (at the $p < .01$ level) with each of the SERVQUAL dimensions: Responsiveness ($r = .44$), Reliability ($r = .63$), Assurance ($r = .57$), Empathy ($r = .46$), and Tangibles ($r = .57$). A multiple regression of the overall satisfaction index onto the five SERVQUAL dimensions yields an R^2 of .78 ($F = 22.71, p < .001$). Appendix A provides the item-to-total correlations, which range from .53 to .79. These three analyses indicate substantial convergent validity for SERVQUAL in nursing homes.

Criterion-Related Validity

Criterion-related validity refers to comparing test or scale scores with one or more external variables or criteria that are known or believed to measure the attribute under study.[41] Do customers' perceptions of service quality correlate with government agencies' assessments? The numbers of deficiencies and complaints pertaining to the 41 nursing homes was collected from the state's Bureau of Quality Compliance as an alternative measure of service quality. Complaints are filed when the bureau receives a written or verbal complaint. A deficiency refers to a state violation given a nursing home when a governmental survey team reviews the home and finds it out of compliance with a nursing home regulation. The correlation coefficient between complaints filed in 1990 and deficiencies noted in 1990 is high ($r = .61, p < .001$). The reliability of such measures has not been demonstrated, even though they are often used in research.[42,43]

Correlations reported in Table 3 between complaints filed and the five factors of SERVQUAL are all negative and statistically significant. Correlations between deficiencies noted and the satisfaction measures are all negative, and four out of six are statistically significant. Thus, nursing homes with deficiencies and complaints noted by governmental agencies also tend to be perceived by customers as offering lower service quality.

Customers were asked a behavioral question of whether they had recommended the nursing home to someone else. The t tests comparing the SERVQUAL dimensions and the customers' recommending behavior exhibit highly significant differences (see Table 4). Satisfied customers are much more likely to recommend that particular nursing home than are dissatisfied customers. These correlations and t tests indicate the criterion-related validity of SERVQUAL as adapted for use with nursing homes.

DISCUSSION AND CONCLUSION

The reliability and validity of the SERVQUAL instrument is demonstrated in this study of customers' perceptions of service quality in nursing homes. Family members' perceptions of service quality correlate significantly with complaints filed with the state's regulatory agency, and with deficiencies noted by them. Scores on the SERVQUAL

Table 3. Correlations between Complaints or Deficiencies and Customers' Perceptions of Service Quality

Service quality dimensions	Complaints filed (N = 38)	Deficiencies noted (N = 39)
Responsiveness	−.46‡	−.36§
Reliability	−.42§	−.16
Assurance	−.40§	−.24*
Empathy	−.51‡	−.36§
Tangibles	−.25*	−.16
Overall Index	−.41§	−.30†

*p < .10; †p < .05; §p < .01; ‡p < .001.

Table 4. Comparisons of Customers Who Recommend the Nursing Home to Those Who Do Not Recommend It

SERVQUAL	Recommended		t Test
	Yes*	No†	
Responsiveness	5.31 (1.54)	4.50 (1.60)	4.64§
Reliability	6.37 (.73)	5.71 (1.19)	5.79§
Assurance	6.30 (.83)	5.77 (1.03)	4.86§
Empathy	6.17 (1.23)	5.43 (1.50)	4.88§
Tangibles	6.33 (.75)	5.85 (.98)	5.27§

*Number of responses ranged from 227–244.
†Number of responses ranged from 117–132.
§p < .001.

dimensions correlate strongly with scores on a separate index of overall satisfaction with nursing service. The t-tests were significant for all five SERVQUAL dimensions when comparing whether or not customers had recommended the nursing home to other people.

Standardized measurement scales enable researchers to compare the results of studies across organizations in the same service industry.[44] Comparisons within various health care settings ought to be conducted with greater caution. Differences on subscale scores between this study and studies conducted in hospital settings[5,6] point out differences between nursing homes and hospitals. Another issue to be concerned with is the different job levels studied within an organization. Our study focuses specifically on nursing staff, which includes registered nurses, licensed practical nures, and nurses' aides. A few comments by the family members in our study indicated that they would have preferred an opportunity to distinguish between the nurses and the nurses' aides. In the hospital studies, this issue of reference job becomes even more problematic because the term *employees* seems to include everyone from the housekeeping staff to the physicians. A client's or family member's perception of the different professional groups may be very different. Studying service quality in nursing homes enables researchers to examine situations characterized by multiple, ongoing interactions between the family member and the employee. In nursing homes, unlike in hospitals, physicians play a minor role in the outcomes of patients, and nursing staff exercise substantial discretion in performing their jobs.

To improve the generalizability of our findings, it would be useful for future research to conduct a replication using a random sample of skilled nursing facilities throughout the

United States. We know very little about possible differences between the people who chose to respond and those that did not participate. Based on uncompleted surveys returned with notes on them, we conjecture that many of the people who did not respond felt they were not sufficiently informed to complete the survey (some of the most recent admissions), or they lived far away and could not visit frequently, or the person was not an immediate relative (spouse, child, or sibling) and participated relatively less in the clients' care. In other words, our data may tend to describe those customers who are more informed and involved in assessing service quality.

Considering that the majority of residents still come to a nursing home for nursing care, and considering that nursing service is the largest department in a nursing home, logic suggests that it is the area where a home should concentrate its survey efforts. Other means of surveying can be employed to detect concerns with different areas. For example, an interview format could be used on those issues, such as food service, where clients and family members can critique tangible items. For services such as pharmacy, with which families may not directly interact, surveys addressed to nursing and medical staff might be appropriate. For some services, such as physical therapy, patient outcomes can be measured.

For assessing nursing services, the SERVQUAL instrument used in this study appears to be an appropriate tool. Any of the service–quality dimensions could be used alone if one has severely limited time or money for conducting surveys. This study has created norms data specifically for nursing homes. Other nursing administrators can compare their homes' scores with those reported in this study. Lower scores on any of the SERVQUAL dimensions might signal the existence of potential problems within an organization.

While gathering information on SERVQUAL, administrators should consider also surveying employees on known antecedents of service quality such as organizational commitment and role conflict[45] and consider organizational antecedents such as size and ownership.[46] Babakus and Mangold[5] suggested that SERVQUAL be utilized by employees to measure how they think clients perceive the quality of the service they render. Gaps between family members' and employees' perspectives could point out the need to educate staff and monitor customer satisfaction on an ongoing basis. SERVQUAL could also be used longitudinally within organizations to measure the changes in perceived service quality that occur when initiating new programs or changes in perceptions over time.

REFERENCES

1. Parasuraman, A., Zeithaml, V.A., and Berry, L.L. *SERVQUAL: A Multiple-Item Scale for Measuring Customer Perceptions of Service Quality (Report No. 86-108).* Cambridge, MA: Marketing Science Institute (1986).

2. Lewis, B.R. "Quality in the Service Sector: A Review." *The International Journal of Bank Marketing* 7 (1989): 4–12.

3. Bojanic, D.C. "Quality Measurement in Professional Services Firms." *Journal of Professional Services Marketing* 7 (1991): 27–36.

4. Wong, S.M., and Perry, C. "Customer Service Strategies in Financial Retailing." *The International Journal of Bank Marketing* 9 (1991): 11–16.

5. Babakus, E., and Mangold, W.G. "Adapting the SERVQUAL Scale to Hospital Services: An Empirical Investigation." *Health Services Research* 26 (1992): 767–86.

6. O'Connor, S.J. "Service Quality, Service Marketing and the Health Care Consumer: A Study Assessing the Dimensions of Service Quality and Their Influence on Patient Satisfaction and Intention to Return." PhD dissertation, University of Alabama, Birmingham, 1988.

7. Saleh, F., and Ryan, C. "Analyzing Service Quality in the Hospitality Industry Using the SERVQUAL Model." *The Service Industries Journal* 11 (1991): 324–45.

8. Davies, M.A. "On Nursing Home Quality: A Review and Analysis." *Medical Care Review* 48 (1991): 129–66.

9. Parasuraman, A., Zeithaml, V.A., and Berry, L.L. "SERVQUAL: A Multiple-Item Scale for Measuring Consumer Perceptions of Service Quality." *Journal of Retailing* 64 (1988): 12–40.

10. Reidenbach, R.E., and Sandifer-Smallwood, B. "Exploring Perceptions of Hospital Operations by a Modified SERVQUAL Approach." *Journal of Health Care Marketing* 10 (1990): 47–55.

11. Donabedian, A. *Explorations in Quality Assessment and Monitoring,* vol. 3, *The Methods and Findings of Quality Assessment and Monitoring: An Illustrated Analysis.* Ann Arbor, MI: Health Administration Press, 1985, p. 5.

12. Rubin, H.R. "Can Patients Evaluate the Quality of Hospital Care?" *Medical Care Review* 47 (1990): 267–326.

13. Davies, A.R., and Ware, J.E. *Involving Consumers in Quality of Care Assessment: Do They Provide Valid Information (Report No. P-7400).* Santa Monica, CA: Rand Library Collection, 1987.

14. Davies, A.R., and Ware, J.E. "Involving Consumers in Quality of Care Assessment." *Health Affairs* 7 (1988): 33–48.

15. Gerbert, B., and Hargreaves, W.A. "Measuring Physician Behavior." *Medical Care* 24 (1986): 838–47.

16. Hall, J.A., and Dornan, M.C. "Meta-analysis of Satisfaction with Medical Care: Description of Research Domain and Analysis of Overall Satisfaction Levels." *Social Science and Medicine* 27 (1988): 637–44.

17. Locker, D., and Dunt, D. "Theoretical and Methodological Issues in Sociological Studies of Consumer Satisfaction with Medical Care." *Social Science and Medicine* 12 (1978): 283–92.

18. Ware, J.E., Davies-Avery, A., and Stewart, A.L. "The Measurement and Meaning of Patient Satisfaction." *Health and Medical Care Services Review* 1 (1978): 3–15.

19. Bennett, R. "Evaluation Index: Resident's Satisfaction with Residential Facility." In *Health Program Evaluation and Demography,* eds. D.J. Mangen and W.A. Peterson. Minneapolis, MN: University of Minnesota Press, 1984.

20. McCaffree, K.M., and Harkins, E.B. "Satisfaction with Nursing Home Scale." In *Health Program Evaluation and Demography,* eds. D.J. Mangen and W.A. Peterson. Minneapolis, MN: University of Minnesota Press, 1984.

21. Kane, R.L., et al. *Predicting the Course of Nursing Home Patients: A Process Report.* Santa Monica, CA: Rand, 1982.

22. Kruzich, J.M., Clinton, J.F., and Kelber, S.T. "Personal and Environmental Influence on Nursing Home Satisfaction." *The Gerontologist* 32 (1992): 342–50.

23. Kleinsorge, I.K., and Koening, H.F. "The Silent Customers: Measuring Customer Satisfaction in Nursing Homes." *Journal of Health Care Marketing* 11 (1991): 2–13.

24. Gustafson, D.H., et al. "The Quality Assessment Index (QAI) for Measuring Nursing Home Quality." *Health Services Research* 25 (1990): 97–127.

25. Mount, J.K. "Nursing Home Responsiveness to Research Requests: Results of a Field Study." *The Gerontologist* 32 (1992): 414–19.

26. Gerety, M.B., et al. "Medical Treatment Preferences of Nursing Home Residents: Relationship to Function and Concordance with Surrogate Decision-Makers." *Journal of the American Geriatric Society* 41 (1993): 953–60.

27. Rohrer, J.E., et al. "Patterns of Change in Functional Status in Extended Care." *Health Services Research* 23 (1988): 495–509.

28. Eagle, V.F., and Graney, M.J. "Predicting Outcomes of Nursing Home Residents: Death and Discharge Home." *Journal of Gerontology: Social Sciences* 48 (1993): S269–75.

29. Shaughnessy, R.W., Schlender, R.E., and Kramer, A.M. "Quality of Long-Term Care in Nursing Homes and Swing-Bed Hospitals." *Health Services Research* 25 (1990): 65–96.

30. Lewis, M.A., et al. "Changes in Case Mix and Outcomes of Readmissions to Nursing Homes Between 1980 and 1984." *Health Services Research* 24 (1990): 713–28.

31. Hu, T., et al. "Cost Effectiveness of Training Incontinent Elderly in Nursing Homes: A Randomized Clinical Trial." *Health Services Research* 25 (1990): 455–77.

32. Bowers, B., and Becker, M. "Nurses' Aides in Nursing Homes: The Relationship Between Organization and Quality." *The Gerontologist* 32 (1992): 360–66.

33. *Wisconsin Nursing Home Directory & Factbook, June 1989*. Madison, WI: Division of Health, Wisconsin Department of Health and Social Service, 1990.

34. *Wisconsin Nursing Home Utilization (1990)*. September. Madison, WI: Division of Health, Wisconsin Department of Health and Social Service, 1991.

35. Babakus, E., and Boller, G.W. "An Empirical Assessment of the SERVQUAL Scale." *Journal of Business Research* 24 (1992): 253–68.

36. Carman, J.M. "Consumer Perceptions of Service Quality: An Assessment of the SERVQUAL Dimensions." *Journal of Retailing* 66 (1990): 33–55.

37. Cronin, J.J., and Taylor, S.A. "Measuring Service Quality: A Reexamination and Extension." *Journal of Marketing* 56 (1992): 55–68.

38. Shewchuck, R.M., O'Connor, S.J., and White, J.B. "In Search of Service Quality Measures: Some Questions Regarding Psychometric Properties." *Health Services Management Research* 4 (1991): 65–75.

39. Parasuraman, A., Berry, L.L., and Zeithaml, V.A. "Refinement and Reassessment of the SERVQUAL Scale." *Journal of Retailing* 67 (1991): 420–50.

40. Cook, T.D., and Campbell, D.T. *Quasi-Experimentation: Design and Analysis Issues in Field Settings.* Boston: Houghton Mifflin, 1979.

41. Kerlinger, F.N. *Foundations of Behavioral Research.* New York: Holt, Rinehart, & Winston, 1986.

42. Nyman, J.A. "Excess Demand, Consumer Rationality, and the Quality of Care in Regulated Nursing Homes." *Health Services Research* 24 (1989): 105–27.

43. Riportella-Mueller, R., and Slesinger, D.P. "The Relationship of Ownership and Size to Quality of Care in Wisconsin Nursing Homes." *The Gerontologist* 22 (1982): 429–33.

44. Fick, G.R., and Brent Ritchie, J.R. "Measuring Service Quality in the Travel and Tourism Industry." *Journal of Travel Research* 30 (1991): 2–9.

45. Steffen, T.M., Nystrom, P.C., and O'Connor, S. "Satisfaction with Nursing Homes: The Design of Employees' Jobs Can Ultimately Influence Family Members' Perceptions." *Journal of Health Care Marketing* 16 (1996): 34–38.

46. Steffen, T.M., and Nystrom, P.C. "Organizational Determinants of Service Quality in Nursing Homes." *Hospital & Health Services Administration* 42 (1997): 179–191.

SERVQUAL Adapted for Nursing Homes ($N = 371–412$)

Item no.	Item-to-total correlation	Description
		TANGIBLES
1	.53	This health care facility has up-to-date equipment.
2	.46	This health care institution has physical facilities that are visually appealing.
3	.54	The nursing staff are well dressed and appear neat.
		RELIABILITY
5	.75	When the nursing staff promises to do something by a certain time, they do so.
6	.75	When someone has problems, the nursing staff are sympathetic and reassuring.
7	.79	The nursing staff are dependable.
8	.71	The nursing staff provide services (such as bathing, food, and medication) at the time promised.
9	.64	The nursing staff keep their records accurately.
		RESPONSIVENESS
10	.59	The nursing staff do not tell exactly when services will be performed.
11	.76	Patients do not receive prompt service from the nursing staff.
12	.74	The nursing staff here are not always willing to help patients.
13	.72	The nursing staff are too busy to respond to requests promptly.
		ASSURANCE
14	.67	You can trust the nursing staff.
15	.64	You feel that what you discuss with the nursing staff is kept confidential.
16	.60	The nursing staff are polite.
17	.68	The nursing staff get adequate support from the facility to do their jobs well.
		EMPATHY
18	.75	The nursing staff do not give individual attention.
19	.77	The nursing staff do not give personal attention.
20	.73	The nursing staff do not know what the patient's needs are.
21	.71	The nursing staff do not have the patient's best interests at heart.

15

Measuring Patient Satisfaction with Medical Rehabilitation

Allen W. Heinemann, Rita Bode, Kristine C. Cichowski, and Edward Kan

THE IMPORTANCE OF MEASURING PATIENT SATISFACTION

Patient satisfaction is widely recognized as an important component of health care outcomes. Perhaps the most respected authority on health care quality, Donabedian, stated, "Patient satisfaction may be considered to be one of the desired outcomes of care, even an element in health status itself. . . . It is futile to argue about the validity of patient satisfaction as a measure of quality. Whatever its strengths and limitations as an indicator of quality, information about patient satisfaction should be as indispensable to assessments of quality as to the design and management of health care systems."[1] Managed care organizations have embraced patient satisfaction as a benchmark of quality care. Self and Sherer[2] present a consensus of quality measure benchmarks that include member satisfaction along with access to care, appropriateness of care, efficiency, technical outcome of care, operating efficiency, accountability, finance, and affordability. Cleary and McNeil[3] reviewed theoretical and empirical work on patient satisfaction with health care. They identified two domains of care quality: technical (i.e., clinical aspects of patient care) and interpersonal (i.e., social–psychological aspects of the patient–clinician relationship). They distinguished two components of patient satisfaction: a cognitive evaluation and an emotional reaction. They used Donabedian's model of structure, process, and outcome of services as the objects of this cognitive and emotional appraisal. The major patient characteristics related to satisfaction include age, gender, and health status, though the relationships between these characteristics and satisfaction are

generally weak. They note that health care provider characteristics such as communication skills, empathy, and caring are the strongest predictors of patient satisfaction.

Ware, Yody, and Adamczyk[4] argue that health status and patient satisfaction are the primary outcomes of interest for rehabilitation care, though the biggest challenge, they believe, is a lack of standardization in measures that would allow outcomes to be compared across programs. A variety of instruments have been developed for use in various health care settings including large medical–surgical chains,[5] a women's hospital,[6] home care,[7] nursing home services,[8] and outpatient services.[9] Fewer instruments have been developed for medical rehabilitation settings. Wilson[10] described a mailed survey for use by patients with physical disabilities; Toczek-McPeake and Matthews[11] developed a survey for clients of a large adult rehabilitation center; McComas, Kosseim, and Macintosh[12] described a questionnaire for mothers of children with disabilities; and Lewinter and Mikkelsen[13] developed an interview for use with patients in a stroke unit.

A multitude of satisfaction-with-health-care measures have been developed, with the consequence that no instrument is widely used. A variety of technical and economic

An earlier version of this manuscript was presented at the Mid-West Objective Measurement Seminar, December 5, 1996, in Chicago, Illinois. Funding was provided in part by the Ralph and Marian Falk Medical Research Trust. Members of the Survey Design Team that developed the satisfaction instrument include Barbara Black, Kristine Cichowski, MS, Bobbie Clark, Anita Halper, MA, CCC-SP, Nancye Holt, MS, RN, Rosemarie King, PhD, RN, Diane Ortolano, MA, PT, Holly Simantel, BS, Gloria Tarvin, MSW, ACSW, Ruth Ann Watkins, MS, OTR/L, and Jane Willemsen, MA, RN.

J Rehabil Outcomes Meas, 1997, 1(4), 52–65

issues has delayed the adoption of a common instrument, including a failure to evaluate components of care that are important to patients,[14] response bias resulting from mailed surveys,[15] and the expense of using interviewers.[16] Despite these difficulties, Rhinehart[17] notes the importance of developing meaningful, reliable, and objective measures of health care organizations' performance that can be compared against a useful benchmark. The Health Policy Advisory Unit[18] used focus groups and found that satisfaction was most strongly related to medical care and information, physical facilities, nontangible environmental factors, quantity of food, nursing care, and visiting arrangements. Attributes of satisfaction identified in a meta-analysis of 221 articles[19] included overall quality, humaneness, technical competence, outcome, facilities, continuity of care, access, informativeness, cost, bureaucracy, and attention to psychosocial problems.

The expectations that patients have of health care are believed to affect the extent of their satisfaction with health care. While such a relationship is widely recognized, expectations are usually inferred from the reported level of satisfaction even though patients may have little experience on which to base their expectations. This is particularly true in rehabilitation, since few patients have previous rehabilitative experience. Ross, Frommelt, Hazelwood, and Chang[20] reviewed theories of consumer behavior and studies examining relationships between expectations and satisfaction. They found support for the hypothesis that initial expectations and subsequent experience determine extent of satisfaction in primary care and mental health despite the variety of ways in which expectations are measured.

The Rehabilitation Institute of Chicago (RIC) assessed patient satisfaction with a mailed questionnaire for several years; concerns about a low response rate and the likelihood that response bias would affect results led to the formation of a task force that was charged with developing a more satisfactory method of assessing patient satisfaction and providing clinicians with feedback about patients' concerns. This report summarizes the results of these efforts and the psychometric properties of a patient satisfaction survey. The objectives of this report are to:

1. Describe the development of a measure of patient satisfaction with medical rehabilitation.
2. Evaluate evidence for the measure's reliability and construct validity.
3. Explore associations between satisfaction and related constructs.

Evidence of construct validity was provided by the coherence of items with an underlying construct of satisfaction. Patterns of satisfaction from various types of respondents, differences across specific impairment groups and age groups, and correlations with functional status were the related constructs of interest.

METHODS

Instrument

An Inpatient Satisfaction Survey was developed by asking patients to propose questions that addressed important components of their rehabilitative experience. They were asked "What questions should we ask to find out how people felt about their stay at RIC?" Fifty patients were interviewed, half during their rehabilitation hospitalization and half by telephone one month after discharge; they were stratified across impairment groups, age, and floors of the hospital. Seven themes emerged from a content analysis of their proposed questions; the themes included:

1. Admission processes (e.g., "Were your fears and anxieties eased when you were admitted?").
2. Medical and nursing care (e.g., "Were you treated with consideration and patience by the staff?").
3. Timeliness of service.
4. Teaching and communication.
5. Staff and therapy effectiveness.
6. Living conditions and environment (e.g., "Did your visitors have a comfortable place to sit?").
7. The discharge process.

The 125 proposed questions were condensed into a 40-item questionnaire and rated on a four-point scale (poor, fair, good, excellent). Table 1 lists the items. The content of many items reflects domains of satisfaction identified in previous studies including communication, care effectiveness, care by specific disciplines, and environmental factors.

Interviewers from the hospital's Outcomes Management Department make up to two telephone calls to all patients one month after discharge in order to complete the questionnaire. Satisfaction information is incorporated in a computerized database that provides integrated feedback to clinical staff about their performance and identifies concerns that require follow-up.

Sample

There were a total of 9,626 discharges from RIC between 1992 and 1996. Interviews were completed for 3,942 of these patients (41 percent). The most frequent reason for not completing an interview was the inability to locate the patient. Of these patients, the majority (85 percent) were admitted to acute rehabilitation for the first time. Women composed 53 percent of the sample; 63 percent of the respondents were the patients themselves, with an additional 33 percent family, 1 percent friends, 1 percent other caregivers, and the remainder unidentified. Age was categorized as: younger than 20 years (10 percent), 20 to 39 (13 percent), 40 to 65 (31 percent), 66 to 79 (31 percent), and 80

Table 1. Items Measurement Report

Obsvd count	Obsvd average	Fair average	Linear measure	Model S.E.	Infit MnSq	Items
3,068	3.4	2.7	.06	.04	1.1	1 Care received on first day
3,371	3.4	2.8	−.09	.03	0.9	2 Patience and consideration shown
3,176	3.4	2.7	.06	.03	0.9	3 Listening to you when you need to talk
3,264	2.9	2.0	1.30	.03	1.2	4 Response time when assistance requested
3,275	3.4	2.8	−.09	.03	1.1	5 Therapies starting on time
3,118	3.4	2.7	.03	.04	0.9	6 Included in decisions about program
3,304	3.4	2.8	−.18	.04	0.7	7 Response to questions
3,340	3.5	3.0	−.78	.04	0.8	8 Skill and knowledge in therapies and treatment
3,294	3.4	2.8	−.18	.04	0.8	9 Explanations of schedules, procedures, therapies
3,303	3.5	2.9	−.47	.04	0.8	10 Encouragement in therapies and self-care
3,034	3.3	2.6	.20	.03	0.8	11 Communications among staff about your care
3,380	3.2	2.4	.68	.03	1.3	13 Living conditions (cleanliness, noise, privacy)
3,258	3.3	2.6	.30	.03	1.4	15 Preparation for going home
3,299	3.4	2.7	.00	.03	1.1	16 Coordination of discharge plans
3,187	3.5	2.9	−.34	.04	0.8	17 Instructions/training received about your care
2,539	3.4	2.8	−.09	.04	1.2	18 Availability of home equipment when needed
3,084	3.3	2.6	.19	.03	0.9	19 Explanation of follow-up procedures
1,433	3.2	2.5	.45	.05	0.9	20 Billing and accounting services
3,367	3.5	2.9	−.38	.04	0.7	21 Care received at RIC
3,319	3.5	3.0	−.62	.04	1.1	22 Physicians
3,347	3.5	2.9	−.39	.04	0.9	23 Nurses
3,168	3.2	2.5	.48	.03	0.9	24 AM Nursing assistants and technicians
3,252	3.2	2.4	.59	.03	1.0	25 PM Nursing assistants and technicians
2,898	3.0	2.1	1.12	.03	1.3	26 Night nursing assistants and technicians
3,053	3.4	2.8	−.04	.04	1.2	27 Social worker
3,315	3.6	3.1	−1.16	.04	1.0	28 Physical therapist
3,201	3.6	3.1	−.93	.04	1.1	29 Occupational therapist
1,341	3.5	2.9	−.33	.06	1.2	30 Speech pathologist
677	3.4	2.8	−.13	.08	0.9	31 Audiologist
1,121	3.4	2.8	−.09	.06	1.0	32 Recreational therapist
1,959	3.3	2.7	.16	.04	1.2	33 Psychologist
368	3.3	2.6	.38	.10	0.9	34 Vocational rehabilitation counselor
1,163	3.4	2.7	.13	.06	1.0	35 Chaplain
1,500	3.3	2.5	.52	.05	1.2	36 Dietitian
706	3.4	2.8	−.07	.08	1.2	37 Prosthetist/orthotist
428	3.4	2.7	.00	.10	1.0	38 Pulmonary rehabilitation therapist
1,955	3.5	2.9	−.29	.05	0.9	39 Volunteers

Obsvd Count	Obsvd Average	Fair Average	Measure	Model S.E.	Infit MnSq	
2,590.9	3.4	2.7	.00	.04	1.0	Mean (Count: 37)
992.2	0.1	0.2	.49	.02	0.2	Standard deviation

Items are listed by the order in which they are asked of patients.
Observed count = number of responses to each item.
Observed average = mean response for each item.
Fair average = mean response for each item adjusted for item difficulty.
Linear measure = item difficulty in logits; item difficulties are anchored at a mean of 0 and a standard deviation of 1.
Model S.E. = Standard error of measurement associated with each linear measure.
Infit MnSq = Mean square fit statistic with expectation of 1. Values greater than 1.2 indicate unexpected noise; values less than 0.8 indicate dependency in the data.

or older (14 percent). Primary impairments included orthopaedic conditions (25 percent), stroke (21 percent), brain injuries (13 percent), spinal cord injuries (12 percent), and a variety of other impairments (29 percent). Patients for whom the identity of the respondents were unknown were excluded from further analysis, as were the relatively small number of patients with a primary impairment of cardiac disease, congenital diseases, and multiple major diagnoses, as well as those who responded to fewer than 10 survey items. The analyses were thus conducted on data from 3,827 patients.

Statistical Analyses

The raw score obtained by summing responses to rating scale items is ordinal in nature, which precludes its use in parametric statistical comparisons because these raw data only allow rank ordering of scores. A measurement procedure that can be used to develop reliable, valid, and interval-scaled measures from ordinal scores is Rating Scale (or Rasch) Analysis.[21] Interval measures have the advantage of equal distances between units of the scale. Transforming ordinal-level scores to interval-level measures allows one to quantify individuals' satisfaction along a linear continuum of satisfaction, make quantitative comparisons within individuals across time, or compare satisfaction between individuals or across groups of individuals using parametric statistics.

Previous research suggests that patient satisfaction is multidimensional. Rasch analysis assumes that a single dimension underlies the responses to a set of purposefully chosen items and provides evidence of the extent to which the set of items meets this assumption. When the evidence for unidimensionality is compelling, the measures derived from the analysis become useful in describing and evaluating patient satisfaction. This psychometric procedure views satisfaction items as a continuum that runs from easy-to-be-satisfied-with to difficult-to-be-satisfied-with. If the items form a single construct, one would expect patients to be more satisfied with the easy-to-be-satisfied-with items and less satisfied with the difficult-to-be-satisfied-with items. Thus, when a patient reports more satisfaction with an item than one would expect based on his or her overall satisfaction level, that response misfits the model. In real life, patients do not always respond as expected, but when a substantial proportion respond unexpectedly to an item, this indicates that the item does not fit with the other items in forming a single construct.

When the fit between each item and the underlying construct is adequate and the range of measured satisfaction in a sample sufficiently large, each patient can be characterized by a single satisfaction measure and each item by an estimate of its difficulty (the item's calibration). Estimates of latent patient satisfaction and item difficulty are not observed directly, but are inferred from the ordinal observations obtained when patients are rated on the item set. Rasch analysis[22] is a probabilistic approach to measure construction and validation that provides estimates of patient satisfaction and item difficulty in log-odds units (logits).

Several criteria are used to judge and improve the adequacy of a measure. The two most frequently used criteria are *person separation* (the range of satisfaction measured by the set of items) and *item misfit* (the extent to which the sample as a whole responds unexpectedly to specific items). In order to measure satisfaction, one needs to assume that patients vary in terms of it. Separation is a function of how much patients vary in their satisfaction relative to how precisely one can measure it. Good separation is an indication that the selected items are sensitive to the presumed differences that exist among patients. The larger the separation, the greater the number of unique levels of satisfaction that can be differentiated among patients. Evidence of acceptable person separation is a separation index of 2 or greater.

Two indicators of item fit are defined. *Infit* indicates the extent to which items close to a patient's satisfaction level are rated consistently with overall satisfaction level, while *outfit* indicates the extent to which items far from a patients' satisfaction level are rated consistent with overall satisfaction level. Item misfit indicates either that persons who were satisfied in general were not satisfied with certain aspects of their stay or that those who were not satisfied in general were satisfied with these particular aspects. A pattern of misfitting items should give users pause to consider whether their construct of satisfaction should be defined differently from what they hypothesized. Large outfits (mean square fits greater than 1.5) may reveal that the item set is used differently for subgroups of patients. Small fit statistics (< .5) generally are not a concern, though they provide insights into how an item set might be shortened by deleting redundant items. Ideal fit is indicated by a mean square value of 1.0. While both infit and outfit are useful indicators of noise, large infit (mean square values greater than 1.5) usually reflects more serious problems in the item's coherence with the measure's underlying construct.

Multifaceted rating scale analysis using Facets[23] allows the simultaneous calibration of various aspects of the items or persons. In this analysis we were interested in calibrating the items (various aspects of satisfaction), rating scale (the distance between poor, fair, good, and excellent), respondents (patients, family members, friends, and other caregivers), impairment groups (stroke, spinal cord injury, etc.), gender, and age groups (categorized into five groups).

RESULTS

Respondent Versus Nonrespondent Characteristics

Respondents differed from nonrespondents in terms of impairment, gender, age, race, and functional status. Patients with traumatic brain injury (37 percent response rate) and burns (32 percent) were less likely to be interviewed, while those with arthritis (48 percent), orthopaedic impairments (48 percent), and major multiple trauma (56 percent) were more likely to be interviewed (X^2[df = 12] = 63.6, $p < .001$). Women (43 percent) were more likely to be interviewed than men (39 percent; X^2[df = 1] = 12.9, $p < .001$). Patients between 20 and 29 years of age were less likely to be interviewed (35 percent), while those between 66 and 79 were more likely to be interviewed (45 percent; X^2[df = 4] = 45.1, $p < .001$). Native Americans (29 percent) and Asian Americans (32 percent) were less likely to be interviewed (X^2[df = 5] = 30.9, p < .001). Finally, patients who were interviewed were admitted and discharged with higher functional status and made larger gains as measured by the FIM^{SM} instrument than patients who were not interviewed t(df = 8,104) = 5.7, p < .001 for admission ratings, t(df = 7,624) = 7.3, p < .001 for discharge, and t(df = 7,378) = 3.3, p = .001 for gain).

Overview of Rating Scale Analyses

Five steps were involved in the analysis of the patient satisfaction items. First, all items were calibrated to identify misfitting items. Second, misfitting items were deleted and estimates of overall patient satisfaction were obtained. Item and step calibration from this step were used for all subsequent analyses. Third, with the items and steps anchored, patients were nested into categories based on various characteristics, and the effects of being in each of these categories were estimated. Fourth, the effect of respondent type was controlled statistically and patient satisfaction was reestimated. Finally, patient satisfaction with and without controlling for respondent type was compared.

In the first analysis, patient characteristics are ignored and items were calibrated to estimate their difficulty level, that is, how easy or difficult it was for patients to report satisfaction considering specific aspects of satisfaction. Items that did not fit the measurement model (i.e., those items to which patients responded unexpectedly based on their responses to the total set of items) were identified.

The analysis showed that three items, *food, safety of belongings,* and *other staff* significantly misfit the model; that is, the item mean square residual was greater than 1.5. Some otherwise satisfied patients were not as satisfied with food and safety as one would have expected. Items such as *other*

staff frequently misfit measurement models because patients do not refer to the same person in responding to the item. Three additional items were included in this calibration to determine their fit with the satisfaction construct: *recommend RIC to others, helpfulness of the stay,* and *expectations met.* While *recommend RIC to others* fit the model, the other two did not. Misfit in terms of whether *expectations were met* could result from unrealistic or idiosyncratic expectations on the part of some patients, while misfit in *helpfulness of stay* reflects a distinct aspect of patients' attitudes.

In the second analysis, misfitting items were deleted and the remaining items were recalibrated. The resulting item continuum is shown in Figure 1. In this map, the items are grouped by content (staff in general, services provided, and specific staff) to illustrate how the items were distributed among similar items in terms of patient satisfaction. For staff in general, patients are most satisfied with their knowledge and skills and least satisfied with response time. For services provided, patients were most satisfied with the instruction and training received and least satisfied with the living conditions. Finally, for specific staff, patients were most satisfied with occupational and physical therapists and least satisfied with night nursing assistants and technicians. Statistics for the satisfaction items are presented in Table 1. The overall fit of the remaining items (1.0) is ideal and indicates that patient satisfaction is unidimensional; that is, all items (both technical and interpersonal) cohere together to form a single scale. Thus, although both components of patient satisfaction are included, dual scales are not necessary. The item reliability of 0.99 for the 37 items is excellent. Category statistics are presented in Table 2. These statistics indicate that patients are able to use the rating scale accurately; that is, the 8 percent of patients who had low overall satisfaction tended to rate the items as "poor" or "fair," the 46 percent with

Table 2. Category Statistics

Category score	Counts used	%	Cum %	Avge meas	Outfit MnSq	Measure	S.E.	Response category name
1	2,004	2	2	−.15	1.8			Poor
2	5,671	6	8	.39	1.3	−1.24	.03	Fair
3	43,816	46	54	1.40	.8	−1.19	.01	Good
4	44,374	46	100	3.58	.9	2.43	.01	Excellent

Response categories are ordered by the manner in which they are asked of patients.
Counts used = number of responses to each category, summed across all items.
Percent and cumulative percent = proportion of responses within each category, and averaged cumulatively.
Average measure = the mean measure (in logits) corresponding to each response category.
Outfit MnSq = mean square fit statistic with expectation of 1. Values greater than 1.2 indicate unexpected noise; values less than 0.8 indicate dependency in the data.
Step calibration measure = the average improvement in total measure corresponding to an increase between consecutive categories.
Standard error = the standard error of measurement associated with each step calibration measure.

```
----------------------------------------------------------------------------------------------------
I  Measr  I +Patients  I -Items                                                        I Scale  I
----------------------------------------------------------------------------------------------------
+   7   + **********  + Staff in General      Services Provided          Specific Staff    +  (4)  +
I       I            I                                                                     I       I
I       I            I                                                                     I       I
I       I            I                                                                     I       I
I       I            I                                                                     I       I
+   6   + *.         +                                                                     +       +
I       I *.         I                                                                     I       I
I       I .          I                                                                     I       I
I       I .          I                                                                     I       I
I       I *.         I                                                                     I       I
+   5   + .          +                                                                     +       +
I       I *.         I                                                                     I       I
I       I *.         I                                                                     I       I
I       I *.         I                                                                     I       I
I       I *.         I                                                                     I       I
+   4   + **.        +                                                                     +       +
I       I **.        I                                                                     I       I
I       I **.        I                                                                     I       I
I       I **.        I                                                                     I       I
I       I **.        I                                                                     I       I
+   3   + ***.       +                                                                     +       +
I       I **.        I                                                                     I   —   I
I       I **.        I                                                                     I       I
I       I **.        I                                                                     I       I
I       I **.        I                                                                     I       I
+   2   + **.        +                                                                     +       +
I       I **.        I                                                                     I       I
I       I **.        I                                                                     I       I
I       I **.        I Response time                                                       I       I
I       I ***.       I                              Night Nursing A&T                       I       I
+   1   + ***.       +                                                                     +       +
I       I *******.   I                                                                     I   3   I
I       I ****.      I           Living conditions       PM Nursing A&T      Dietitian  I       I
I       I **.        I           Billing/accounting services  AM Nursing A&T  Voc Rehab I       I
I       I *.         I Communication about care  Follow-up expln/Prep to go home  Psychologist  Chaplain I  I
*   0   * *.         * Listening/On-time therapy  Home equipment available  Prost/Orthotist  Social Worker *  *
:       :            : Patience and consideration  Included in decisions  Rec Therapist  Pulm Rehab :  :
I       I .          I                           Care on first day                         I       I
I       I .          I Question resp/ Sched expl                        Volunteers  Audiologist I  I
I       I .          I Encouragement      Care/instruction/training rec'd  Nurses  Spch Pathologist I  — I
I       I .          I                                                    Doctors            I       I
I       I .          I Skills and knowledge                                                 I       I
+  -1   + .          +                              Occupational Therapist                  +   2   +
I       I .          I                              Physical Therapist                      I       I
I       I .          I                                                                     I       I
I       I .          I                                                                     I       I
+  -2   + .          +                                                                     +   —   +
I       I .          I                                                                     I       I
I       I .          I                                                                     I       I
I       I .          I                                                                     I       I
+  -3   + .          +                                                                     +       +
I       I .          I                                                                     I       I
I       I .          I                                                                     I       I
I       I .          I                                                                     I       I
I       I .          I                                                                     I       I
+  -4   + .          +                                                                     +  (1)  +
----------------------------------------------------------------------------------------------------
I  Measr  I * = 44    I -Items                                                              I Scale  I
----------------------------------------------------------------------------------------------------
```

Note: Metric maintained by + or I. Spacing expanded with : to show all elements.

Figure 1. Person and item map of patient satisfaction.

higher overall satisfaction tended to rate the items as "good," and the 46 percent with the highest overall satisfaction tended to rate the items as "excellent."

The distribution of patient satisfaction measures is also presented in Figure 1. This distribution is negatively skewed, with the vast majority of patients rating their satisfaction as "excellent," and with the exception of a few ratings of "fair" or "poor," the remainder reporting their satisfaction as "good." Summary statistics for the patient satisfaction measure are presented in Table 3. The person separation (3.66) is more than adequate (adequate defined as values greater than 2.0); the measure has sufficient precision to distinguish five strata of patient satisfaction.

Analyses of Patient Facets

In the subsequent analyses, patients were nested into categories based on characteristics for which differences in satisfaction have been found in earlier studies. These characteristics are age, gender, and impairment group. Because people other than patients responded to the questionnaire, respondent types were also categorized.

The difficulty level of the items needs to be held constant in order to examine the responses of patients nested within each of these characteristics; only then can differences in satisfaction be attributed to group membership. Both item calibrations and the rating scale step structure are anchored (set equal) to the values obtained when individual responses were analyzed. In essence, for each characteristic, patient satisfaction was averaged by category and the average measures were compared across category. Figure 2 shows the map of persons nested within impairment groups, gender, age, and respondent type. Summary statistics for each of these characteristics are presented in Tables 4 to 7. The average effect of belonging to one of these categories is centered at zero. Effects greater than zero indicate greater satisfaction and effects less than zero indicate less satisfaction. Satisfaction levels vary across impairment groups (X^2[df = 9] = 9.7, p

< .01) such that patients with burns are more satisfied and those with pulmonary conditions somewhat more satisfied than other patients. Gender differences in satisfaction were found such that women reported slightly more satisfaction than men (X^2[df = 1] = 131.1, p < .01); however, this difference is so small that it is not meaningful. Differences in satisfaction across age group were found; younger patients are more satisfied than older patients (X^2[df = 4] = 255.7, p < .01). Across respondent types, family, friends, and other caregivers tend to rate patient satisfaction more positively than do patients (X^2[df = 3] = 175.5, p < .01); the difference between patients and other caregivers (almost one-half a logit) is meaningfully significant.

This type of analysis can also provide an estimate of satisfaction after differences in patient characteristics are taken into account. While it is interesting to understand differences across demographic characteristics, it does not make conceptual sense to control for them; however, it does make sense to control for differences based on respondent type. Thus, differences in ratings that are attributable to type of respondent can be eliminated. That is, the finding that other caregivers rated overall satisfaction higher than patients themselves allows us to adjust their ratings downward to reflect the level obtained when patients do their own rating. This residual can be considered an estimate of the rating that would have been obtained if the patients themselves had responded to the survey.

Finally, the residual rating of patient satisfaction was compared to the estimate obtained without controlling for respondent type. The satisfaction of most patients is the same with or without adjusting for respondent type and only a few (those for whom a caregiver responded to the survey) had adjusted overall satisfaction ratings that are less than the original ratings. The correlation between the original and adjusted ratings of 0.999 indicates that while a few ratings decrease, the ordering of patients by satisfaction level is not affected. This finding reflects the fact that relatively few caregivers rated patient satisfaction.

Table 3. Patients Measurement Report

	Obsvd count	Obsvd average	Fair average	Measure	Model S.E.	Infit MnSq
Mean (Count: 3,827)	28.4	3.4	3.4	2.26	.42	1.1
Standard deviation	3.5	0.5	0.5	1.72	.17	0.7

Observed counts = mean number of responses per patient, averaged across all items.
Observed average = mean raw score for each patient.
Fair average = mean raw score for each patient, adjusted for respondent, age, gender, and impairment group.
Measure = the mean measure (in logits) for the sample.
Model S.E. = the standard error of measurement associated with the measure and standard deviation, respectively.
Infit MnSq = mean square fit statistic with expectation of 1.

```
| Meas   + Impairment                                                | +Gender  | +Age    | +Respondent | Scale |
-----------------------------------------------------------------------------------------------------------------
+   3   +                                                       +        +         +            +     (4)  +
|       |                                                       |        |         |            |          |
|       |                                                       |        |         |            |      —   |
|       |                                                       |        |         |            |          |
|       |                                                       |        |         |            |          |
+   2   +                                                       +        +         +            +          +
|       |                                                       |        |         |            |          |
|       |                                                       |        |         |            |          |
|       |                                                       |        |         |            |          |
|       |                                                       |        |         |            |          |
+   1   +                                                       +        +         +            +          +
|       |                                                       |        |         |            |      3   |
|       |                                                       |        |         |            |          |
|       | Burns                                                 |        |         | Caregiver  |          |
|       | Pulmonary D/O                                         |        | 0–19    | Family     |          |
*   0   * Stroke    SCI       Amputee   Brain Injury   * Female  *       * 20–39   * Friends    *          *
:       : Neurological  Orthopaedic  Arthritis  Other   : Male    :       : 40–65   : Patient    :          :
:       :                                                       |        : 66–79   :            :          :
|       |                                                       |        | 80–100  |            |      —   |
|       |                                                       |        |         |            |          |
|       |                                                       |        |         |            |          |
|       |                                                       |        |         |            |          |
+  −1   +                                                       +        +         +            +          +
|       |                                                       |        |         |            |      2   |
|       |                                                       |        |         |            |          |
|       |                                                       |        |         |            |          |
|       |                                                       |        |         |            |          |
+  −2   +                                                       +        +         +            +     (1)  +
-----------------------------------------------------------------------------------------------------------------
| Meas   + Impairment                                                | +Gender  | +Age    | +Respondent | Scale |
```

Note: Metric maintained by + or |. Spacing expanded with : to show all elements.

Figure 2. Item and demographic group map of patient satisfaction.

Validity Evidence

Patient satisfaction now accurately measured can be used to investigate the relationships between satisfaction and functional status and improvement, with whether patients would recommend the hospital to others, how helpful their stays were, and how well their expectations were met. Recall that meeting expectations and helpfulness of the stay did not fit the measurement model established by the satisfaction items; that is, it did not measure the same construct as the satisfaction items. Thus, it is important to understand how satisfaction, helpfulness, and expectations are related.

Patient satisfaction differs with respect to whether or not patients would recommend the facility to others, whether they consider their stays helpful, and whether their expectations were met. One-way analysis of variance was conducted on the measure of patient satisfaction and levels of responses to these three items; patient satisfaction differed by recommendation ($F[\mathrm{df} = 2{,}3816] = 227.3$, $p < .001$), helpfulness of stay ($F[3{,}3811] = 283.3$, $p < .001$), and expectations ($F[2{,}3378] = 219.2$, $p < .001$). Because the variances were heterogeneous across groups, post hoc analyses were conducted using Dunnett's C. The map presented in Figure 3 shows the average satisfaction measures for each group within each of three items. Although all of the differences between groups are statistically significant, interesting patterns result in terms of which groups are substantially more or less satisfied. Patients who are unsure whether they would recommend the facility to others are more similar in satisfaction to those who would not recommend the facility than who would recommend it. The largest gap in satisfaction is between those who felt their stays were very helpful and all the rest. Patients whose expectations were somewhat met are more similar in satisfaction to those whose expectations were met than those whose expectations were not met. Satisfaction was unrelated to linear measures of motor and cogni-

Table 4. Impairment Group Measurement Report

Obsvd Count	Obsvd average	Fair average	Measure	Model S.E.	Infit MnSq	Impairment group
1,050	3.6	3.5	0.34	.06	1.3	11 Burns
2,432	3.4	3.5	0.07	.04	1.8	10 Pulmonary disorder
23,244	3.4	3.4	0.00	.01	1.5	1 Stroke
14,490	3.5	3.4	0.00	.02	1.5	2 Brain dysfunction
5,575	3.4	3.4	0.00	.03	1.5	5 Amputee
10,749	3.4	3.4	0.00	.02	1.6	13 Other impairments
13,243	3.4	3.4	−0.10	.02	1.7	4 Spinal cord dysfunction
2,100	3.4	3.4	−0.10	.04	1.6	6 Arthritis
8,392	3.4	3.4	−0.13	.02	1.7	3 Neurological conditions
25,754	3.4	3.4	−0.04	.01	1.8	8 Orthopedic conditions
10,702.9	3.4	3.4	0.24	.03	1.6	Mean (count: 10)
8,196.6	0.0	0.0	.12	.02	0.2	Standard deviation

Impairment groups are ordered by descending average measure.
Observed counts = number of responses for each impairment group, summed across all items.
Observed average = mean response for all items, summed within impairment group.
Fair average = mean response for all items, adjusted for impairment group differences.
Measure = the mean measure (in logits) for each group, averaged across items.
Model standard error = the standard error of measurement associated with the measure of each impairment group.
Infit MnSq = mean square fit statistic with expectation of 1. Values greater than 1.2 indicate unexpected noise; values less than 0.8 indicate dependency in the data.

tive functional status at admission and discharge as measured by the FIM^{SM} instrument, nor with change in functional status between admission and discharge.

• • •

The objectives of this study were to develop a measure of patient satisfaction with medical rehabilitation, to evaluate evidence for the measure's construct validity, and to explore associations with related constructs. We succeeded in devel-

oping a measure with satisfactory psychometric properties using 37 of the 40 items. Three misfitting items were identified: Satisfaction with food, safety of belongings, and other staff. Cultural and personal dietary preferences may explain dissatisfaction with food. The misfit of overall satisfaction with safety of belongings suggests that while important, some patients are satisfied with their care while being dissatisfied with the safety of their belongings. *Other staff* is too idiosyncratically interpreted to be meaningful; however, asking about other staff does prompt occasional responses,

Table 5. Gender Measurement Report

Obsvd Count	Obsvd average	Fair average	Measure	Model S.E.	Infit MnSq	Gender
50,628	3.5	2.8	.07	.01	1.6	1 Female
56,401	3.4	2.7	−.07	.01	1.7	2 Male
53,514.5	3.4	2.7	.00	.01	1.6	Mean (Count: 2)
2,886.5	0.0	0.0	.07	.00	0.1	Standard deviation

Gender groups are ordered by descending average measure.
Observed Counts = number of responses for each gender group, summed across all items.
Observed average = mean response for all items, summed within gender groups.
Fair average = mean response for all items, adjusted for gender group differences.
Measure = the mean measure (in logits) for each group, averaged across items.
Model standard error = the standard error of measurement associated with the measure of each impairment group.
Infit MnSq = mean square fit statistic with expectation of 1. Values greater than 1.2 indicate unexpected noise; values less than 0.8 indicate dependency in the data.

Table 6. Age Measurement Report

Obsvd Count	Obsvd average	Fair average	Measure	Model S.E.	Infit MnSq	Age group
11,447	3.5	2.8	.22	.02	1.6	1 0–19
14,289	3.4	2.7	−.03	.02	1.7	2 20–39
33,819	3.4	2.7	.01	.01	1.7	3 40–65
33,247	3.4	2.7	−.05	.01	1.6	4 66–79
14,227	3.4	2.7	−.15	.02	1.6	5 80–100
21,405.8	3.4	2.7	.00	.01	1.6	Mean (count: 5)
9,956.5	0.0	0.1	.12	.00	0.0	Standard deviation

Age groups are ordered by descending average measure.
Observed counts = number of responses for each age group, summed across all items.
Observed average = mean response for all items, summed within age groups.
Fair average = mean response for all items, adjusted for age group differences.
Measure = the mean measure (in logits) for each group, averaged across items.
Model standard error = the standard error of measurement associated with the measure of each impairment group.
Infit MnSq = mean square fit statistic with expectation of 1. Values greater than 1.2 indicate unexpected noise; values less than 0.8 indicate dependency in the data.

which provide useful feedback. The overall fit of 37 items indicates that patient satisfaction is unidimensional in that all items (both technical and interpersonal) cohere together to form a single scale. Thus, although both components of patient satisfaction are included, dual scales are not necessary.

While *recommending the facility to others* fits the satisfaction construct, helpfulness of stay and expectations met did not. *Helpfulness of the stay* is a distinctly different construct than satisfaction. Patients could report a low level of helpfulness while being satisfied with their care overall. Expectations are unlikely to be based on prior experience, given that only 15 percent had a previous rehabilitation stay. Nevertheless, satisfaction was related to all three. Patients who were

most satisfied were those who would recommend the facility to others, felt their stays were very helpful, but whose expectations may have been only somewhat met.

Differences in satisfaction across type of respondent were found. Other caregiver ratings were more favorable than family member and friend ratings, which in turn were greater than patient ratings. It is important to adjust for type of respondent in order to minimize this source of bias. Closeness to the patients' experience during rehabilitation may account for this phenomenon. Whatever the source of bias, patients provide the best source of information about their own satisfaction.

Consistent with earlier studies, age was related to satisfaction: greater age was associated with lower levels of satisfac-

Table 7. Respondent Measurement Report

Obsvd Count	Obsvd average	Fair average	Measure	Model S.E.	Infit MnSq	Interviewee
69,421	3.4	2.7 A	.00	.01	1.7	1 Patient
35,610	3.5	2.8	.15	.01	1.6	2 Family
997	3.4	2.8	.07	.06	1.0	3 Friends
1,001	3.5	2.9	.42	.06	1.2	4 Caregiver
26,757.3	3.5	2.8	.16	.04	1.4	Mean (count: 4)
28,396.9	0.0	0.1	.16	.03	0.3	Standard deviation

Respondent groups are ordered by descending average measure.
Observed counts = number of responses for each respondent group, summed across all items.
Observed average = mean response for all items, summed within respondent groups.
Fair average = mean response for all items, adjusted for respondent group differences.
Measure = the mean measure (in logits) for each group, averaged across items.
Model standard error = the standard error of measurement associated with the measure of each impairment group.
Infit MnSq = mean square fit statistic with expectation of 1. Values greater than 1.2 indicate unexpected noise; values less than 0.8 indicate dependency in the data.

```
----------------------------------------------------------------------------------------------------
| Meas    | +Recommend RIC?          | +Helpful stay?        | +Expectations met?          | Scale  |
----------------------------------------------------------------------------------------------------
+   4    +                          +                       +                            +  (4)  +
|        |                          |                       |                            |       |
|        |                          | Stay very helpful     |                            |       |
|        |                          |                       | Expectations met           |       |
+   3    + Would recommend RIC      +                       +                            +       +
|        |                          |                       |                            |       |
|        |                          |                       |                            |   —   |
|        |                          |                       | Expectations somewhat met  |       |
+   2    +                          +                       +                            +       +
|        |                          |                       |                            |       |
|        |                          | Stay helpful          |                            |       |
|        |                          |                       |                            |       |
+   1    +                          + Stay somewhat helpful +                            +       +
|        |                          |                       |                            |   3   |
|        |                          |                       | Expectations not met       |       |
|        | Unsure about recommending RIC |                  |                            |       |
|        |                          |                       |                            |       |
*   0    *                          * Stay not at all helpful *                          *       *
|        |                          |                       |                            |       |
|        | Would not recommend RIC  |                       |                            |   —   |
|        |                          |                       |                            |       |
+  −1    +                          +                       +                            +       +
|        |                          |                       |                            |   2   |
|        |                          |                       |                            |       |
|        |                          |                       |                            |       |
+  −2    +                          +                       +                            +  (1)  +
----------------------------------------------------------------------------------------------------
| Meas    | +Recommend RIC?          | +Helpful stay?        | +Expectations met?          | Scale  |
----------------------------------------------------------------------------------------------------
```

Figure 3. Map of global outcomes related to patient satisfaction.

tion. Factors that might explain this finding include the relatively youthful nature of the staff and a greater experience base of older patients that leads them to have higher expectations.

Two factors found to be related to satisfaction in earlier studies which were not found in this sample were gender and health status. We found a statistically significant but not meaningful difference between men and women in satisfaction. Functional status, a close cousin of health status, as well as gains in functional status, were unrelated to satisfaction. The finding that severity of disability and extent of functional gains are unrelated to satisfaction with care has important clinical, policy, and research implications. This finding discredits the stereotype that persons with more severe disabilities are less likely to report satisfaction. Further, satisfaction can be high even when functional gains are minimal.

It appears that patients' satisfaction derives from benefits other than functional gains.

Several limitations of this study should be considered. First, all patients received rehabilitation at one facility; hence, our certainty about how well this item set will work at other rehabilitation hospitals and units is limited. Certainly the item content is relevant, though the relative difficulty and fit of the items in other settings may vary. Our confidence in generalizing conclusions about satisfaction level is limited by the follow-up of only 41 percent of the patients; nonrespondents differed from respondents in terms of impairment, gender, age, race and functional status. The telephone interview format also can introduce bias. Respondents may have been unwilling to express dissatisfaction to a representative of the hospital who could identify them personally. Many patients continue to receive outpatient care and may worry about prejudicing their care providers. However, the alternative of using a mailed survey with a low response rate and considerable missing data appears more problematic than the assessment methodology adopted here.

Future studies could evaluate changes in satisfaction over time and as program innovations are introduced. For example, a reorganization of patient care was introduced after these data were collected. Effects of the reorganization on satisfaction will be important to assess. The analyses also identify patients for whom the item set measures satisfaction in an idiosyncratic manner. Clinicians could use these results to target patients with unexpected patterns of satisfaction in order to be more responsive to their unique expectations. Finally, the result of these analyses provides a way to shorten the instrument without reducing the precision of satisfaction measurement.

In summary, we derived a psychometrically sound, interval-level measure of patient satisfaction that corrects for bias introduced by different respondent types, that relates meaningfully to theoretical models of patient satisfaction, and is useful in assessing changes over time or after program changes. The measure assesses a wide range of satisfaction, and individual items cohere well together even though the distribution of responses for this sample is strongly biased in a favorable direction. The instrument assesses both technical and interpersonal aspects of care, consistent with major theoretical approaches and allows administrators, clinicians, and researchers to assess an important component of rehabilitation outcomes.

REFERENCES

1. Donabedian, A. "The Quality of Care: How Can It Be Assessed?" *Journal of the American Medical Association* 260 (1988): 1,743–48.

2. Self, D.R., and Sherer, R. "Quality Measures in Health Care." *Health Marketing Quarterly* 13, no. 4 (1996): 3–15.

3. Cleary, P.D., and McNeil, B.J. "Patient Satisfaction as an Indicator of Quality of Care." *Inquiry* 25 (Spring 1988): 25–36.

4. Ware, P.J., Yody, B.B., and Adamczyk, J. "Assessment Tools: Functional Health Status and Patient Satisfaction." *American Journal of Medical Quality* 11, no. 1 (1996): S50–S53.

5. Nelson, E.C., et al. "The Patient Judgment System: Reliability and Validity." *Quality Review Bulletin* 16, no. 6 (1989): 185–91.

6. Cleary, P.D., et al. "Patient Assessments of Hospital Care." *Quality Review Bulletin* 16, no. 6 (1989): 172–79.

7. Westra, B.L., et al. "Development of the Home Care Client Satisfaction Instrument." *Public Health Nursing* 12, no. 6 (1995): 393–99.

8. Zinn, J.S., Lavizzo-Mourey, R., and Taylor, L. "Measuring Satisfaction with Care in the Nursing Home Setting: The Nursing Home Resident Satisfaction Scale." *Journal of Applied Gerontology* 12, no. 4 (1993): 452–65.

9. Rubin, H.R., et al. "Patient's Ratings of Outpatient Visits in Different Practice Settings: Results from the Medical Outcomes Study." *Journal of the American Medical Association* 270, no. 7 (1993): 835–40.

10. Wilson, K.G., et al. "Consumer Satisfaction with a Rehabilitation Mobile Outreach Program." *Archives of Physical Medicine and Rehabilitation* 76, no. 10 (1995): 899–904.

11. Toczek-McPeake, A., and Matthews, M. "Quality Management: A Survey of Client and Career Satisfaction with Speech Pathology and Physiotherapy Services in a Rehabilitation Setting." *Journal of Cognitive Rehabilitation* 13, no. 5 (1995): 12–18.

12. McComas, J., Kosseim, M., and Macintosh, D. "Client-Centered Approach to Develop a Seating Clinic Satisfaction Questionnaire: A Qualitative Study." *American Journal of Occupational Therapy* 49, no. 10 (1995): 980–85. ·

13. Lewinter, M., and Mikkelsen, S. "Parents' Experience of Rehabilitation After Stroke." *Disability and Rehabilitation* 17, no. 1 (1995): 3–9.

14. Avis, M., Bond, M., and Arthur, A. "Satisfying Solutions? A Review of Some Unresolved Issues in the Measurement of Patient Satisfaction." *Journal of Advanced Nursing* 22 (1995): 316–22.

15. Gallagher, J. "Rebuttal—Invalid Patient Surveys: Not A Bargain At Any Price." *Journal of Health Care Marketing* 9, no. 1 (1989): 69–71.

16. Petersen, M.B.H. "Useful Data." *Journal of Nursing Quality Assurance* 2, no. 3 (1988): 25–35.

17. Rhinehart, E. "Evaluating Performance in Managed Care." *Managed Healthcare* 6, no. 3 (1996): 24.

18. The Health Policy Advisory Unit. *The Patient Satisfaction Questionnaire.* Sheffield, England: Sheffield University, 1989. As described by Avis, M., Bond, M., and Arthur, A. "Satisfying Solutions? A Review of Some Unresolved Issues in the Measurement of Patient Satisfaction." *Journal of Advanced Nursing* 22 (1995): 316–22.

19. Hall, J., and Dornan, M. "What Patients Like about Their Medical Care and How Often They Are Asked: A Meta-Analysis of the Satisfaction Literature." *Social Science and Medicine* 27 (1988): 935–39.

20. Ross, C.K., et al. "The Role of Expectations in Patient Satisfaction with Medical Care." *Journal of Health Care Marketing* 7, no. 4 (1987): 16–26.

21. Rasch, G. "Probabilistic Models for Some Intelligence and Attainment Tests." Copenhagen: Danmarks Paedogogiski Institute, 1960; Chicago: University of Chicago Press, 1980.

22. Wright, B.D., and Masters, G.N. "Rating Scale Analysis: Rasch Measurement." Chicago: MESA Press, 1982.

23. Linacre, J.M., and Wright, B.D. *Facets: Many-Facet Rasch Analysis.* Chicago: MESA Press, 1996.

16

Understanding and Assessing Consumer Satisfaction in Rehabilitation

Steven E. Simon and Adele Patrick

Satisfaction with health services has received increasing attention since the 1970s. However, most of the substantive research has centered on medical and mental health care, with less reported specifically in rehabilitation. In order to assist those who wish to effectively manage consumer satisfaction in rehabilitation settings, this article uses cross-disciplinary theory, and research to answer five questions related to understanding, measuring, using and developing this concept:

1. Why is a focus on consumer satisfaction important?
2. What is consumer satisfaction, and how can it be defined as a concept and psychological construct?
3. What are the pertinent issues related to measuring consumer satisfaction?
4. How can consumer satisfaction be measured and evaluated so that the right information is obtained for the purposes defined?
5. What rehabilitation research is needed to develop and effectively use consumer satisfaction information?

WHY IS CONSUMER SATISFACTION IMPORTANT?

Improving Services and Appropriate Service Utilization

During the 1990s, many organizations, including those in health-related services, adopted continuous improvement principles from the total quality movement.[1-3] Such approaches associate improved processes with higher quality services that better meet the needs and expectations of customers, thus leading to increased satisfaction. In this framework, consumer satisfaction is viewed as one indicator of service quality. In fact, Pekarik and Wolff also note a trend

J Rehabil Outcomes Meas, 1997, 1(5), 1–14

toward use of client satisfaction as a core quality assurance indicator in managed care.[4] In addition, the role of satisfaction as a stimulus for more functional service utilization has received support from studies that find associations between patient satisfaction and medical compliance behaviors, as well as with choices regarding whether to use expert versus self care.[5,6] Similarly, in rehabilitation, satisfaction could have impact on whether consumers continue with and complete programs. Appropriate utilization of public rehabilitation services, particularly by minorities, is a salient issue that is related to the 1992 Rehabilitation Act Amendments' requirements for the measurement of consumer satisfaction.[7]

Accounting for the Effectiveness of Services Provided

Programs usually need to show results consistent with the purposes of services offered, in order to justify continued funding, or to demonstrate program effectiveness to prospective customers. This is particularly significant now for managed care and contracted providers, as well as for public rehabilitation agencies. In addition, program accreditation requirements, such as The Commission on Accreditation of Rehabilitation Facilities (CARF) standards,[8] or requirements of the law (Rehabilitation Act),[9] require collection of client satisfaction information partially as a way of demonstrating program effectiveness.

Attracting and Retaining Private Sector Customers

In the private sector, satisfaction may lead customers to initiate or continue services,[5,6,10] thus making it an important component of successful business. In fact, as Jones and Sasser suggest, it may not be sufficient to simply satisfy customers in order to retain them; it may be important to provide the *most* satisfactory service among one's competitors.[11]

Engendering Positive Attitudes Toward Public Service Systems

Providers of public rehabilitation services usually do not compete for customers. Since consumers often have only a single option, they depend on government administrators and elected representatives to make services responsive. Although dissatisfied consumers cannot switch providers, they can create added work through complaints, and they can exert political pressure for change. Thus, an incentive exists for public providers to at least *avoid* dissatisfied consumers. On a more positive note, recent government reengineering initiatives, for example, as generated by the Vice President's National Performance Review[12] and the total quality movement, have placed an emphasis on better and more satisfactory service similar to what consumers have expected from the private sector.

WHAT IS CONSUMER SATISFACTION?

In order to effectively assess and use consumer satisfaction information, it is necessary to understand the meaning of the concept. This section reviews definitional theory and research, leading to a developmental model, a definition of consumer satisfaction, and parameters for operationally defining consumer satisfaction for assessment purposes.

Definitional Theory

The experience of consumer satisfaction (or dissatisfaction) involves a subjective reaction to some external reality. Thus, when we measure consumer satisfaction we are measuring both the external reality and the individual. As noted later, this dual nature of the concept could have implications for choice of a measurement approach, or even for using satisfaction information for change.

What Is the Nature of the Subjective Reaction?

From a psychological perspective, satisfaction has been generally viewed as an affective phenomenon, that is, a state of pleasantness, well-being, or gratification.[13] For example, Lawler indicates that since the 1930s job satisfaction has referred to affective attitudes or orientations to jobs.[14] Similarly, Weirs describes job satisfaction in terms of an "affective (emotional) reaction to elements of the work environment."[15] In the study of life satisfaction or subjective well-being, satisfaction is viewed in such terms as a global evaluation of one's life in positive terms, or pleasant emotional experience.[16]

Of the few in-depth analyses of the consumer satisfaction concept in health services, conclusions have been based mainly on information borrowed from social psychology, job satisfaction, and marketing theories. Linder-Pelz, after reviewing attitude theory and job satisfaction literature, infers that "satisfaction is a positive attitude."[17] Specifically, she defines patient satisfaction as "positive evaluations of distinct dimensions of the health care." In effect, she suggests that satisfaction is an *affect,* the result of social psychological determinants including "perceptions, evaluations, and comparisons." According to Linder-Pelz, these determinants involve the "interaction or discrepancy relation" among five hypothesized antecedent perception and attitude variables: expectations, value, entitlement, occurrences, and interpersonal comparisons. However, in subsequent research involving the first four of these factors, Linder-Pelz found weak relationships for most individual variables or variable interactions with satisfaction. Expectations appeared to be the most important antecedent, but it accounted for only 8 percent of the patient satisfaction variance.[18]

Pascoe, integrating models of marketing researchers, defined patient satisfaction as "a health care recipient's reaction to salient aspects of the context, process, and result of their service experience."[19] He essentially views satisfaction as an evaluation comparing the prominent aspects of the service experience to a subjective standard. The comparison involves a cognitive evaluation and an emotional reaction to the structure, process, and outcome of services. The nature of the subjective standard is described by Pascoe as "any one, or a combination, of the following: a subjective ideal, a subjective sense of what one deserves, a subjective average of past experience in similar situations, or some minimally acceptable level."

Fitzpatrick and Hopkins in a review of survey research on patient evaluations of health care found patients' views treated as attitudes (defined as generalized dispositions along a favorable-unfavorable continuum).[20] Such attitudes "are affective, shaped by 'emotional orientations' (per Segall and Burnett[21] as cited in Fitzpatrick and Hopkins) towards health care and fairly undiscriminating with regard to the instrumental outcomes of their encounters with health care. Judgments of outcomes are determined by patterns of expectations formed by the habituation of experience." However, in a study using standardized interviews of outpatients treated for headaches, Fitzpatrick and Hopkins subsequently found that prior expectations were tentative and not a likely basis from which varying satisfaction might emerge; nor were emotional orientations a substantial basis for evaluation.[20]

The work of Linder-Pelz, Pascoe, and Fitzpatrick and Hopkins is helpful in clarifying the affectual nature of consumer satisfaction. However, the cognitive evaluation process and its relation to satisfaction-related affect remains unclear.

The External Reality

A subjective consumer satisfaction response reflects the result of cognitive processing (perception and evaluation) of service encounters. These encounters include real events and attributes that take place in the context of a particular service spectrum. The service spectrum represents a system level, type of program, process segment(s), and scope of service to which the consumer is exposed and which are relevant for satisfaction assessment purposes. For example, a hospital rehabilitation medicine department may wish to measure patient satisfaction with vocational services. The service spectrum of interest is defined as predischarge vocational evaluation and counseling services for inpatients in a spinal cord injury program:

> System level: rehabilitation medicine department
> Program type: inpatient spinal cord injury
> Process segment: predischarge
> Scope of service: vocational evaluation and counseling services

In order to accurately understand the meaning of consumer satisfaction experiences, the full service spectrum to which they apply should be precisely defined.

Definitional Research

This section reviews research conducted in medical, mental health, and rehabilitation on the empirically derived structure of consumer satisfaction.

Global Satisfaction

Some studies have identified a general unidimensional, bipolar (satisfied to dissatisfied) factor presumed to represent overall satisfaction with services. Examples of instruments available to measure this factor in rehabilitation include the Client Satisfaction Questionnaire (CSQ),[22] the Scale of Client Satisfaction,[23] and the Vocational Evaluation Satisfaction Scale (VESS).[24] Most of these instruments measure satisfaction indirectly through assessing judgments or opinions regarding such factors as whether needs or expectations have been met, or by assessing factual information. Although such instruments do seem to measure a useful global reaction construct that shows unidimensional factor structure, high measured internal consistency of items, and moderate correlations with other similarly developed instruments, evidence that they truly measure the *satisfaction* construct does not seem clear.

The Two-Factor Approach

Some research suggests that instead of experiencing global reactions along a bipolar unidimensional continuum from satisfaction to dissatisfaction, people experience reactions to some stimuli along a high to low (or neutral) *positive attitude* (or satisfaction) dimension and others along a high to low (or neutral) *negative attitude* (or dissatisfaction) dimension.[16,25–28] For example, Cryns and colleagues identified

two second-order factors, positive and negative attitude, which in their study accounted for about half of the common variance of geriatric HMO patients' attitudes toward health care.[25] In effect, low ratings on positive attitude items, such as amount of care received at the HMO compared to other plans and quality of care on short notice, were related to *lack* of positive attitude, such as apathy or disengagement, rather than to negative attitude. Positive ratings on those items were associated with satisfaction. On the other hand, low ratings on negative attitude items such as worries about getting the right kind of care when needed or being put on hold by the switchboard before they know what you want, were associated with dissatisfaction. However, high ratings on those items were not particularly associated with positive attitude.

Although the two-factor approach to global satisfaction is logically appealing, most of its support comes from research on mood and subjective well-being; and from unsubstantiated job satisfaction theory. Support in the former area is strong; however, consumer satisfaction appears to be a different construct, which is not so much a personality trait as an affect in response to external stimuli. The limited findings thus far supporting a two-factor approach could be due to anomalies in questionnaire design.

Consumer Satisfaction as a Multidimensional Construct

Numerous researchers have examined satisfaction as a multidimensional phenomenon. For example, in medical care, a literature review by Ware, Snyder, Wright, and Davies,[29] and meta analysis by Hall and Dornan[30] resulted in identifying a variety of patient satisfaction dimensions. Several notable individual factor analysis studies have also been done in medical, mental health, and rehabilitation settings that help clarify the multidimensional nature of consumer satisfaction.[25,27,29,31–33] Unfortunately there is limited agreement on dimensions identified across studies, perhaps owing to differences in measurement strategies, instrumentation, and data analysis, as well as setting-specific differences. A potentially significant contributing factor may also relate to whether professional "expert" or consumer input defines inventory items from which satisfaction domains are empirically derived. Although early research tended to depend mainly on input from professionals, recent studies[25,27,29] seem more likely to use focus group or other direct consumer feedback. The latter approach appears to support better validity of the dimensions identified.

Summarizing from the studies, the following dimensions seem most frequently identified:

1. Patient/staff relationships[25,27,29–32]
2. Quality of care[25,29–31,33]
3. Technical competence/skill of practitioner[25,27,29,30,31,33]
4. Access to care and services[25,29–32]

Less frequently noted are:

5. Continuity of service by same provider[25,29]
6. Financial factors[25,29,30]
7. Physical environment and facilities[27,29,30]

Relationships Among Global and Specific Dimensions

Some studies suggest a hierarchical relationship among general and specific satisfaction dimensions. For example, Cryns and colleagues found 14 primary factors, two second-order general factors, and a third-order general factor.[25] In regression analysis, Miller found that specific factors identified accounted for a substantial portion of overall satisfaction variance ($R^2 = 0.56$).[32] Greenfield and Attkisson also found the factors they identified to consistently show high loadings on their general satisfaction marker.[31]

Global Satisfaction and Service Experiences

From a more fundamental perspective, the level of specific service experiences reported by consumers can explain global satisfaction responses. The association between these experiences and satisfaction responses provides a basis for empirically identifying and then measuring modifiable service factors of importance to consumers in each unique setting or program. For example, if perceived timeliness of intake interviews and perceived amount of courtesy shown to clients by support staff independently account for substantial portions of overall satisfaction variance, measuring consumer experiences in those areas can help determine strategies for satisfaction improvement. This approach has been used to measure consumer satisfaction in business and industry,[34] and in hospitals,[35] as well as to explain satisfaction variance among vocational rehabilitation consumers. For example, a Texas Rehabilitation Commission study[36] found consumer experiences in five specific vocational rehabilita-tion service delivery areas to explain about 38 percent of the variance in overall satisfaction.

Conclusions

Several important conclusions emerge from the available data.

First, consumer satisfaction appears to be an affect that is both a response (dependent variable) to service experiences and a stimulus (independent variable) for consequential (future) action. On the basis of what is known, a broad "chain of events" model proposing the point at which a satisfaction response is experienced is shown in Figure 1. The affective response follows the service experience and may change with additional service experiences. Each service experience consists of cognitively processed information derived from service encounters that take place within the service spectrum. Service encounters consist of an interface between consumers and the service environment, resulting in service attributes and events. Cognitive processing involves perception and evaluation (interpretation) of the service attributes and events, as well as the context in which they occur. Although not shown in Figure 1, satisfaction responses also seem likely to be influenced by prior experience and other predispositional factors, as well as by new information, all of which may influence cognitive processing. At present, the full nature of causes and effects, their mechanisms, and their relationship to satisfaction are unclear. Also, although the model is depicted as linear to illustrate a proposed typical sequence of events, in reality the development of satisfaction responses over time may be less predictable. For example, a satisfied consumer who receives outside information that he or she is paying too much for services may suddenly become a dissatisfied consumer (after new cognitive processing) without having any further service encounters.

Second, consumer satisfaction is likely to contain a unidimensional, bipolar (satisfied to dissatisfied) global dimension

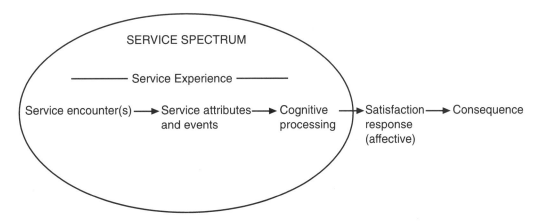

Figure 1. Chain of events model for consumer satisfaction.

that is potentially inclusive of common variance from separate positive and negative bipolar global dimensions. Specific satisfaction dimensions can also be identified that share some common variance with the global dimension (e.g., quality of care, timeliness of services). Multiple dimensions are likely to generalize less across settings as specificity of the service spectrum and dimensions assessed increases. For example, studies on satisfaction with the overall mental health service system might identify a global and several broad categories. However, studies on satisfaction with mental health services provided through HMOs, and further, those provided by a specific HMO might show somewhat different patterns of multidimensional categories.

Third, domain content of satisfaction dimensions to be assessed should represent areas of service experience important to consumers *as defined by consumers.* This approach supports content valid measurement and user involvement in service delivery planning.[37-41] An exception would be domain content for the most global aspect of service, such as "In an overall sense, how satisfied were you with the services provided?" Such content could reasonably be defined by service providers or evaluators. Alternately, global content could also be defined by items representing the full range of important consumer-defined service experiences.

Fourth, consistent with the model in Figure 1, levels of consumer satisfaction may be explained in terms of the degree to which specific service experiences that are defined as important by consumers are perceived as present (or absent) during the total service experience.

Finally, the more precisely the relevant service spectrum can be defined and differentiated, the more valuable satisfaction information is likely to be. For example, in rehabilitation, the medical and vocational rehabilitation service processes are substantially different. Even different phases of these services are substantially different in context, content, process, and outcome. From a definitional perspective, differentiation clarifies the field of experience to which satisfaction and its explainers refer. From a psychometric point of view, precise definition should minimize measurement error.

Table 1 integrates the above conclusions for use in operationally defining satisfaction for assessment purposes. Using this table, one would first define the pertinent service spectrum. The dimensions of interest and their domains, domain content, and source of domain content then form the basis for defining and assessing satisfaction for the desired purposes.

A Definition of Consumer Satisfaction

Based on the theory, research, and consequent conclusions, we can now define consumer satisfaction as *a level of pleasantness, well-being or gratification felt in reaction to a total specified service experience or to its important components.* This definition limits satisfaction to the affectual portion of the "chain" in Figure 1. "Specified" refers to the relevant service spectrum defined by the assessor. "Important components" refer to any single or category (dimension) of service experiences within the total specified service experience that are salient to the consumer.

WHAT ARE THE PERTINENT MEASUREMENT ISSUES?

This section discusses special measurement issues pertinent to the selection and design of satisfaction surveys.

Table 1. Parameters for Operationally Defining Consumer Satisfaction for Assessment Purposes

Service Spectrum	Dimensions	Domain	Domain Content	Source of Domain Content
System level	Global (unidimensional)	Single area representing total service experience within service spectrum	Highly global items; or Sampling of items representing full range of salient service experiences within the service spectrum	Evaluator Consumer input from service experience
Program type				
Process segment				
Scope of service	Global (2-factor)	Two broad areas representing total service experience within service spectrum	Undefined at current stage of research	Consumer input from service experience
	Multidimensional	Multiple areas representing most important dimensions of total service experience within service spectrum	Salient service experiences	Consumer input from service experience

Objective Scale Design Issues

Satisfaction questionnaires usually consist of objective items, opportunities for subjective responses, or both. Objective measurement scaling can be described in terms of stimulus-centered, subject-centered response,[42-44] and external criterion methods.[43] In stimulus-centered scaling, systematic response variation (by respondents) is attributed to differences among referent stimuli, such as effectiveness of different world leaders, stressfulness of work events, or satisfactoriness of services rendered. Subject-centered scaling attributes variation in responses (to stimuli) to differences among respondents, such as in abilities or attitudes. Response scaling addresses both stimulus and people variation. Finally, external criterion methods measure the relationship of subject variation (in response to stimuli), to variation of the same subjects on a criterion, in an attempt to maximize prediction. As described earlier, this approach has been used in associating overall satisfaction with contributing service experiences.

The above methods involve different assumptions that may influence the choice of scaling approaches. For example, for stimulus scaling, Dawis suggests the Thurstone method, Q sort, and rank order approaches.[43] For subject centered scales, *rating* approaches such as Likert scale procedures and the semantic differential are recommended. Nunnally, on the other hand, suggests the Q sort, semantic differential, and a variety of other rating scales as appropriate in both subject and stimulus scaling.[44] However, when using rating scales for stimulus-centered situations, he suggests the major assumption "that individual differences are not important in judgments or preferences in relation to the particular set of stimuli" must be met. In effect, subjects must be considered "replicates of one another." For external criterion scaling, rating scale methods appear to be appropriate.[43]

In *satisfaction evaluation,* it is often assumed that variation in consumer responses is due to differences in stimuli. For example, administrators use average satisfaction ratings of services (stimuli) for decisions regarding service changes that will improve satisfactoriness (e.g., training to improve telephone skills of support staff). Using this rationale, stimulus-centered scaling methods would seem most appropriate. However, approaches such as the Thurstone method, Q sort, or rank order methods are rarely used in measuring satisfaction. In one reported attempt, Pascoe and Attkisson developed the Evaluation Ranking Scale for assessing patient satisfaction.[45] Although it appears to be an effective evaluation technique, it requires special training to administer and score, and individual (rather than paper and pencil) administration. Thus, costs of administrative overhead may make its use impractical.

If satisfaction variation is viewed more as a function of consumer interpretations than of true stimulus differences (although then would service providers be expected to change satisfaction by changing consumer interpretations, rather than services?), or if justification for meeting Nunnally's assumption can be demonstrated, then subject-centered methods would be considered appropriate. In reality, subject-centered methods tend to be almost exclusively used (e.g., rating scales) in satisfaction measurement, probably because of familiarity and ease of scale construction, rather than due to theoretical considerations.

Actually, a case could potentially be made for the importance of both stimulus and subject variation in satisfaction measurement. Under those circumstances, response-centered methods would be most appropriate. However, their complexity and unfamiliarity due to limited use in applied situations is likely to inhibit development in the near future. Recognizing that theoretical scale choice issues will not be resolved in this article, the remainder of this section will focus on the more common rating scale approach.

Types of Rating Scales

A wide variety of rating scales and their variations are described well by several authors.[35,44,46,47] These scales usually consist of a statement ("Overall, I was satisfied with the services received") followed by categories of equal appearing intervals on which to respond (e.g., Fully Agree, Mostly Agree, Slightly Agree, Slightly Disagree, Mostly Disagree, Fully Disagree; or Fully Disagree 1 2 3 4 5 Fully Agree). *Summated rating* scales, which sum the rating scores on a number of items (to give a single total score) on a unidimensional factor such as global satisfaction, or on each of several multidimensional factors, may be used. Sometimes multiple scales, each consisting of a single item and constructed with attention to producing highly reliable responses, may be used, particularly as predictor or explanatory variables in external criterion methods.

Positive Response Tendencies

Scores on objective satisfaction scales are usually influenced by positive response tendencies. Resulting high satisfaction levels, lack of score variability, and restriction of score range have led researchers to question the validity and usefulness of such measures.[6,19,20,30,37-39,45,49-54] These researchers suggest that spuriously high scores may result from scale characteristics such as lack of sensitivity, lack of discrimination ability, or ceiling effects; or consumer response patterns such as failure of dissatisfied consumers to respond, acquiescent response sets, and the desire to present oneself in a socially desirable manner.

Several researchers have explored the effects of specific questionnaire and scale design characteristics on positive response tendencies. For example, Schul and Schiff found that if general satisfaction is probed first, it reflects negative information more than if it is assessed last.[55] Sabourin and

Leichner[53] and Peterson and Wilson[52] determined that items worded toward satisfaction (such as "how satisfied are you with . . .") seem to result in positive answers, while items worded toward dissatisfaction seem to result in negative answers. However, this was not corroborated on an objective measure used in a study by Perrault and colleagues.[27] Such conflicting findings may suggest value in using neutrally worded questions that allow for *affective* response choices.

With respect to graphic scale design, Devlin, Dong, and Brown noted that failure to include a midpoint or neutral category forces a (usually positive) choice and that two-point scales result in more positive bias than four-point scales.[46] They also found that placing negative categories to the left helps cancel the tendency to respond positively. Westbrook (1980) found that the D-T scale, which uses extreme anchors of delighted and terrible, reduced the problem of high reported levels of satisfaction resulting from lack of instrument sensitivity. The ranking method, as used in the Evaluation Ranking Scale,[45] was found to reduce positive response problems, also supporting the theoretical value of ranking methods for stimulus scaling.

Response Set Bias

This refers to the tendency of subjects to respond in a particular manner without regard to what scales are attempting to measure. While positive response tendencies can be due to a bias toward acquiescence, other response sets include the tendency to select only extreme or neutral responses, or to respond to subsequent items on a survey using the same category (e.g., moderately satisfied) that one used on prior items, or to use the response on a prior item as a basis for responding to a subsequent item.[35,47]

As with positive response tendencies, other types of response set bias can be controlled to some extent through scale or instrument construction. For example, Stratmann and colleagues suggest that tendencies to use the same categories of response and to respond to subsequent items based on responses to prior items increase as the number of points in a scale increases.[35] As a remedy, they suggest using the smallest number of response categories (two). However, based on an extensive theoretical literature review, Cox suggests that two or three response categories cannot transmit enough information, and result in frustration and stifling of respondents.[42] He recommends using no more than nine response categories, with five to nine being optimal. Other simple possibilities for reducing response set bias include using different levels of scaling for different items (e.g., two-point, five-point, seven-point), keeping surveys short, and avoiding the same type of scale for too many consecutive questions.

Rating Scale Reliability

When constructing rating scales, both the number of items measuring an attitude (satisfaction in this case) and the number of steps in item scales appear to affect reliability. According to Nunnally, reliability increases as the number of scale steps increase, up to 20.[44] However, there is a leveling effect at about seven steps, with little additional gain after 11 steps. He suggests that when only one item is used to measure attitudes, it is wise to have at least ten scale steps. When scores are summed over a number of items, however, the number of scale steps becomes less important. Cronbach, on the other hand, warns that increasing the number of response alternatives simply to increase reliability could decrease validity due to the emergence of response set bias.[56]

Scale Discrimination Power

It is important for satisfaction rating scales to be able to discriminate effectively among different levels of the characteristics measured (e.g., satisfactoriness of services, extent to which service experiences occurred). Poorer discrimination results in loss of information and understated or erroneous data analysis and evaluation. For example, Cohen shows that dichotomization of variables results in substantial loss of statistical power and explanation of variance.[57] Based on Cohen's research, Devlin, Dong and Brown suggest using at least three scale points.[46]

Multicollinearity

In external criterion methods, multicollinearity, that is, high correlations among referent independent variables, reduces the probability of identifying valid explainers of criterion variance. It also inhibits the ability to reliably identify comparative importance of explainers of the criterion.

Stratmann and colleagues suggest reducing multicollinearity through question design.[35] Specifically, they recommend using events or problems as the independent variables, designing items to be independent of one another based on selection from the full range of events and problems related to the criterion (overall satisfaction) as identified in focus groups, and using two-point scales to reduce response set bias and halo effect.

Selecting the Best Scale Design for Objective Measures

If one views satisfaction measurement strictly from a stimulus-centered perspective, a ranking or other non–rating scale method is probably the best scale design for objective measures. If a rating scale approach can be justified, then alternatives exist on the basis of the importance of issues considered above. To further help with such decisions, Devlin, Dong, and Brown considered 10 possible formats in identifying the best alternatives based on minimal response bias, respondent interpretation and understanding, discriminating power, ease of administration, ease of use by respondents, and credibility and usefulness of results.[46] Their best recommendations are a 5-point scale that can be used to measure *expectations* (1 = much better, 2 = better, 3 = just as, 4 = worse, 5 = much worse); and a 4-point scale that can be used to measure *requirements* (1 = exceeded, 2 = met, 3 = nearly met, 4 = missed). They note that these scales consistently result in high reliabilities (coefficient alphas of .80–.90) and high validities (Multiple R of .60–.80) with effective performance on the factors they identified. The expectations and requirement scales might best be used to measure satisfaction indirectly within the cognitive processing phase of the chain of events model of consumer satisfaction (see Figure 1 and section on Global Satisfaction above).

For directly measuring satisfaction, the D-T Scale (1 = Terrible, 2 = Unhappy, 3 = Mostly dissatisfied, 4 = Mixed [about equally satisfied and dissatisfied], 5 = Mostly satisfied, 6 = Pleased, 7 = Delighted) appears to show reasonable retest reliability, validity, and less negative skewing than other scales.[58] Also, Devlin, Dong and Brown describe two satisfaction scales that manage positive response bias well, but which are limited in discriminating high end performance (1 = very satisfied, 2 = satisfied, 3 = somewhat satisfied, 4 = dissatisfied, 5 = very dissatisfied; and 1 = very satisfied, 2 = satisfied, 3 = neither, 4 = dissatisfied, 5 = very dissatisfied).

For measuring the extent to which service experiences (see Figure 1) were perceived to occur, the Stratmann et al. model of two response categories (no–yes),[35] specifically recommended for this purpose, is a possibility. However, scales with more response categories (e.g., 5–9) may show more desirable psychometric properties.

Subjective Response Alternatives

Open-ended response choices allow respondents to provide information that might not be assessed or that might be inhibited in objective formats. This may be helpful in obtaining more in-depth information, in combating positive response tendencies, and in further interpreting objective results. However, use and interpretation of such qualitative information is fraught with hazards. For example, there are no standardized protocols to classify and analyze the information. Also, when open-ended questions are added to objective inventories, response rate to subjective items may be low (e.g., 20 percent) and some respondents may provide more information than others (similar to a group with a few very verbal members). How does one decide what is important and what is a function of the services measured rather than personal issues of a few respondents? In addition, when response rates are low, comments may be biased. For instance, perhaps only dissatisfied (or satisfied) consumers are responding. Other issues are the types of questions to ask, whether to ask for written responses or to do interviews (a costly alternative), and when asking for written responses on an objective survey, where to place the open-ended questions to encourage responses and avoid biases.

Limited research has been conducted on the use of qualitative consumer satisfaction assessment. Several studies exploring its value in overcoming positive response tendencies have been equivocal, although some new knowledge has emerged. For example, in a review of research about attitudes towards mental health hospitalization, Weinstein found that qualitative studies characterized patient attitudes in negative (dissatisfaction) terms.[59] In a study that compared qualitative and quantitative approaches, Greenley and colleagues found that respondents answered closed and open-ended questions with similar levels of (high) satisfaction.[60]

Polowczyk and colleagues in a study of patient satisfaction with health care services, found that patient satisfaction interviews by other patients may have allowed more openness or truthfulness, reducing acquiescent response set.[61] Perrault and colleagues also used a trained interviewer procedure to compare satisfaction results against those found using standard general satisfaction scales with psychiatric outpatients.[27] They found that open-ended questions phrased in positive or neutral terms ("service aspects for which you are satisfied," "how is the clinic functioning") resulted in as much as or more negative skewing (positive responses) than on objective scales. However, when questions were phrased negatively ("service aspects for which you are not satisfied," "what would you like to change"), a majority of patients responded with negative comments. They concluded that, with qualitative measures, how questions are focused seems to influence the types of answers provided. However, based on the results of Polowczyk and colleagues and Perrault and colleagues, it is difficult to determine whether nonthreatening personal interviews or the nature of the questions are most significant.

At this point, it can be concluded that qualitative information should be collected and used with caution. While interview techniques are costly for routine assessment, they can (along with focus groups) be used on a periodic basis to obtain in-depth information. On a routine basis, it may be worthwhile to include open-ended items that focus separately on positive and negative factors, in objective surveys, while making certain that administration is perceived by consumers as occurring in a nonthreatening context. Where to place such questions may also be relevant, since some respondents may have a tendency to avoid taking time to write out responses at the end of an inventory unless they have very strong feelings to express. Recent Department of Veterans Affairs satisfaction research[62] suggests the value of including an opportunity for an open-ended response after each objective item and for more general comments at the end of the survey.

HOW CAN WE MEASURE AND EVALUATE SATISFACTION FOR REHABILITATION PURPOSES?

This section suggests how to use satisfaction theory and a sound assessment approach to identify or construct satisfaction survey instruments.

Measurement Alternatives

As can be inferred from the chain of events model in Figure 1, satisfaction responses can be measured directly from a dimensional perspective as global affect (overall satisfaction) or as multidimensional affects (satisfaction with important areas of service [defined by consumers] such as quality of services, financial aspects, and physical setting). Using an external criterion–based perspective, we can also identify and directly measure the extent to which service experiences viewed by consumers (and empirically verified) as important to satisfaction responses exist when services are received. This would provide a method to both measure satisfaction level and evaluate its meaning on the basis of contributing service variables.

Attempts can also be made to measure satisfaction indirectly, as has been done in survey instruments mentioned earlier. For example, questions about whether needs or expectations were met with respect to global service experiences (such as "To what extent has this program met your needs") may indirectly assess global satisfaction. In fact, indirect questions ranging from judgments about specific services received, to the condition of physical facilities (e.g., clean bathrooms), to consequences of satisfaction affect (e.g., "Based on your experiences would you refer a friend to this program?") have also been used on surveys to measure global satisfaction. On some surveys, both direct and indirect indicator questions are included. However, since surveys using indirect questions may not always target factors associated with satisfaction affect, and thus require more rigorous construct validation, this article will focus on suggestions for constructing direct measures of global and multidimensional satisfaction.

Selecting a Measurement Alternative Based on Purpose

Some purposes for measuring satisfaction require only a general satisfaction indicator. For example, for marketing uses, a reliable, global indicator may be sufficient to show that most program consumers are satisfied. On the other hand, many purposes for using satisfaction instruments necessitate assessing *what can be changed* to enhance consumer satisfaction. This requires measuring specific areas of satisfaction known to be important to consumers; or both overall satisfaction and the service experiences that contribute most to overall satisfaction variation (external criterion–based method).

Measuring Global and Multidimensional Satisfaction

Koch and Merz reviewed several standard instruments that measure global satisfaction and which may be appropriate for use in rehabilitation.[63] In particular, the eight-question version of the Client Satisfaction Questionnaire (CSQ-8) is general enough for most settings. Although it has tendencies toward indirectly measuring global satisfaction and encouraging positive response bias, its overall psychometric properties are acceptable and well researched.

Referring to Table 1, we suggest that construction of new global satisfaction instruments in rehabilitation contain either highly global items, or a sample of items representing the full range of service experiences perceived as important by consumers. Highly global items can be constructed by evaluators using five- to nine-point satisfaction scales to assess the broadest aspects of service (for example: "How satisfied are you with all of the services you received?" "What is your feeling about the quality of services provided?" "How satisfied are you with the way our staff treated you?"). After testing a larger item pool, reduction to a summated scale consisting of four or five items demonstrating high internal consistency reliability, plus content and construct validity, should result.

When sampling the range of service experiences, a summated scale can be constructed with item content based on focus group or other consumer input from the service spectrum of interest. Using five- to nine-point satisfaction scales, each item should measure level of satisfaction with a service experience identified as important. The range of items surveyed should represent the entire domain of important experiences; for example, "To what extent were you satisfied with the time it took to be seen by a counselor for the first time?" and "How do you feel about the distance you must travel to get to the rehabilitation office?" This type of inventory may require more items than the highly global scale described above, in order to cover the full satisfaction domain and to achieve high internal consistency reliability.

If a multidimensional scale is desired, a large sample of items representing the entire domain of satisfaction experiences may be administered to an appropriate sample of consumers and subjected to factor analysis in an attempt to identify independent reliable item groupings that represent multidimensional categories of satisfaction. Summated scales constructed from these item groupings may then be used with norms or repeated administrations over time to determine specific areas for intervention and change. At present, we are aware of no standard multidimensional surveys for rehabilitation.

External Criterion–Based Satisfaction Measurement

The external criterion–based procedure may have some advantages over multidimensional satisfaction measurement. For example, it allows for high specificity in identifying service characteristics that can be changed to improve satisfaction. Also, when developed using multiple regression techniques, it can provide information on perceived provider performance of the most important (empirically derived) consumer-experienced service factors with respect to overall satisfaction, as well as the comparative importance of those factors (to consumers). On the other hand, measures developed using this method may generalize less across settings than multidimensional satisfaction measures.

External criterion-based surveys can be developed using a broad prototype methodology as follows:

1. Define the applicable service spectrum.
2. Conduct focus groups to identify service experiences judged important by consumers (e.g., timely appointments, competent treatment modalities used by therapist, easy geographical access to facility).
3. Construct a pool of questions to reliably assess (a) degree to which important service experiences were present, and (b) level of overall satisfaction (several highly global items).
4. Administer the final questionnaire to a large sample of consumers.
5. Do statistical analysis (e.g., intercorrelation analysis, factor analysis, analysis of internal consistency, reliability of item groupings, multiple regression analysis) to identify the composite of single items and reliable item groupings (of service experiences), with low multicollinearity that account for the most overall satisfaction variance.
6. Develop revised (shortened) questionnaire to measure overall satisfaction and only those service experiences identified as most important in the statistical analysis.
7. Do retest reliability study, and replication study to validate original findings.

Criterion-based measures can be used for diagnostic purposes. For base rate information, the questionnaire should be administered to a large group of consumers. Scores can then be calculated for each scale (or item) representing service experiences, and for overall satisfaction. Subsequent group administrations may then be used to evaluate service experience scale and overall satisfaction scores against the base rate data. For example, if scores decline significantly on overall satisfaction, it would then be determined whether any service experience scales have declined as well. Service change strategies would then be considered for those specific areas.

When criterion-based measures are constructed and validated, partial regression coefficients can be also used to assess comparative importance of service experiences. For example, using the product of beta coefficients and problem frequency, Stratmann and colleagues describe an "impact index" that can prioritize problems for intervention on a scale of 0–100.[35]

Using Open-Ended Auestions

Objective inventories should usually include open-ended questions to clarify objective responses and counteract overly positive response tendencies. Suggestions for such questions include:

1. Add space for open-ended comments after each question.
   Example—Any comments?_____
2. Ask one positively and one negatively phrased open-ended question at the end of the survey. Examples: What aspects of service were you most satisfied with? What aspects of service were not satisfactory? What aspects of service would you change?

WHAT ADDITIONAL SATISFACTION RESEARCH IS NEEDED IN REHABILITATION?

Within health-related areas, additional research is needed to clarify both theoretical and measurement issues related to consumer satisfaction. This is even more the case in rehabilitation where such topics have received sparse attention.

As begun in this article, continued development and testing of a comprehensive model of consumer satisfaction is needed as a basis for understanding satisfaction as both an effect of experiences and a cause of future action. The cognitive processing that takes place in formulating satisfaction responses particularly needs better empirically based explanation. Empirical information is also needed to explain the impact of consumer satisfaction on rehabilitation outcomes and how satisfaction affects the rehabilitation process. For example, are satisfied clients more likely to complete programs and achieve better functional capacity, satisfactory employment, greater independence, more autonomy, or a better quality of life?

Satisfaction constructs also need better definition and clarification. For example, can important multidimensional satisfaction factors that generalize across rehabilitation settings be identified? To what extent can the more specific external criterion approach to measurement identify generalizable factors that account for enough overall satisfaction variance across rehabilitation settings to be useful for change purposes? Also, clarification is needed regarding whether global satisfaction is a unidimensional factor, a two-factor construct, or some combination.

Studies continue to be needed in satisfaction measurement. The potentials of stimulus and response scaling methods should be explored and evaluated to determine whether they offer better results than subject-centered approaches. If they do, practical measurement methods that fit such models need to be developed. With respect to rating scales, more research is needed to identify scale characteristics that consistently counteract positive response tendencies and other response bias, while demonstrating reliable measurement. Studies to better identify how to structure and use open-ended questions to get the most valid information and to minimize bias are also needed.

• • •

Focus on satisfaction in rehabilitation is important in order to improve services, for accountability, and to make initiating and completing services more attractive to consumers. Satisfaction can be viewed as an affective unidimensional (global) response or as multidimensional affective responses to service experiences; and as a stimulus (or stimuli) for consequential actions. Although global or multidimensional consumer satisfaction may be measured directly or indirectly, the external criterion-based approach offers advantages in terms of diagnosing and impacting on specific service characteristics that account for overall satisfaction. Further research is needed to more fully clarify satisfaction theory, its practical correlates for rehabilitation, and valid measurement approaches.

REFERENCES

1. Deming, W.E. *Out of the Crisis.* Cambridge, MA: Institute of Technology for Advanced Engineering Study, 1986.
2. Lubeck, R.C., and Davis, P.K. "W.E. Deming's 14 Points for Quality: Can They Be Applied to Rehabilitation?" *Journal of Rehabilitation Administration* 15, no. 4 (1991): 216–21.
3. Nelson, E.C., et al. "The Patient Judgment System: Reliability and Validity." *Quality Review Bulletin* 15 (1989): 185–91.
4. Pekarik, G., and Wolff, C.B. "Relationship of Satisfaction to Symptom Change, Follow-up Adjustment, and Clinical Significance." *Professional Psychology: Research and Practice* 27, no. 2 (1996): 202–208.
5. Hulka, B.S., and Zyzanski, S.G. "Validation of a Patient Satisfaction Scale: Theory, Methods, and Practice." *Medical Care* 20, no. 6 (1982): 649–53.
6. Ware, J.E. Jr., and Davies, A. "Behavioral Consequences of Consumer Dissatisfaction with Medical Care." *Evaluation and Program Planning* 6 (1983): 291–97.
7. Americans with Disabilities Act of 1990, 42 U.S.C. 12101 (1992).
8. The Rehabilitation Accreditation Commission. *Standards Manual and Interpretive Guidelines for Employment and Community Support Services.* Tucson, AZ: CARF, 1997.
9. Rehabilitation Act of 1973, 29 U.S.C. 701 (1993).
10. Zastowney, T.R., Roghmann, K.J., and Cafferata, G.L. "Patient Satisfaction and the Use of Health Services." *Medical Care* 27, no. 7 (1989): 705–23.
11. Jones, T.O., and Sasser, W.E. "Why Satisfied Customers Defect." *Harvard Business Review* (Nov.–Dec. 1995): 88–99.
12. Gore, A. *Creating a Government that Works Better and Costs Less: Report of the National Performance Review.* Washington, DC: Government Printing Office, 1993.
13. Chaplin, J.P. *Dictionary of Psychology.* New York: Dell, 1985.
14. Lawler, L.L. *Motivation in Work Organizations.* San Francisco, CA: Jossey-Bass, 1994, pp. 78–112.
15. Weirs, H.M. "Learning Theory in Industrial and Organizational Psychology." In *Handbook of Industrial and Organizational Psychology,* vol. 1, ed. M.D. Dunnette and L.M. Hough. 2nd edition. Palo Alto, CA: Consulting Psychologists Press, Inc., 1990.
16. Diener, E. "Subjective Well-Being." *Psychological Bulletin* 95, no. 3 (1984): 542–75.
17. Linder-Pelz, S. "Toward a Theory of Patient Satisfaction." *Social Science in Medicine* 16 (1982a): 577–82.
18. Linder-Pelz, S. "Social Psychological Determinants of Patient Satisfaction: A Test of Five Hypotheses." *Social Science in Medicine* 16 (1982b): 583–89.
19. Pascoe, G.C. "Patient Satisfaction in Primary Health Care: A Literature Review and Analysis." *Evaluation and Program Planning* 6 (1983): 185–210.
20. Fitzpatrick, R., and Hopkins, A. "Problems in the Conceptual Framework of Patient Satisfaction Research: An Empirical Exploration." *Sociology of Health and Illness* 5, no. 3 (1983): 297–311.
21. Segall, A., and Burnett, M. "Patient Evaluation of Physician Role Performance." *Social Science and Medicine* 14 (1980): 269–78.
22. Larsen, D.L., et al. "Assessment of Client/Patient Satisfaction: Development of a General Scale." *Evaluation and Program Planning* 2 (1979): 197–207.
23. Wright, G.N., Reagles, K.W., and Butler, A.J. "An Expanded Program of Vocational Rehabilitation: Methodology and Description of Client Populations." *Wisconsin Studies in Vocational Rehabilitation.* Series 2, Monograph XI. Madison, WI: University of Wisconsin Regional Rehabilitation Research Institute, 1970.
24. Sabin, M.C., Cuvo, A.J., and Musgrave, J.R. "Developing a Client Satisfaction Scale in a Vocational Evaluation Setting." *Vocational Evaluation and Work Adjustment Bulletin* 30, no. 4 (1987): 107–13.
25. Cryns, A.B., et al. "The Hierarchical Structure of Geriatric Patient Satisfaction: An Older Patient Satisfaction Scale Designed for HMOs." *Medical Care* 27, no. 8 (1989): 802–16.
26. Herzberg, F., Mausner, B., and Snyderman, B. *The Motivation to Work.* New York: Wiley, 1959.
27. Perrault, M., et al. "Patient Satisfaction with Outpatient Psychiatric Services." *Evaluation and Program Planning* 16 (1993): 108–18.
28. Watson, D., and Tellegen, A. "Toward a Consensual Structure of Mood." *Psychological Bulletin* 90, no. 2 (1985): 219–35.
29. Ware, J.E., et al. "Defining and Measuring Patient Satisfaction with Medical Care." *Evaluation and Program Planning* 6 (1983): 247–63.
30. Hall, J.A., and Dornan, M.C. "Meta-analysis of Satisfaction with Medical Care: Description of Overall Satisfaction Levels." *Social Science in Medicine* 27, no. 6 (1988): 637–44.
31. Greenfield, T.K., and Attkisson, C.C. "Steps Toward a Multifactorial Satisfaction Scale for Primary Care and Mental Health Services." *Evaluation and Program Planning* 12 (1989): 271–78.
32. Miller, R.R., Jr. "Dimensions of Service Satisfaction with Clinic Visits in a Group Practice HMO: The Service Cycle Model." *Evaluation and Program Planning* 15 (1992): 395–401.
33. Winter, P.L., and Keith, R.A. "A Model of Outpatient Satisfaction in Rehabilitation." *Rehabilitation Psychology* 33, no. 3 (1988): 131–42.
34. Collins, C. "Profiles: Five Minutes with J.D. Power III." *The Magazine of Continental Airlines* (October 1996): 22–4, 26.
35. Stratmann, W.C., et al. "Patient Satisfaction Surveys and Multicollinearity." *Quality Management in Health Care* 2, no. 2 (1994): 1–12.
36. Schwab, A.J., Smith, T.W., and DiNitto, D. "Client Satisfaction and Quality Vocational Rehabilitation." *Journal of Rehabilitation* (Oct./Nov./Dec. 1993): 17–23.
37. Avis, M., Bond, M., and Arthur, A. "Satisfying Solutions? A Review of Some Unresolved Issues in the Measurement of Patient Satisfaction." *Journal of Advanced Nursing* 22 (1995): 316–22.

38. Clark, C., Scott, E., and Krupa, T. "Involving Clients in Programme Evaluation and Research: A New Methodology for Occupational Therapy." *Canadian Journal of Occupational Therapy* 60, no. 4 (1993): 192–99.

39. Elbeck, M., and Fecteau, G. "Improving the Validity of Measures of Patient Satisfaction with Psychiatric Care and Treatment." *Hospital and Community Psychiatry* 41, no. 9 (1990): 998–1001.

40. Nelson, C.W. "Patient Satisfaction Surveys: An Opportunity for Total Quality Improvement." *Hospital and Health Services Administration* 35, no. 3 (1990): 409–27.

41. Lebow, J.L. "Research Assessing Consumer Satisfaction with Mental Health Treatment: A Review of Findings." *Evaluation and Program Planning* 6 (1983): 211–36.

42. Cox, E.P. III. "The Optimal Number of Response Alternatives for a Scale: A Review." *Journal of Marketing Research* 17 (1980): 407–22.

43. Dawis, R.V. "Scale Construction." *Journal of Counseling Psychology* 34, no. 4 (1987): 481–89.

44. Nunnally, J. *Psychometric Theory.* New York: McGraw-Hill, 1978.

45. Pascoe, G.C., and Attkisson, C.C. "The Evaluation Ranking Scale: A New Methodology for Assessing Satisfaction." *Evaluation and Program Planning* 6 (1983): 185–210.

46. Devlin, S.J., Dong, H.K., and Brown, M. "Selecting a Scale for Measuring Quality." *Marketing Research* 5, no. 3 (1993): 12–17.

47. Kerlinger, F.N. *Foundations of Behavioral Research.* 2nd ed. New York: Holt, Rinehart and Winston, Inc., 1973.

48. Berger, M. "Toward Maximizing the Utility of Consumer Satisfaction as an Outcome." In *The Assessment of Psychotherapy Outcome,* ed. M.J. Lambert, E.R. Christensen, and S.S. Dejuliio. New York: Wiley, 1983, pp. 56–80.

49. Bornstein, P.H., and Bychtarik, R.G. "Consumer Satisfaction in Adult Behavior Therapy: Procedures, Problems, and Future Perspectives." *Behavior Therapy* 14 (1983): 191–208.

50. Essex, D.W., Fox, J.A., and Groom, J.M. "The Development, Factor Analysis, and Revision of a Client Satisfaction Form." *Community Mental Health Journal* 17, no. 3 (1981): 226–35.

51. Holcomb, W.R., et al. "The Development and Construct Validation of a Consumer Satisfaction Questionnaire for Psychiatric Inpatients." *Evaluation and Program Planning* 12 (1989): 189–94.

52. Peterson, R.A., and Wilson, W.R. "Measuring Customer Satisfaction: Fact and Artifact." *Journal of the Academy of Marketing Science* 20 (1992): 61–71.

53. Sabourin, S., and Leichner, P. "Patient Satisfaction with Outpatient Psychiatric Services: Qualitative and Quantitative Assessments." *Evaluation and Program Planning* 16 (1993): 109–18.

54. Tanner, B.A., and Webb, S. Jr. "A Validity Scale for the SHARP Consumer Satisfaction Scales." *Evaluation and Program Planning* 8 (1985): 147–53.

55. Schul, Y., and Schiff, M. "Measuring Satisfaction with Organizations: Predictions from Information Accessibility." *Public Opinion Quarterly* 57 (1993): 536–51.

56. Cronbach, L.J. "Further Evidence on Response Sets and Test Design." *Educational and Psychological Measurement* 10 (Spring 1950): 3–31.

57. Cohen, J. "The Cost of Dichotomization." *Applied Psychological Measurement* 7, no. 3 (1983): 249–53.

58. Westbrook, R.A. "A Rating Scale for Measuring Product/Service Satisfaction." *Journal of Marketing* 44 (1980): 68–72.

59. Weinstein, R.M. "Patient Attitudes Toward Mental Hospitalization: A Review of Quantitative Research." *Journal of Health and Social Behavior* 20 (1979): 237–58.

60. Greenley, J.R., et al. "Patient Satisfaction with Psychiatric Inpatient Care: Issues in Measurement and Application." *Research in Community and Mental Health* 5 (1985): 303–19.

61. Polowczyk, D., et al. "Comparison of Patient and Staff Surveys of Consumer Satisfaction." *Hospital and Community Psychiatry* 44, no. 6 (1993): 589–91.

62. Simon, S.E. Unpublished raw data on development of vocational rehabilitation surveys, 1997.

63. Koch, L.C., and Merz, M.A. "Assessing Client Satisfaction in Vocational Rehabilitation Program Evaluation: A Review of Instrumentation." *Journal of Rehabilitation* 61, no. 4 (1995): 24–30.

PART III

Orthopedic Rehabilitation Outcomes

17

The Reliability and Validity of the Orthopedic Rehabilitation Outcome Scale

Dennis L. Hart, Craig A. Velozo, Jin-Shei Lai, and Edward A. Dobrzykowski

THE PROBLEM OF OUTCOME SCALES

The measurement of effectiveness outcomes in health care can be difficult. There are literally hundreds of ways to measure outcomes from a variety of perspectives, many of which have merit and have demonstrated predictive power.[1–9] Broadly speaking, outcomes can include patient morbidity, mortality, health status, and satisfaction.[10] A comprehensive outcomes measurement system designed today typically includes patient-reported measures, clinician-reported measures, and pertinent demographic (population-specific) indicators.

In orthopedic rehabilitation, there are patient-reported outcome scales that have varying degrees of validity, reliability, and sensitivity to change. Examples of these scales include the Oswestry Low Back Pain Questionnaire,[11] the Neck Disability Index,[12] the Lysholm scale,[13] and the Shoulder Pain and Disability Index.[14] All of these scales are "disease" specific; that is, they were developed to be responsive to change in patients' perceptions of their functional abilities in spite of their low back, neck, knee, and shoulder syndromes, respectively. Although these scales are sensitive to changes in patients' perception of their functional abilities, the challenge in orthopedic rehabilitation is to develop a generic, non–disease-specific outcome scale that uses a consistent methodology and is reliable and valid across the common patient groups seen in acute orthopedic clinics regardless of pathology. Without a generic scale, orthopedic outcomes measurements would require a different disease-specific scale for each diagnostic group, which presents numerous logistical and operational problems.

Because outpatient orthopedic rehabilitation spans a considerable variety of conditions, the typical method for therapist documentation of patient progress is the measure of physical impairment rather than the functionally based measures. Functional measures are now preferred by insurance companies.[15] Clinicians such as physical therapists and occupational therapists have been trained to use such impairment measures as strength, range of motion, endurance, gait, sensation, edema, posture, and so on to document at initial evaluation and demonstrate change throughout treatment. However, these "traditional" impairment measures, which are well known to clinicians, do not adequately quantify the patient's progress toward functional treatment goals, and there may not be a direct relationship between a positive improvement in a measure of physical impairment and a concomitant improvement in function.

DESCRIPTION OF A SCALE

A generic orthopedic outcome scale was developed by National Rehabilitation Centers in Brentwood, Tennessee, in the late 1980s in response to the request for standardized outcomes scales from the insurance companies. The standardized scale accommodated computerized clinical documentation and was used to support the corporate therapists. Over the years, the scale evolved, but needed scientific testing for reliability and validity. National Rehabilitation Centers (presently the Rehability Corporation, Brentwood, Tennessee) contracted with Formations in Health Care, Inc. (presently Medirisk Inc., Chicago, Illinois) to perform the field testing of the reliability and validity of this measurement tool. The purpose of this article is to describe the reliability and validity testing of the orthopedic rehabilitation outcome scale for acute rehabilitation patients from that field test.

There are three steps required to complete the scale: patient examination, functional goal setting, and scale quantification.

J Rehabil Outcomes Meas, 1997, 1(1), 1–7

Patient Examination

During the patient examination, each pertinent measure of physical impairment and functional deficit is quantified. Pertinence is defined by the therapist. The measures of physical impairment are evaluated by traditional methods. The functional deficits are evaluated through directed patient questioning and patient report.

Functional Goal Setting

Each deficit in impairment and function is then examined with "the end in mind" to determine the functional goal of treatment. In other words, how much improvement do the therapist and patient believe they can attain by the end of treatment? The therapist who finds a reduction in shoulder flexion (e.g., 120 degrees), for example, could use the AMA *Guides To the Evaluation of Permanent Impairment* to determine the expected amount of flexion (180 degrees).[16] If the therapist and patient believe they will attain the full 180 degrees, the goal becomes 180 degrees of shoulder flexion before the end of treatment. If, on the other hand, the unaffected shoulder flexes to 140 degrees, and the therapist and patient believe 140 degrees is expected on the affected shoulder, then the goal becomes 140 degrees of flexion. If there was a preexisting shoulder adhesive capsulitis, and 125 degrees is the best they expect, 125 degrees of flexion becomes the goal.

As another example, if the patient reports difficulty sitting more than two hours because of low back pain, then the therapist should ask how much sitting does the patient need and expect to have following treatment. If the patient needs to sit six hours at work, then six hours becomes the functional goal.

Scale Quantification

The ratings for each physical impairment and each functional deficit are then quantified in a standard manner. In the first example, the goal of treatment is 180 degrees of flexion. The current measurement is 120 degrees. The scale becomes the percent of current over expected: $(120/180) \times 100 = 67$ percent. The orthopedic outcome scale utilizes 25 percent increments of change as a standard. The therapist selects 0 percent (< 25 percent), 25 percent (25 percent to < 50 percent), 50 percent (50 percent to < 75 percent), 75 percent (75 percent to < 100 percent) or 100 percent (100 percent). Therefore, the 67 percent becomes a scale of 50 percent. In the second example, the current flexion is 120, and the expected goal is 140. The percent is 86 percent, or a scale of 75 percent. In the example of the low back pain, the current functional measure is 2 hours, and the expected goal is 6 hours. This is a $(2/6) \times 100 = 33$ percent for a scale of 25 percent.

The pertinent measures are monitored (remeasured) throughout treatment and at discharge. The measures are compared with the expected functional goal at each measurement. With the functional goals established at the initial visit, the resultant "outcome" is the quantifiable change in the scales between the initial evaluation, status measurement, and last visit, which should be the discharge visit. In this manner, the scales are independent of any specific treatment techniques and clinical skills.

TESTING THE OUTCOME SCALE

A pilot test of the new orthopedic rehabilitation outcome scale was performed to evaluate its validity and reliability. Rehability Corporation hired Formations In Health Care, Inc., an outcomes research and database firm, to solicit orthopedic rehabilitation outpatient facilities nationally to participate in the research project. The facilities represented programs that were hospital based, publicly owned, or in private practice. At least one clinician representative from each facility was identified and attended a mandatory training session of the outcome scale. A comprehensive training manual explaining the orthopedic rehabilitation outcome scale and data collection methodology was provided. All clinicians participating in the pilot test completed a competency-based certification examination at the conclusion of the training session.

Clinician representatives were permitted to train additional clinician raters at their facilities. Following this step, data collection was initiated. During a preliminary test period of three weeks in March and April 1994 at Rehability, and nine weeks from February to April 1995 in the expanded national effort, clinicians collected information on orthopedic patients in their facilities who initiated and completed their rehabilitation during this time period. In order to minimize the introduction of subject selection bias, all consecutive orthopedic patients seen in the facilities were asked to participate in the research.

ANALYSIS

Ratings at admission and discharge were analyzed using one parameter Item Response Theory (IRT). This methodology has recently been used to validate a number of physical function scales in rehabilitation.[17–23] Rasch, one application of IRT, allows the identification of three important characteristics of multi-item instruments: (1) unidimensionality, (2) a hierarchical item continuum, and (3) reproducibility.[24] Unidimensionality represents whether an instrument comprises a single dominant construct, even though multiple attributes are measured. Rasch analysis determines this through fit statistics (infit and standardized z scores). This characteristic is a necessary precursor to combining the items to obtain a total score for an assessment. A hierarchical continuum represents a structure in which items of a unidimensional construct progress from easy to difficult in a hypothesized fashion. Finally, reproducibility is an indication of how well the order of item difficulty remains stable across different samples of patients and different test occasions (e.g., admission to discharge).

ASSESSING RESPONSES TO THE SCALE

Forty-two clinical facilities in the United States participated on a voluntary basis. A total of 300 patients was included (Table 1). Subjects represented a wide distribution of diagnostic categories. The majority (32%) involved back and neck disorders, followed by 22 percent lower extremities (LE) disorders (LE fractures/dislocations/strains and knee disorders). All other disorders represent 4–7.33 percent of the sample. The mean patient age was 44.1 years, with a range of 11.7–83.2 years. There were 128 males (43%) and 172 females (57%).

ADMISSION RESULTS

All of the impairment items were analyzed separately at admission (initial evaluation) and at discharge. In contrast to traditional statistics, Rasch analysis calculates an expected model and then determines how well the data fit the model. For purposes of this study, items were considered to form a unidimensional construct if they had less than 35 percent more noise in the data than modeled (infit mean square $\leq$ 1.35 and standardized z score $\geq$ 2.0).[25]

At admission, all of the items did not meet the criterion of unidimensionality. Edema showed an infit mean square (MnSq) of 1.35 and an associated standardized z score (STD) of 2.6. Sensation showed an infit MnSq of 1.57 and associated STD of 2.6. These items "misfit" the Rasch model because a number of persons received unexpected scores on these items. Therefore, edema and sensation were removed from the scale, and the analysis was run again. The results are presented in Table 2 in order of item difficulty. Measures for the items are presented in logits (log-odd units), which are the natural log of the performance of the item relative to the performance of the total set of items.[26]

With the removal of edema and sensation, all the items fit the first desirable characteristic of multi-item instruments, unidimensionality. In addition, the instrument generally met the second criterion, hierarchical item continuum. The hierarchy of item difficulty presented in Table 2 (top items more difficult than lower items) appears to be consistent with clinical observations. Endurance appears to be the most difficult item for these patients. In addition, active range of motion appears to be more difficult than passive range of motion, as expected. The representation of gait as the easiest item may be due to the proportionally low number of patients with lower extremity involvement (22%: combination of LE fractures/dislocations/strains and knee disorders in Table 1) in contrast to patients with upper extremity or back involvement (46.33%: combination of back/neck disorders, shoulder disorders, and UE fractures/dislocations/strains in Table 1). The majority of patients who have back or upper extremity involvement may have little difficulty with gait.

The overall metrics at admission approached acceptable criterion for this instrument for construct validity. Person separation reliability, which is close in formulation to traditional internal reliability coefficients, was 0.75 (generally, acceptable levels are 0.80 and above). In addition, the instrument was well matched to the sample under study with the average person ability measures only 0.80 ± 1.28 higher than the average difficulty level of the items.

DISCHARGE RESULTS

A similar analysis was run on discharge data. Edema again appeared erratic (MnSq = 1.59, STD = 2.3). In contrast to admission, sensation at discharge fit the criterion for unidimensionality. For purposes of comparing admission and dis-

Table 1. Participating Patient Population

Diagnoses	n	Percent
Back/neck disorders	96	32.00
LE fractures/dislocations/strains	38	12.67
Knee disorders	28	9.33
Other joint disorders	22	7.33
Shoulder disorders	21	7.00
UE fractures/dislocations/strains	19	6.33
Muscle/soft tissue disorders	15	5.00
Osteoarthrosis	12	4.00
Other	16	5.33
Unknown	33	11.00
Total	300	100

Table 2. Admission Items Statistics In Measure Order (Difficult to Easy)

Item	Measure		Infit	
	Logits	Error	MnSq	STD
Endurance	.65	.09	.91	−1.0
Active range of motion	.30	.08	.77	−3.2
Strength	.06	.08	1.08	.9
Passive range of motion	.09	.08	.78	−2.7
Posture	−.43	.09	1.30	2.8
Gait	−.49	.09	1.24	2.2

charge measures, both edema and sensation were removed from the scale and the analysis was run again. The results are presented in Table 3.

All items at discharge represented a unidimensional construct as indicated by infit mean squares less than 1.35 and associated z scores less than 2.0. The hierarchical continuum again was consistent with clinical observations, with endurance being the most difficult item and active range of motion being more difficult than passive range of motion. The item hierarchy at discharge also indicated that the instrument met the third important desirable characteristic of reproducibility. That is, the hierarchy of item difficulties at discharge was the same as was found for admission.

The instrument at discharge showed moderate measurement qualities. Person separation reliability was 0.67. At discharge the instrument was not well matched to the sample under study with the average person ability measures 2.39 ± 1.45 logits higher than the average item difficulty. While the latter finding suggests that the instrument is "too easy" for patients at discharge, this should be expected. Patients generally should receive high ratings at discharge, indicating good rehabilitation and the achievement of clinical goals.

To further investigate the instrument value in detecting change in patient status, admission and discharge scores of patients ($n = 141$) were compared. To ensure that the instrument was used in the same manner from admission and discharge, we applied a method of "anchoring" the discharge measures by step measure and item calibration at admission.[27] Figure 1 is a plot of each patient's score (in logits) at admission (x axis) and discharge (y axis). Points that lay along the center diagonal indicate that patient measures do not change from admission and discharge. The two dashed lines represent the 95 percent confidence interval. Therefore, only points lying outside the dashed lines represent patients that "significantly" improved (above the top dashed line) or significantly became worse (below the bottom dashed line). As can be seen in the figure, approximately half of the patients showed significant improvements and no patients showed significant decrements on the orthopedic outcome scale.

Table 3. Discharge Items Statistics In Measure Order (Difficult to Easy)

Item	Measure		Infit	
	Logits	Error	MnSq	STD
Endurance	1.12	.16	1.27	1.6
Active range of motion	.40	.15	.65	−2.7
Strength	.09	.16	1.14	.9
Passive range of motion	−.04	.18	.70	2.0
Posture	−.38	.20	1.25	1.2
Gait	−1.20	.23	.97	1.1

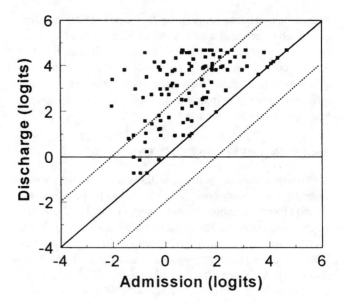

Figure 1. Orthopedic scores: Admission/discharge comparison.

EXAMINING THE FINDINGS

The findings from this study indicate that items of strength, active range of motion, passive range of motion, endurance, posture, and gait can be combined to create a unidimensional scale. In addition, these items form a reasonable hierarchy. While the scale only approaches reasonable construct validity criteria, it appears to be adequately sensitive to monitor patient improvement from admission to discharge.

While the "final" set of items worked well together to form a unidimensional construct, edema and sensation were erratically scored relative to the rest of the items on the scale. A possible reason for this erratic scoring is the relevance of these items to the sample under study. For example, the majority of patients who presented with back and neck disorders do not characteristically present with edema. Therefore, it is likely that therapists evaluating these patients had difficulty obtaining meaningful values for edema. Items that lack clarity or are inappropriate for the sample under study are likely to be erratically scored.

The hierarchical order of the items also should have had some relationship to the sample under study. While the order we found fit some general rationale, this rationale did not fit with all diagnostic groups in the sample. For example, the finding that endurance represented a difficult item is consistent with the common clinical observation that endurance is one of the more challenging areas for rehabilitation for most diagnostic groups. In contrast, the finding that gait was the easiest item does not have such convincing rationale. While for patients with upper extremity injuries or back pain, gait is likely to represent a relatively easy activity, this is not likely the case with patients who have lower extremity disorders.

For the latter diagnosis, one would expect that gait would be one of the more difficult items on the scale. In future studies, it may be more sound to separate patients with upper and lower extremity disorders, since we would hypothesize that these groups would use the scale differently (i.e., gait should represent a "hard" item for someone with a lower extremity problem and represent an "easy" item for someone with a hand injury). It is possible that the overall measurement qualities of the instrument will improve if it is used with a more homogeneous sample.

There are positive implications in the identification of a unidimensional construct. A single value can be calculated and used as a basis for the measurement of functional outcome from the clinician perspective through the use of readily available impairment ratings. Identification of a single construct permits the "quantification" of outcome and a method to demonstrate treatment effectiveness in orthopedic patients. There is simplification of data reporting in a process of outcomes management. Also, there is the potential to compare patient-reported and clinician-reported measures of outcome.

The theoretical basis of the orthopedic rehabilitation outcomes scale requires a clinical paradigm shift away from the common measurement and tracking of physical impairment to a three-part decision process: (1) make a measurement (physical impairment and functional deficit), (2) set a functional goal for each measurement, and (3) determine how far away from the goal the patient is, so the measurement can be scaled in a standard manner. This new paradigm is independent of specific clinical techniques and provides a standard format in which most patients with acute orthopedic problems can be assessed. The strengths of the paradigm are its reliance on functional goals, measurements, and its generic scope. Because there is "fair" reliability, the next step is to improve the operational definitions for the remaining variables. This should improve the reliability of the instrument.

Finally, while the scale showed only moderate measurement qualities (e.g., construct validity), it appeared to be adequately sensitive to detect "significant" changes in the sample under study. As presented, approximately 50 percent of the patients showed significant improvements and no patients showed significant decrements. While it is likely that therapist-generated measures would be biased in showing patient improvement, the finding that improvements can be detected with the orthopedic rehabilitation outcome scale is promising.

•　　•　　•

An orthopedic rehabilitation outcome scale that includes commonly accepted measures of physical impairment and functional deficits used in the clinical evaluation and rehabilitation of acute orthopedic patients has been developed. Through the combined efforts of clinicians in a multisite national study, the orthopedic rehabilitation outcome scale was evaluated and was demonstrated to be reliable, valid, and responsive to change in outpatient orthopedic patients. The orthopedic rehabilitation outcome scale, when used in conjunction with additional clinician- and patient-reported measures and a risk adjustment mechanism, should permit valid outcome comparisons of clinicians, facilities, and programs. The scale is now included in the Medirisk, Inc. Orthopedic Rehabilitation Outcome Scale.

REFERENCES

1. Gordon, H.S., and Rosenthal, G.E. "Impact of Marital Status on Outcomes in Hospitalized Patients. Evidence from an Academic Medical Center." *Archives of Internal Medicine* 155, no. 22 (1995): 2465–71.

2. McCarthy, M.L., et al. "Functional Status Following Orthopedic Trauma in Young Women." *Journal of Trauma* 39, no. 5 (1995): 828–36.

3. Friedman, E., and Thomas, S.A. "Pet Ownership, Social Support, and One-Year Survival after Acute Myocardial Infarction in the Cardiac Arrhythmia Suppression Trial (CAST)." *American Journal of Cardiology* 76, no. 17 (1995): 1213–17.

4. Reisine, S., McQuillan, J., and Fifield, J. "Predictors of Work Disability in Rheumatoid Arthritis Patients. A Five-Year Follow-Up." *Arthritis and Rheumatology* 38, no. 11 (1995): 1630–7.

5. Idler, E.L., and Kasl, S.V. "Self-Ratings of Health: Do They Also Predict Change in Functional Ability?" *Journal of Gerontology* 50, no. 6 (1995): S344–53.

6. Jin, R.L., Shah, C.P., and Svoboda, T.J. "The Impact of Unemployment on Health: A Review of the Evidence." *Canadian Medical Association Journal* 153, no. 5 (1995): 529–40.

7. Mahler, D.A., and Mackowiak, J.I. "Evaluation of the Short-Form 36-Item Questionnaire To Measure Health-Related Quality of Life in Patients with COPD." *Chest* 107, no. 6 (1995): 1585–89.

8. Lerner, D.J., et al. "Job Strain and Health Related Quality of Life in a National Sample." *American Journal of Public Health* 84, no. 10 (1994): 1580–85.

9. Mahler, D.A., et al. "Impact of Dyspnea and Physiologic Function on General Health Status in Patients with Chronic Obstructive Pulmonary Disease." *Chest* 102, no. 2 (1992): 395–401.

10. Benson, D.P. *Measuring Outcomes in Ambulatory Care.* Chicago: American Hospital Association Publishing, 1992.

11. Fairbank, J., et al. "The Oswestry Low Back Pain Disability Questionnaire." *Physiotherapy* 66, no. 8 (1980): 271–73.

12. Vernon, H., and Mior, S. "The Neck Disability Index: A Study of Reliability and Validity." *Journal of Manipulative and Physiologic Therapeutics* 14 (1991): 409–15.

13. Tegner, Y., and Lysholm, J. "Rating Systems in the Evaluation of Knee Ligament Injuries." *Clinical Orthopaedics and Related Research* 198 (1985): 43–48.

14. Williams, J.W., Holleman, D.R., and Simel, D.L. "Measuring Shoulder Function with the Shoulder Pain and Disability Index." *Journal of Rheumatology* 22, no. 4 (1995): 727–32.

15. Stewart, D.L., and Abeln, S.H. *Documenting Functional Outcomes in Physical Therapy.* St. Louis, MO: Mosby, 1993.

16. Engelberg, A.L., ed. *Guides to the Evaluation of Permanent Impairment.* 3d ed. Chicago, IL: American Medical Association, 1988.

17. Dobel, S.E., et al. "Functional Competence of Community-Dwelling Persons with Multiple Sclerosis Using the Assessment of Motor and Process Skills." *Archives of Physical Medicine and Rehabilitation* 75 (1994): 843–51.

18. Haley, S.M., McHorney, C.A., and Ware, J.E. "Evaluation of the MOS SF-36 Physical Functioning Scale (PF-10): I. Unidimensionality and Reproducibility of the Rasch Item Scale." *Journal of Clinical Epidemiology* 47 (1994): 671–84.

19. Heinemann, A.W., et al. "Relationships between Impairment and Physical Disability as Measured by the Functional Independence Measure." *Archives of Physical Medicine and Rehabilitation* 74 (1993): 566–73.

20. Wright, B., and Linacre, M. "Reasonable Mean-Square Fit Values." *Rasch Measurement Transactions* 8 (1994): 370.

21. Silverstein, B., et al. "Applying Psychometric Criteria to Functional Assessment in Medical Rehabilitation: II. Defining Interval Measures." *Archives of Physical Medicine and Rehabilitation* 73 (1991): 507–18.

22. Velozo, C.A., et al. "Differences in Functional Scale Discrimination at Admission and Discharge: Rasch Analysis of the Level of Rehabilitation Scale-III (LORS-III)." *Archives of Physical Medicine and Rehabilitation* 76, no. 8 (1995): 705–12.

23. Whiteneck, G.G., et al. "Quantifying Handicap: A New Measure of Long-Term Rehabilitation Outcomes." *Archives of Physical Medicine and Rehabilitation* 73 (1992): 519–26.

24. Haley, McHorney, and Ware, "Evaluation of the MOS SF-36 Physical Functioning Scale (PF-10)."

25. Wright and Linacre, "Reasonable Mean-Square Fit Values."

26. Haley, McHorney, and Ware, "Evaluation of the MOS SF-36 Physical Functioning Scale (PF-10)."

27. Linacre, J.M., and Wright, B.D. *A User's Guide to BIGSTEPS.* Version 2.6. Chicago, IL: MESA Press, 1995, pp. 51–56.

18

The Focus On Therapeutic Outcomes (FOTO) Outpatient Orthopedic Rehabilitation Database: Results of 1994–1996

Edward A. Dobrzykowski and Terri Nance

Focus On Therapeutic Outcomes, Inc. (FOTO; Knoxville, Tennessee), was created in 1992 from a desire to create a standardized outcome measurement and reporting system for rehabilitation of outpatients with orthopedic dysfunction. The goal of FOTO was to demonstrate rehabilitation effectiveness and efficiency in outpatient orthopedic practice. FOTO is a privately owned outcomes measurement research and database company and is independent from providers and payers of outpatient rehabilitation services.

The FOTO orthopedic outcomes measurement system for outpatient rehabilitation comprises patient health status and patient satisfaction measures, reports of the types of clinician treatments performed, and patient demographic and descriptive indicators. There are additional measures that evaluate the level of goal achievement; staffing mix during the episode of care; and efficiency measures of cost, number of visits, and duration of treatment. Referral source and payer source information are included. This article reports specifically on patient health status, patient satisfaction, cost, visits, and episode length observed in a select sample from the FOTO database during 1994–1996.

The FOTO orthopedic outcomes measurement system collects data at the initiation (first visit) and conclusion (last visit) of the rehabilitation episode. Interim data (interval measures) are optional and may be used by the clinician to assess progress during rehabilitation.

EFFECTIVENESS MEASURES

The patient health status measure included in the FOTO system is the Medical Outcomes Study SF-36 (Medical Out-

comes Trust, Boston, Massachusetts). The patient-reported SF-36 comprises 36 questions and has demonstrated reliability and validity in a variety of ambulatory patient populations.[1-5] Eight domains (subscales) make up the SF-36 health status survey: bodily pain, role limitations—physical, physical functioning, role limitations—emotional, energy/fatigue, mental health, social functioning, and health perceptions. The usual time for completion is 10–15 minutes, and the survey requires a minimum reading level of the eighth grade. The SF-36 is valid for patients 14 years of age and older. Patients may complete the survey themselves or be interviewed.

[In January 1996, FOTO made a change from inclusion of the SF-36 to the SF-12, while continuing to include all items of the physical functioning domain of the SF-36. The SF-12 retains approximately 90 percent of the explanation of patient variance demonstrated by the SF-36,[6] and reduces respondent burden to a completion time of 5 minutes.]

The initial design of the FOTO system included both the patient-reported SF-36 and "condition-specific" measures for low back, neck, and knee disorders, which were completed concurrently by each patient. The condition-specific measures utilized were the Oswestry Low Back Disability Questionnaire,[7] the Neck Disability Index,[8] and the Lysholm Scale[9] with low back, neck, and knee disorders, respectively. These conditions represented on average 50 percent to 75 percent of the total patient population in most outpatient orthopedic rehabilitation facilities.

During early collection of data in 1993–1994, FOTO demonstrated a correlation and similar magnitudes of change in health status with the aforementioned condition-specific questionnaires and the SF-36.[10,11] As a result, the use of the condition-specific questionnaires was discontinued in favor of the more broadly applicable general health status survey, SF-36. The benefit in this conversion to use of the SF-36 without the additional condition-specific measures was a

J Rehabil Outcomes Meas, 1997, 1(1), 56–60

significant reduction in respondent burden and item size of the FOTO system.

The patient satisfaction measures can be completed on an interval basis and at discharge. Patients rate their care over the course of treatment in nine areas as "very satisfied," "somewhat satisfied," "neither satisfied nor dissatisfied," "somewhat dissatisfied," or "very dissatisfied." The areas evaluated by the patient include information and treatment regarding their condition, overall care, convenience in scheduling and location, waiting time, phone contact, and overall experience.

EFFICIENCY MEASURES

At the time of patient discharge, information on cost, the number of outpatient visits, and episode length (days) is recorded. Cost is defined as the net adjusted cost at the time of billing, reflecting discounts with managed care agreements.

Database Characteristics (1994–1996)

A sampling of the FOTO database from 1994–1996 was assessed, which included 24,303 patient episodes. Descriptions will be made of the typical facility and clinician profiles. The results of facility effectiveness for patient health status (known as the Outcomes Index, Value Index, Utilization Index) and patient satisfaction (Patient Satisfaction Index) in six impairment categories (lumbar spine, cervical spine, shoulder, arm/hand, hip/leg, and other) will be described. The results of facility efficiency will also be described, including cost, number of visits, and episode length in six impairment categories. In addition, the mean number of visits by payer source (Medicare, Medicaid, workers' compensation, health maintenance organization [HMO], preferred provider organization [PPO], indemnity, litigation, self-pay, other) will be described in the six impairment categories.

Facility Profiles

A total of 384 facilities in 34 states reported outcomes data. The average outpatient orthopedic rehabilitation facility was open for 49 hours weekly and employed the equivalent of 3.0 physical therapists (PTs), 0.87 physical therapist assistants (PTAs), 0.77 occupational therapists (OTs), 0.07 certified occupational therapy assistants (COTAs), 0.26 athletic trainers (ATs), and 1.89 clinical support staff.

Clinician Profiles

There was a total of 1,404 clinicians in the database, which includes 1,055 women (75%) and 345 men (25%) (4 did not specify gender). The number of clinicians with entry level baccalaureate degrees was 937 (67%), followed by 231 (16%) with entry level master's degrees. The average years of direct patient care experience was 9.42 years.

Patient Profiles

There was a total of 24,303 patients, of which 58% were female and 42% were male. The mean age of patients was 44.8 years, with a range of 18–93 years.

Effectiveness Results

Outcomes Index

FOTO reports an indicator of change in patient-reported health status known as the outcomes index (OI). The OI is similar to effect size. The benefits to the use of the OI are in providing clinicians a description of the magnitude of change, comparing changes in other scales and with benchmarks that signify clinically meaningful changes, or with changes obtained with another treatment regimen or in another group of patients.[12] The OI is calculated as follows:

$$\frac{\text{Health status score (discharge)} - \text{Health status score (admission)}}{\text{Standard deviation of health status score (admission)}}$$

The OI reports an average of the total change of scores from six of the domains of the SF-36: bodily pain, role limitations—physical, physical functioning, energy/fatigue, mental health, and social functioning. The FOTO OI is reported by impairment group in Table 1.

Value Index

FOTO reports an index on the value of the health status change achieved for the costs of the rehabilitation incurred over an episode of care, known as the value index (VI). The FOTO VI is calculated as follows:

$$\frac{\text{Outcome index}}{\text{Episode cost}}$$

Episode is defined in days from the initiation until the conclusion of rehabilitation. The cost is defined as the net cost incurred following any initial adjustment for managed care contracts. For example, a patient's total cost is $1,000. As the patient belongs to a PPO, which provides for a 20 percent discount, the net billed cost is $800. The FOTO VI is reported by impairment group in Table 1.

Utilization Index

FOTO reports an index on the value of the health status change achieved for the number of visits incurred per episode, known as the utilization index (UI). The UI is calculated as follows:

$$\frac{\text{Outcome index}}{\text{Number of visits}}$$

The FOTO UI is reported for each impairment group in Table 1.

Table 1. Index by Impairment Category

Impairment	OI	VI	UI	PSI
All categories	54.8	55.9	55.5	94.8
Arm/hand	48.3	47.7	45.8	95.6
Cervical spine	55.9	60.1	60.9	93.9
Lumbar spine	63.1	70.1	70.7	94.2
Hip/leg	57.4	56.7	55.1	95.2
Shoulder	49.7	45.5	44.2	95.3
Other	49.1	47.7	48.0	95.0

Patient Satisfaction Index

FOTO reports an index of patient satisfaction using nine indicators previously described. The patient satisfaction index (PSI) is calculated as an average of each response and is weighted by the total number of questions answered by the patient. The FOTO PSI is reported for each impairment group in Table 1.

Efficiency Results

The mean number of visits for patients across all impairment groups and payers was 8.0 visits. For the six impairment categories, the mean number of visits is listed in Table 2. The mean number of visits for each payer source is listed in Table 3.

The mean cost per patient episode across all impairment groups was $811. For the six impairment categories, the average costs are listed in Table 2.

The mean episode duration for patients across all diagnoses and payers was 29 days. For the six impairment categories, the mean costs are listed in Table 2.

DISCUSSION

The providers that contract with FOTO and contribute outcomes information have for perhaps the first time been able to quantify the effectiveness and efficiency of outpatient orthopedic rehabilitation using a standardized measurement system on a national basis. The SF-36 and SF-12 health status surveys are rapidly becoming the "gold standard" as general health status measures with broad utility in ambulatory practice. The OI, VI, and UI were created to simplify the reporting and understanding of health status and cost results.

An analysis of 24,303 patient episodes from the FOTO orthopedic rehabilitation database was described and reviewed. A total of 384 practices in 34 states were contributors to the FOTO database. The profile of a typical patient is 44 years of age, is seen for eight visits, during an episode length of about one month, at a cost of $811.

In return for outcomes data generated at the provider site and sent to FOTO, a quarterly report is generated for the provider by FOTO, listing indicators of both efficiency and effectiveness. In reporting of this nature, trending of outcome results over time is apparent and assists in the rehabilitation provider's management and monitoring of practice variation.

The utilization information presented in the FOTO database with a range of seven to nine visits regardless of impairment category begs the question: Is provider utilization being much more controlled by the payer, rather than the specific condition? The influence of managed care and cost containment efforts in health care is readily apparent. The FOTO database demonstrates a utilization pattern that "clinically" should elucidate more variation in results.

The payer source utilization means for all categories (Table 3) range from 5.3 visits for self-payment by patients to 10.2 visits for patients on workers' compensation. The self-payment and HMO payer source data reflect lower utilization levels as expected with increased payment responsibility by patients and costs absorbed by providers. FOTO data on higher utilization levels for workers' compensation patients reflect trends seen in the insurance industry. Further study is needed to evaluate the effect of both restrictive and liberal utilization rates on health status outcomes and subsequent impact on rates of recidivism. Only then will the true cost of rehabilitation be determined.

There are limitations to the analysis and interpretation attributed to outcomes data. Providers are required to enroll all pa-

Table 2. Mean Visits, Duration, and Cost

Impairment	Visits	Duration (days)	Cost ($)
All categories	8	29	811
Arm/hand	9	30	858
Cervical spine	8	29	772
Lumbar spine	7	25	746
Hip/leg	9	31	823
Shoulder	9	33	898
Other	9	29	781

Table 3. Mean Visits by Payer Source

Source	Visits
Indemnity	8
Medicare	9
PPO	8
Medicaid	6.6
HMO	5.7
Workers' compensation	10.2
Litigation	9.5
Self-pay	5.3
Other	7.3

tients seen with musculoskeletal dysfunction in their practices. The knowledge of discharge timing for outpatients presents challenges in the collection of patient-reported data at discharge. Selection bias can be detected in a facility report with a preponderance of missing information from that facility.

In the comparisons of outcomes among outpatient rehabilitation providers, a mechanism must exist for the consideration of case mix factors, often referred to as risk adjustment. The method for risk adjustment attempts to control for variation represented by elements outside of provider control, such as patient comorbidities, severity of the condition, age of the patient, and region of the country. The FOTO database information as presented in this article is not risk adjusted. [FOTO is presently risk adjusting data for provider management reports, using age, impairment group, and admission health status score.] Work is underway to further understand additional factors that both contribute to risk and assist in the prediction of outcome variance in the FOTO database.

• • •

The process of outcomes management in outpatient orthopedic rehabilitation, as in other parts of the health continuum, is becoming absolutely essential. Providers have demonstrated the utility of FOTO outcomes information in continuous quality improvement, meeting program evaluation and accreditation requirements, marketing, and demands for outcomes information from managed care organizations. The growing need for outcomes information, such as that provided by the FOTO orthopedic outcomes measurement system and database, will continue to assist providers in their monitoring of results, response for professional accountability, and ability to link "economic" outcomes such as visits and cost with "functional" health status and patient satisfaction.

REFERENCES

1. McHorney, C.A., et al. "The Validity and Relative Precision of MOS Short- and Long-Form Health Status Scales and Dartmouth COOP Charts: Results from the Medical Outcomes Study." *Medical Care* 30, suppl. 5 (1992): MS253–265.

2. Ware, J.E., Kosinski, M., and Keller, S.D. "A 12-Item Short-Form Health Survey: Construction of Scales and Preliminary Tests of Reliability and Validity." *Medical Care* 34, no. 3 (1996): 220–33.

3. Jenkinson, C., Wright, L., and Coulter, A. "Criterion Validity and Reliability of the SF-36 in a Population Sample." *Quality of Life Research* 3, no. 1 (1994): 7–12.

4. Lyons, R.A., Perry, H.M., and Littlepage, B.N. "Evidence for the Validity of the Short-Form 36 Questionnaire (SF-36) in an Elderly Population." *Aging* 23, no. 3 (1994): 182–84.

5. Ruta, D.A., et al. "The SF-36 Health Survey Questionnaire: I. Reliability in Two Patient-Based Studies." *Quality Health Care* 1995 (in press).

6. Ware et al., "A 12-Item Short-Form Health Survey."

7. Fairbank, J.C.T., et al. "The Oswestry Low Back Pain Disability Questionnaire." *Physiotherapy* 66, no. 8 (1980): 271–73.

8. Vernon, H., and Mior, S. "The Neck Disability Index: A Study of Reliability and Validity." *Journal of Manipulative and Physiological Therapeutics* 14 (1991): 409–15.

9. Tegner, Y., and Lysholm, J. "Rating Systems in the Evaluation of Knee Ligament Injuries." *Clinical Orthopaedics and Related Research* 198 (1985): 43–48.

10. Jette, D.U., and Jette, A.M. "Physical Therapy and Health Outcomes in Patients with Spinal Impairments." *Physical Therapy* 76, no. 9 (1996): 930–41.

11. Jette, D.U., and Jette, A.M. "Physical Therapy and Health Outcomes in Patients with Knee Impairments." *Physical Therapy* 76, no. 11 (1996): 1178–87.

12. Jette and Jette, "Physical Therapy and Health Outcomes in Patients with Spinal Impairments."

19

Physical Therapy Treatment of Low Back Pain: A Report of Outcomes According to Three Types of Patient Classification

Michael A. O'Hearn

APPROACHING A CLASSIFICATION SCHEME

The use of physical therapy in the treatment of low back pain (LBP) accounts for approximately 25 percent of all patients seen in outpatient clinics.[1] A recent survey of 1,200 physicians showed that more than 80 percent believed physical therapy to be effective in the treatment of LBP, despite a lack of scientific evidence supporting its effectiveness.[2] In fact, a recently released report by the federal Agency for Health Care Policy and Research (AHCPR) rated many specific physical therapy modalities as "not recommended" for treatment of LBP based on the lack of conclusive scientific evidence.[3]

There is, however, increasing scientific evidence supporting the use of physical therapy as a *whole* in the short-term treatment of LBP. Di Fabio and others[4] in studying 42 workers' compensation patients with low back pain showed that 90 percent of the patients without signs of a discogenic injury returned to work within four weeks from the commencement of treatment. Gill and others,[5] reporting on a case series of 50 patients, showed 74 percent of all patients had returned to work by the end of a six-week physical therapy program. In both studies patients demonstrated both clinical and functional improvement. Despite the favorable outcomes of these studies, more research is needed. Perhaps the fundamental challenge to researchers is that 80 percent of LBP is undiagnosable.[6] This makes it difficult for researchers to place patients in categories. Without valid classifications of patients it is difficult to compare outcomes for different types of treatment and assist clinicians to develop critical pathways for patient management.

Many health care professionals have their own classification schemes for patients with LBP, often approaching it from a "tissue model" where they look to find an anatomical structure at fault based on patient history and the physical evaluation. The subsequent diagnoses are vague conditions such as "facet joint syndrome," "trigger points," and "myofascial pain."[7,8] Recognizing this problem, the Quebec task force (QTF) for low back pain recommended the implementation of a simpler method of classification based on location of pain and/or presence of unquestionable pathology detected in clinical evaluation and confirmed on imaging techniques.[9] DeRosa and Porterfield[8] agree with this concept and present a modified version of the Quebec recommendations suitable for physical therapists.

An alternative classification scheme within physical therapy is to categorize patients with LBP according to treatment. Hence a patient with LBP that is relieved with extension exercises is classified as having "extension syndrome." Delitto and others[10,11] present an elaborate but complicated scheme. Such a classification scheme assists the physical therapist in planning treatment, but it does not necessarily allow effective communication with other health professionals treating the patient and, as Rothstein[12] has pointed out, may preclude the patient from a different treatment by isolation in the treatment assigned classification.

Physical therapists often informally classify patients according to the expected outcome of treatment. Outcome expectations may be influenced by duration of symptoms and the insurance status of the patient. Many therapists believe that a patient who is receiving workers' compensation or has an injury of long duration will not improve as much as a patient with an acute injury and no issues of possible secondary gain. Thus a de facto classification is already being made, despite a lack of evidence to support these assumptions.

J Rehabil Outcomes Meas, 1997, 1(3), 23–31
© 1997 Aspen Publishers, Inc.

The author thanks Dr. A.L. Millar of Andrews University for her assistance in the preparation of this manuscript.

Such informal classification of patients may influence the quality of the physical therapy received, especially if expectations are too low.

The purpose of this paper is to report the outcome of patients with LBP according to three types of classification. The classifications used were a modified Quebec task force classification, duration of symptoms, and insurance status. Within these three groups the outcomes of number of treatments, Oswestry score,[13] forward bending, and straight leg raise were measured and compared.

SUBJECTS

Two hundred and sixty-three consecutive patients (109 male, 154 female) referred to physical therapy, with ages ranging from 11 to 91, were included in this study. Patients were referred from 59 different medical or osteopathic physicians. All patients had low back pain or symptoms thought to be arising from the lumbosacral spine, representing 24 different diagnoses. The diagnosis of low back pain or lumbosacral strain represented 49 percent of the total diagnoses. Almost all patients were from Berrien county in southwest Michigan. The only patients excluded from this study were those referred for once-only instruction in home exercises, or the prescription of a TENS unit where no follow-up was anticipated. If any of these patients returned for follow-up, they were included in the study.

PROCEEDING WITH THE STUDY

Data Collected

Prior to the initial evaluation, patients completed the Oswestry Low Back Pain Disability Questionnaire. This disease-specific, reliable, and valid tool has common use in the evaluation of LBP.[13,14,15] The Oswestry measures the effect of back pain on activities of daily living. Items included are the common functional activities that are often adversely affected by LBP, such as sitting, walking, standing, sleeping, lifting, and self care. This questionnaire was chosen because of its specificity and ease of administration. Patient response is scored out of 100. Higher scores indicate higher perceived patient disability. Any item questions omitted by the patient resulted in the overall score being converted into a percentage.

The patient was then evaluated by a physical therapist using that therapist's own evaluation style, but also measuring straight leg raise (SLR) and forward bending (FB). SLR was recorded in degrees using an inclinometer placed on the patients' tibia. FB was recorded in centimeters of fingertips to the floor using a tape measure or a carpenter's ruler. Each measurement was taken at the immediate onset of either lower extremity or back pain. Intratester and intertester reli-

ability of such measures has been demonstrated by previous research. [16,17,18] To ensure reliability of taking measurements, we gave inservicing, written instructions, and introduced competency testing for all clinicians taking measurements. Competency testing consisted of both an open book written quiz requiring clinicians to classify hypothetical patients, and observation of correct measuring of FB and SLR. We believe that these simple reliable measures (Oswestry, FB, SLR) would be valid in showing the change in status of a patient's low back pain. They are easy to perform and are usually part of the standard evaluation of LBP. Also there was the need to keep to a minimum the amount of data to be collected to ensure staff compliance. The same data was also collected again at discharge.

Patient Classification

Following evaluation, patients were classified according to a scheme similar to one as suggested by the QTF.[9] This scheme generally uses location and duration of symptoms unless an X-ray, magnetic resonance imaging (MRI), or computer tomography (CT) scan enables a conclusive diagnosis. Table 1 shows the criteria for each of the nine classifications that we chose to use in our modified scheme.

The rationale for using such a classification is based on the premise that current tissue-at-fault, a priori, clinical classifications are unduly influenced by examiner bias adversely influencing validity. The original Quebec classification was modified slightly to suit a physical therapy practice and the type of patients seen. We have added an extra category for symptom location as suggested by DeRosa and Porterfield.[8] This is the B4 category of extremity pain being more severe than the actual back pain. The observation has been that many patients with this condition have a poorer outcome.[8] Reliability for this classification has not been achieved by formal study but established by inservicing, written instructions provided to all therapists, and formal competency testing. All classifications were checked at discharge by this author by review of patient notes.

Of the nine classifications, the most difficult to reach a consensus on was the classification of chronic low back pain (B8). Many clinicians make this classification according to duration of symptoms, usually greater than three to six months. However, as DeRosa and Porterfield[8] have indicated, the true definition of chronic pain should relate to the demonstration of abnormal illness behavior, and not relate to the duration of symptoms. Due to the recurrent nature of LBP in highly functioning individuals, the label *chronic* may be overly utilized. We arbitrarily chose 10 criteria that are commonly reported in the literature[19,20] as relating to abnormal illness behavior in patients with LBP, defining chronic back pain as being the presence of a minimum of 6 out of 10 of these criteria. These criteria are listed in Table 1.

Table 1. Criteria for Classification Using the Modified Quebec Classification Scheme

Modified Quebec classification	Criteria for classification
B1	Low back and/or buttock pain, area includes T12 to the gluteal fold. No neurological signs or symptoms in the lower extremity. This category includes those with pain in the iliosacral area.
B2	Low back pain with radiation into the proximal extremity (above the knee).
B3	Low back pain with radiation or symptoms into the distal extremity (below the knee).
B4	Low back pain with lower extremity pain, but the extremity pain being greater than the proximal symptoms.
B5	Low back pain due to a herniated intervertebral disc. Patient has neurological signs and diagnosis is confirmed by CT scan or MRI.
B6	Postsurgical low back and /or lower extremity pain, less than 6 months since surgery (such as laminectomy, discectomy, or fusion).
B7	Postsurgical low back and/or lower extremity pain, greater than 6 months since surgery.
B8	Chronic low back pain. Patients have a minimum of 6 of the following 10 criteria. 1. Off work and/or need help with most of home duties. 2. Oswestry score greater than 75. 3. Complains of whole leg giving way. 4. History of previous failed treatment. 5. Lies down greater than once per day because of increased pain. 6. Reports that pain is 5/5 on daily basis on the numerical analogue scale. 7. Pain on initiation of rotation. 8. Pain on gentle axial loading. 9. Excessive superficial tenderness on palpation. 10. Reports of having to attend the emergency room because of recurrent LBP.
B9	Other. This group included vertebral body fractures, spinal stenosis, and other conditions. It did not include fractures of the transverse processes or spondylolisthesis.

Following the initial modified Quebec classification, patients were also grouped according to duration of symptoms. The three categories of symptom duration chosen were those as recommended by the QTF[9]: less than seven days, seven days to seven weeks, and greater than seven weeks. We chose duration of symptoms as a classification to see if time between onset of symptoms and commencement of physical therapy was associated with a poorer outcome. If the back pain was recurrent, the date of the most recent exacerbation was used to give this classification. The third classification used was insurance status. We intended to test the commonly held perception that those patients that may have issues of secondary gain have a poorer outcome than those patients who have no such apparent gain. The patients were classified into one of six different insurance groups at commencement of treatment: commercial (e.g., Blue Cross), workers' compensation, Medicare, Medicaid, automobile, and private pay. The private pay group included patients who did not have insurance either because they were denied coverage from their carrier or they were uninsured from the outset.

Treatment

The clinic employs seven physical therapists, with a mean experience of 5.7 years. All therapists are well trained in current concepts of back care, including lumbar stabilization, joint mobilization, and osteopathic manual therapy. Assisting in patient care were four certified athletic trainers, a physical therapist assistant, and a physical therapy technician. The facility has a sports medicine focus with a well equipped gymnasium and an aquatic therapy pool. All staff were very compliant in the collection of data. Treatment frequency was usually two to three times per week. Physical therapy provided was either specified by the referring physician or determined by the evaluating physical therapist.

All of the clinical measures (Oswestry, FB, SLR) were recorded at initial evaluation and again at discharge on specific forms and entered on a PC database program (Paradox v.5.0, Borland Intl. Inc.). Criteria for discharge was either goals being met, treatment discontinued by the referring physician, or self discharge by the patient. If a patient was unavailable for collection of data at discharge, then it was assumed that no progress had been made and the most recent measurements were recorded, assuming that no further progress had been made.

Data Analysis

Significance of change within each classification for the clinical measures of forward bending, straight-leg raise, and Oswestry score was performed using paired t-tests with alpha set at 0.05. Data analysis was performed on a PC spreadsheet (Quattro Pro v.6.0, 1994 Novell Inc.). Between-group differences and effect size were analyzed using a repeated measures analysis of variance (ANOVA) and a multivariate analysis of variance (MANOVA), using SPSS software (6.1).

OUTCOMES

The outcomes of the patients in the modified Quebec task force classification (QTFC) are shown in Table 2. This shows that the majority of patients (79.5 percent) fall into the first three groups. There were only two patients who had clinical as well as special imaging evidence of lumbar disc herniation (B5). One patient in the "other" group (B9) had a spinal tumor originally undiagnosed by the referring physician. There were several instances of missing data in the analysis of the outcomes. This was often due to lack of compliance on behalf of the patient, or the treating clinician forgetting to record the data, or an incorrect entry into the PC database. The missing data does not seem to have influenced the overall results.

Paired t-tests showed significant change ($p < 0.05$) for all clinical measures in groups B1 to B3. The other five categories of patients (B4–B9) accounted for only 20.5 percent of the patients in this classification. In general these groups appeared to have worse outcomes compared to groups B1–B3 by not demonstrating within-group change. Though the B4 group (leg pain greater than low back pain) showed significant decreases in Oswestry score ($p = 0.0125$), there was no significant change in FB or SLR ($p = 0.21, 0.11$). The patient groups of B6–B9 showed no significant improvement in any clinical measure except for the Oswestry score in the B6 group (postsurgery < 6 months), which reduced to a mean of 26.3 +/– 10.5 from 44.0 +/– 7.3 ($p = 0.021$). Between-group analysis showed significant difference between groups in the modified Quebec classification for the variables of Oswestry score ($p = 0.006$) and SLR ($p = 0.002$). Table 2 showed that the chronic pain classification (B8) had an initial mean 64.6 +/– 13.4, compared to the nonreferred LBP group, which had a mean of 36.9 +/– 17.9. The chronic pain group also had a

Table 2. Outcome According to the Modified Quebec Task Force Classification (means and standard deviations). (Missing observations are recorded in parentheses.)

Modified QTFC	Age	No. Rx	Initial Oswestry	Final Oswestry	Initial Forward Bending	Final Forward Bending	Initial SLR	Final SLR
B1 (n = 99)	41.5+/–18.2 (42 males, 57 females)	7.9 +/–7.9	36.9+/–17.6	27.7+/–21.0*	24.1+/–19.2	18.8+/–17.7* (3)	58.1+/–23.3	67.0+/–19.1* (10)
B2 (n = 33)	41.5+/–16.3 (9 males, 24 females)	8.4+/–6.4	43.4+/–15.8	28.8+/–19.4*	29.8+/–19.0	23.8+/–19.1* (1)	56.3+/–19.5	63.5+/–16.5* (7)
B3 (n = 77)	49.1+/–16.3 (30 males, 40 females)	9.9+/–5.1	44.2+/–16.9	34.8+/–16.0*	26.8+/–17.5	21.3+/–17.6* (3)	49.4+/–18.7	53.5+/–20.1* (8)
B4 (n = 15)	47.9+/–16.8 (8 males, 7 females)	9.7+/–6.0	35.6+/–15.0	24.8+/–16.4*	21.0+/–16.7	17.9+/–16.8** (0)	57.8+/–26.4	64.4+/–23.5** (1)
B5 (n = 2)	37 (32,42) (1 male, 1 female)	2.5 (2,3)	24,46	24,46 (N\A)	6,0	6,0 (N\A)	15,80	15,80 (N\A)
B6 (n = 6)	53.2+/–11.3 (3 males, 3 females)	10.8+/–4.4	44.0+/–7.3	26.3+/–10.5*	29.4+/–17.2	24.8+/–12.9** (1)	40.0+/–30.8	45.0+/–28.7** (2)
B7 (n = 16)	51.2+/–13.4 (7 males, 9 females)	7.0+/–4.0	38.9+/–16.0	34.4+/–17.9**	31.5+/–20.5	29.5+/–19.3** (4)	49.9+/–23.8	48.8+/–27.0** (0)
B8 (n = 7)	39.4+/–4.8 (3 males, 4 females)	9.9+/–8.0	64.6+/–13.4	62.9+/–14.1**	41.4+/–25.4	40.3+/–25.1** (0)	25.8+/–26.8	25.8+/–26.8** (1)
B9 (n = 8)	46.5 +/–25.5 (3 males, 5 females)	7.5+/–5.0	54.1+/–19.8	49.8+/–20.6**	27.5+/–24.2	26.7+/–24.9** (2)	43.2+/–33.0	43.2+/–33.0** (2)

*Change in score significant beyond the level of 0.05 probability.
**Change not significant at 0.05 level of probability.

significantly reduced SLR, with a mean of 25.8 +/– 26.8 degrees on initial evaluation. With the dependent variable of number of treatments required, there was a trend noted in the modified Quebec classification: the further pain was referred down the extremity, the more treatment occurred. Patients who had back pain with radiation into the distal extremity (B3) required a mean of 9.9 +/– 5.1 treatments, whereas those with nonradiating symptoms (B1) required a mean of 7.9 +/– 7.9 treatments. These trends were not statistically significant.

Outcomes for patients grouped according to duration of symptoms are presented in Table 3. Significant improvement in all the clinical measures was found within all three groups of patients. There was a trend indicating that the shorter the duration of symptoms, the fewer the treatments that would be required. The "acute" group required only 6.5 +/– 4.0 treatments, whereas the longer duration groups required a mean of 8.3 +/– 7.0 and 9.2 +/– 7.5 treatments. This trend was not statistically significant.

In the classification of patients according to insurance (Table 4), there were significant decreases in Oswestry score for all groups except private pay ($p = 0.39$). For the clinical measures of FB and SLR there was no significant improvement for Medicaid, auto insurance, or private pay patients. Though the commercial insurance group had a mean discharge Oswestry score of 23.3 +/– 20.6 compared to 29.6 +/– 18.9 in the workers' compensation group, the difference was not considered to be significant. The highest Oswestry score on discharge was with the Medicaid group (44.8 +/– 20.4). The mean ages for this classification did not seem to be unusual compared to the other patient groupings, except Medicare patients had a mean age of 70.9 +/– 7.9 years. An ANOVA showed the most significant difference ($p < 0.000$) was number of treatments. The lowest number of treatments

was the commerically insured with a mean of 5.5 +/– 5.4, while the autoinsurance group was 17.9 +/– 20.0.

A repeated-measures ANOVA was also used to analyze before and after differences. This identified a significant difference in the pre and post measures of SLR ($p < 0.022$), with the three independent variables of class, duration, and time together. There were no differences for FB or Oswestry over time.

Data was also analyzed using the ANOVA controlling for effect size as suggested by recent physical therapy literature.[21,22] The effect sizes were small, ranging from 0.25 to 0.60, with the ANOVA showing SLR to be significantly different.

DISCUSSION

The evaluation of the outcomes presented in this paper show that in our clinic the majority of patients with low back pain show both functional and clinical improvement over the course of their physical therapy. These findings are not meant to be a substitute for a blinded controlled study, nor do they demonstrate any continuance of improvement beyond the period of treatment. The measured outcomes may have been the same with less or no treatment. Physical therapy *as a whole* seems to be beneficial in the short-term management of patients with low back pain. Our results showed that within the modified QTF classification, those patients with persistent lower extremity pain were associated with a poorer outcome. The lack of demonstrated improvement in FB and SLR in B4 patients (leg pain greater than back pain), according to Maitland,[23(p.126)] is possibly associated with nerve root irritation. DiFabio and others[4] showed that those patients with disc injuries showed no significant change in FB, SLR, or Oswestry score. Gill and others[5] in their series

---

Table 3. Outcome According to Duration of Symptoms (means and standard deviations). (Missing observations are recorded in parentheses.)

Symptom Duration	Age	No. Rx's	Initial Oswestry	Final Oswestry	Initial Forward Bending	Final Forward Bending	Initial SLR	Final SLR
< 7 days (n = 20)	34.4+/–13.9 (10 males, 10 females)	6.5+/–4.0	32.9+/–15.0	24.3+/–18.2*	28.2+/–21.2	20.5+/–17.7* (0)	52.6+/–22.0	65.4+/–19.3* (2)
7 days– 7 weeks (n = 111)	45.1+/–17.1 (43 males, 68 females)	8.3+/–7.0	42.3+/–16.6	27.3+/–20.8*	25.0+/–19.2	17.6+/–17.5* (5)	55.1+/–23.7	63.3+/–23.7* (11)
> 7 weeks (n = 132)	46.5+/–16.5 (55 males, 77 females)	9.2+/–7.5	40.6+/–17.4	34.1+/–19.1*	24.6+/–19.7	21.9+/–19.8* (10)	54.3+/–22.8	58.8+/–21.3* (20)

*Significant at a probability level of less than 0.05.
**Not significant at the 0.05 level.

Table 4. Outcome According to Insurance (means and standard deviations). (Missing observations are recorded in parentheses.)

Insurance	Age	No. Rx's	Initial Oswestry	Final Oswestry	Initial Forward Bending	Final Forward Bending	Initial SLR	Final SLR
Commercial (n = 82)	38.3+/–14.2 (32 males, 50 females)	5.5+/–5.4	37.1+/–18.8	23.3+/–20.6*	23.1+/–20.9	17.4+/–18.9* (6)	56.2+/–25.9	62.9+/–23.8* (14)
Workers' Comp. (n = 96)	40.9+/–9.8 (55 males, 41 females)	8.0+/–5.7	38.9+/–17.0	29.6+/–18.9*	26.9+/–18.3	21.0+/–18.0* (3)	53.3+/–21.1	61.9+/–22.3* (6)
Medicare (n = 47)	70.7+/–9.7 (11 males, 36 females)	8.9+/–5.4	44.1+/–11.8	34.7+/–16.3*	19.0+/–16.9	14.1+/–15.0* (5)	54.2+/–24.1	58.4+/–23.2* (8)
Medicaid (n = 22)	34.9+/–9.6 (6 males, 16 females)	6.0+/–4.8	49.8+/–16.6	44.8+/–20.4*	32.1+/–18.7	31.1+/–19.8** (0)	52.5+/–21.1	56.7+/–19.2** (3)
Auto. (n = 11)	42.2+/–16 (5 males, 6 females)	17.9+/–20.0	38.0+/–14.3	29.1+/–18.9*	29.8+/–20.6	30.7+/–19.9** (1)	58.3+/–22.4	60.6+/–23.3** (1)
Private (n = 5)	43.8+/–20.3 (5 females)	8.2+/–7.6	45.8+/–23.1	36.2+/–26.6**	22.0+/–25.4	22.0+/–25.4** (0)	59.0+/–19.6	68.0+/–21.4** (0)

*Significant at a probability level of less than 0.05.
**Not significant at the probability level of less than 0.05.

of 50 patients showed that the persistence of leg pain may be associated with a poorer outcome. In our series of patients we had only two patients with confirmed disc herniation and associated neurological signs. Perhaps many of our B4 patients had low-grade disc injuries and our classification scheme was not sensitive enough to detect the difference. A problem that we encountered was lost contact with the patient after discharge from physical therapy. Further follow-up may have resulted in reclassifying of some patients.

Other groups to perform poorly within the modified QTFCS were those classified as having chronic pain syndrome and postlumbar surgery patients. Neither of the postsurgical groups (B6, B7) showed any significant improvement in either FB or SLR within their group. The B6 group (less than six months from surgery) showed significant improvement in Oswestry score, whereas the B7 group did not. However, the small numbers in each group warrant cautious interpretation of these results. The lack of change in FB or SLR may owe to the treatment emphasis in these patients. The philosophy of this clinic is to focus on improving stability and strength in post-surgical patients; therefore range of motion (ROM) measures such as FB and SLR may not be sensitive and specific enough to detect clinical change. The clinic does not have a dynamometer to measure trunk strength and we were unaware of any reliable, inexpensive alternative test. Perhaps recording trunk strength would have shown a correlation with the decreasing Oswestry scores in these and other pa-

tients that showed improved Oswestry scores but no change in the ROM measures that were employed.

There was a poor response of the chronic pain patients (B8) to treatment, but there were only seven patients that matched the criteria used. We have a sports and orthopedic clinic lacking the multidisciplinary approach (e.g., psychological counseling) that is thought to be required when dealing with this patient group. Our treatment emphasis with these patients was improving function through improving physical conditioning in conjunction with biomechanical counseling. Our poor results with these patients suggests that we should consider referral to a more appropriate clinic after initial evaluation.

In regard to classifying patients according to duration of symptoms, one point of interest is the low number of patients with symptoms of less than seven days duration (n = 20). This is despite clinic policy of commencing treatment within two working days of every new referral. Informal discussion with some of our referring physicians and attention to patient history indicate that in our locale physicians prefer to treat acute LBP with limited rest and nonsteroidal anti-inflammatory medication. Our area also has a prominent chiropractic community, with many potential patients seeking chiropractic care for the treatment of acute LBP.

Approximately 50 percent of our patients had symptoms for longer than seven weeks, thus being beyond the normal spontaneous resolution time of six weeks. Though these patients demonstrated improvement in the outcomes of interest, improvement could only be regarded as modest. Our data showed a further trend: the longer the symptom duration, the higher the Oswestry score on discharge. The mean Oswestry score on discharge for the "greater than seven weeks" group was 34.1. Our experience with the Oswestry is that such a score would not enable a person to work in a job where there was any repetitive lifting or bending. Di Fabio and others,[4] in their study of workers' compensation patients, found at discharge from physical therapy that those classified as a "disc" injury had 45 percent rate of return to work, with a mean Oswestry of 38, compared to the "mechanical" pain group that had a 90 percent rate of return to work, with the mean Oswestry at discharge being 23. Therefore, even though there is a significant decrease in Oswestry score for patients whose symptoms last beyond seven weeks, it may not be of a sufficient decrease for the patient to return to full work or home duties. The change in means for the other two groups seems to be more clinically significant, though this was not statistically significant.

Of the patient grouping by insurance, Medicaid patients tended to have the worst outcome. Medicaid patients had a mean number of six treatments, but did not improve significantly in the measures of SLR or FB. Medicaid patients had the highest mean Oswestry score on initial evaluation (49.8) and showed statistical ($p = 0.038$) but not clinical significance in decrease of Oswestry score. The mean score on discharge was 44.8, with such a score, according to Fairbank and others,[13] representing a "severe disability." Thus we consider the decrease in score by five points to not be clinically significant. Also with the Medicaid group there was no difference in FB or SLR. The difference in Oswestry scores amongst insurance groups was not statistically significant. The tendency in our data is partially supported by Jette and Jette,[21] where low income, lower levels of education, and unemployment were associated with a poorer outcome in a large series of patients ($N = 739$) with low back pain. The tendency towards a poor outcome in Medicaid patients could be difficulty in adherence to a physical therapy rehabilitation program. Follow-up studies in our clinic show that up to 62 percent of these patients self-discharge from physical therapy before reaching their goals. We have also constructed a treatment "compliance ratio," which has been added to our database for the last 83 patients. This is a simple percentage of number of physical therapy appointments *kept,* divided by the number actually *made.* In the Medicare patients this percentage is 89 percent, while in the Medicaid group it is 65 percent. This indicates that individual goals are not being met for these patients. Goal setting should be a joint effort between patients and physical therapists, with clear explanation of the importance of treatment compliance.

• • •

The results of our series of 263 patients show that the majority will improve in the course of their physical therapy with both improved function, as measured by the Oswestry questionnaire, and improved ROM, demonstrated by changes in FB and SLR. Poorer outcomes seem to be associated with patients that have predominant leg pain. Postlumbar surgery patients, patients with chronic pain syndrome, and Medicaid patients also seem to be associated with less than favorable results. The physical therapist needs to consider these factors when assessing rehabilitation potential of the patient with low back pain.

REFERENCES

1. Jette, A.M., and Davis, K.D. "A Comparison of Hospital-based and Private Outpatient Physical Therapy Practice." *Physical Therapy* 71, no. 5 (1991): 366–75.

2. Cherkin, D.C., et al. "Physician Views about Treating Low Back Pain." *Spine* 20, no. 1 (1995): 1–10.

3. Rothstein, J.M., Delitto, A., and Scalzitti, D.A. "Understanding AHCPR Clinical Practice Guideline No. 14: Acute Low Back Problems in Adults." American Physical Therapy Association Guide. *PT Magazine* (September 1995): 2–24.

4. Di Fabio, R.P., Mackey, G., and Holte, J.B. "Physical Therapy Outcomes for Patients Receiving Workers' Compensation Following Treatment for Herniated Lumbar Disc and Mechanical Low Back Pain Syndrome." *Journal of Orthopedic and Sports Physical Therapy* 23, no. 3 (1996): 180–87.

5. Gill, C., et al. "Low Back Pain: Program Description and Outcome in a Case Series." *Journal of Orthopedic and Sports Physical Therapy* 20, no.1 (1994): 11–16.

6. Spratt, K.F. "A New Approach to the Low-Back Physical Examination." *Spine* 15 (1990): 96–102.

7. Deyo, R. "Practice Variations, Treatment Fads, Rising Disability. Do We Need a New Clinical Research Paradigm?" *Spine* 18, no. 15 (1993): 2153–62.

8. DeRosa, C.P., and Porterfield, J.A. "A Physical Therapy Model for the Treatment of Low Back Pain." *Physical Therapy* 72, no. 4 (1992): 261–72.

9. Spitzer, W.O. "Diagnosis of the Problem (the Problem of Diagnosis), Scientific Approach to the Assessment and Management of Activity Related Spinal Disorders: a Monograph for Clinicians, Report of the Quebec Task Force of Spinal Disorders." *Spine* 12 (suppl.) (1987): 16–21.

10. Delitto, A., et al. "A Treatment-Based Classification Approach to Low Back Pain: Identifying and Staging Patients for Conservative Treatment." *Physical Therapy* 75, no. 6 (1995): 470–80.

11. Delitto, A., et al. "Evidence of Use of an Extension Mobilization Category in Acute Low Back Syndrome: A Prescriptive Validation Pilot Study." *Physical Therapy* 73, no. 4 (1993): 216–18.

12. Rothstein, J. Editor's note: "Patient Classification." *Physical Therapy* 7, no. 4 (1993): 214–15.

13. Fairbank, J.C.T., et al. "The Oswestry Low Back Pain Disability Questionnaire." *Physiotherapy* 66 (1980): 271–73.

14. Deyo, R., et al. "Outcome Measures for Studying Patients with Low Back Pain." *Spine* 19 (Suppl.) (1994): 2032S–36S.

15. Kopec, J.A., and Esdaile, J.M. "Functional Disability Scales for Back Pain." *Spine* 20 (1995): 1943–49.

16. Matyas, T.A., and Bach, T.M. "The Reliability of Selected Techniques in Clinical Arthrometrics." *Australian Journal of Physiotherapy* 31, no. 5 (1985): 175–95.

17. Gauvin, M.G., Riddle, D.L., and Rothstein, J.M. "Reliability of Clinical Measurements of Forward Bending Using a Modified Fingertip-to-Floor Method." *Physical Therapy* 70, no. 7 (1990): 443–47.

18. McCombe, P.F., et al. "Reproducibility of Physical Signs in Low Back Pain." *Spine* 14, no. 9 (1989): 908–18.

19. Waddell, G., et al. "Chronic Low-Back Pain, Psychologic Distress, and Illness Behavior." *Spine* 9 (1984): 209–13.

20. Waddell, G., et al. "Objective Clinical Evaluation of Physical Impairment in Chronic Low Back Pain." *Spine* 17, no. 6 (1992): 617–28.

21. Jette, D.U., and Jette, A.M. "Physical Therapy and Health Outcomes in Patients with Spinal Impairments." *Physical Therapy* 76, no. 9 (1996): 930–45.

22. Stratford, P.W., Binkley, J.M., and Riddle, D.L. "Health Status Measures: Strategies and Analytic Methods for Assessing Change Scores." *Physical Therapy* 76, no. 10 (1996): 1109–23.

23. Maitland, G.D. *Vertebral Manipulation.* 5th ed. London: Butterworth-Heinemann, 1986.

20

The Effect of Timely Onset of Rehabilitation on Outpatient Orthopedic Practice: A Preliminary Report

Alphonso L. Amato, Edward A. Dobrzykowski, and Terri Nance

The duration of time from the patient's injury to the initiation of rehabilitation has been inferred as having an effect upon the eventual outcome. Clinicians have speculated that more favorable outcomes would result from more rapid onset of a patient's rehabilitation postinjury. It is taught that the appropriate acute treatment, including the use of therapeutic modalities, brief periods of immobilization and rest, exercise, and patient education assists in the protection of the injury while promoting healing. Beginning exercise regimens earlier within protected range of motion is hypothesized to result in less diminution of strength, residual loss of functioning, and morbidity, although because of the natural history of some clinical problems[1] and concerns about practice variations,[2] some authors caution against clinical rationale without statistical support.

There are several factors that contribute to the period of time that elapses prior to the initiation of outpatient orthopedic rehabilitation. Factors include a patient's reluctance to seek care, either from the belief that the injury will improve on its own; that the personal time for rehabilitation is not available; or that the health care is not affordable. Other potential impediments to timely initiation of rehabilitation are the new "gatekeepers," usually primary care physicians (PCPs) or rehabilitation case managers. They restrict authorization for patient access to health care services and administer rigid control over provider utilization in an attempt to control cost. Additionally, in some geographic locations, onset may be delayed due to the scarce availability of rehabilitation providers.

The measurement of patient outcomes in outpatient orthopedic rehabilitation is a process that considers patient-reported information (health-related quality of life, or HRQL, and satisfaction), clinician-reported information (functional gains and treatments performed), and administrative efficiency data (visits, duration, costs). Confounding variables, however, will influence the dependent variable, and must be controlled by design of statistical application before the results can be utilized. These variables can include but are not limited to age, diagnosis, severity of condition, extent of comorbidities, socioeconomic status, the number of prior occurrences, and the timing of the onset of rehabilitation. The process of measurement and control for these variables in the determination of outcomes is known as risk adjustment.[3]

The actual outcome benefit attributable to the timeliness of rehabilitation onset is of interest to the health care provider, payer, and patient. There are several positive implications if an enhanced outcome effect can be demonstrated through improved efficiency in referrals to orthopedic rehabilitation and expediency in the initiation of care. Physicians may be more apt to refer patients sooner status post musculoskeletal injury or surgery, payer systems may provide benefit plans that encourage and incentivize early use of rehabilitation, and there may be increased support for the public's direct access to rehabilitation providers and availability of patient reimbursement without the necessity for PCP referral. If an enhanced outcome effect cannot be demonstrated, then more rigid control of rehabilitation provider utilization may be warranted.

The purpose of this preliminary review is to investigate outcomes as the time between onset of musculoskeletal disorders and rehabilitation, and the age of the patient varies. Patients in rehabilitation services in outpatient orthopedic practice were studied. The outcome measures evaluated were patient HRQL, patient satisfaction, the number of outpatient visits, and cost. The method chosen to address this inquiry was the examination of a sample of the Focus On Therapeutic Outcomes, Inc. (FOTO, Knoxville, Tennessee)

J Rehabil Outcomes Meas, 1997, 1(3), 32–38

orthopedic rehabilitation outcomes database. The FOTO outcomes database sample consisted of 24,196 patient episodes of outpatient orthopedic rehabilitation, collected from 384 facilities located in 34 states, during 1995 and 1996. The selected FOTO database outcome measures were patient HRQL, patient satisfaction, the number of visits, episode length (days), and the cost of rehabilitation. Efficiency was measured in number of visits, cost, and episode length. Effectiveness was measured in health status (using an outcomes index and a values index), and in satisfaction. Patients were classified into three age groups: all patients; patients less than 45 years of age; and patients equal to or greater than 45 years of age, respectively. Also captured in the data set were the date of injury onset, the date of initiation of rehabilitation, and the date of conclusion of rehabilitation. The levels of acuity (time from onset of condition until beginning rehabilitation) evaluated were: 0–7 days, 8–15 days, 16–30 days, 31–60 days, 61–90 days, 91–120 days, and 121+ days.

DESCRIPTION OF OUTCOME EFFICIENCY MEASURES

Each occasion a patient is seen for treatment in outpatient rehabilitation is defined as a visit. Visits are reported in the FOTO system as the mean number of visits per episode (defined as the time from initiation until conclusion of rehabilitation). The mean number of visits per group (total; patients less than 45 years of age; patients equal to or greater than 45 years of age) is calculated by dividing the total number of visits in each impairment group by the total number of patients in the same group. The rationale for the inclusion of this particular indicator is to assist providers in the management of their utilization, while beginning to study factors that influence practice variation in the number of visits. What is the appropriate level of resources and number of visits to achieve an optimal outcome result in musculoskeletal rehabilitation? Is the total number of patient visits in a particular episode of care influenced by the timing of the onset of rehabilitation services, positing a relationship to the date of injury? Patients seen for the first time by a rehabilitation provider with a more chronic injury or delayed onset of rehabilitation may have experienced considerable strength and loss of range of motion, become generally debilitated, and may be depressed.[4]

The measurement of actual rehabilitation cost for many service providers is an arduous process, ranging from the administration of numerous payer plans posing varying levels of reimbursement, the inclusion of rehabilitation costs with nonrehabilitation costs, and the increasing prevalence of capitation methods of reimbursement. There must, however, be reasonable accuracy in cost reporting for valid comparisons among providers.

A cost method that reports total gross charges would artificially inflate the true cost to the health care system, and not reflect the actual revenue the provider receives for services rendered. Very few rehabilitation providers today receive their full "list" charges. A more appropriate method for the measurement and comparison of cost among providers is the recording of the revenue received. For example, a patient's total (list) cost is $1,200. As the patient belongs to a preferred provider organization (PPO) that provides for a 25 percent discount, the net billed cost is $900. The net billed cost of $900 should be entered in the FOTO database.

The FOTO database and measurement protocol defines cost as the revenue providers expect to receive, which follows any preliminary payer contractual adjustments (reductions). As a result, the enhanced confidence in the cost noted provides more accurate comparisons by payer type (indemnity plan, preferred provider arrangement, workers' compensation, Medicare, Medicaid, health maintenance organization, litigation, patient self pay). The FOTO outcomes management report represents cost as the mean total revenue in an episode of rehabilitative care.

The effect of timing of rehabilitation onset on the number of visits and cost will be evaluated in patients with musculoskeletal dysfunction.

DESCRIPTION OF OUTCOME EFFECTIVENESS MEASURES

The measurement and reporting of functional outcomes and patient HRQL in rehabilitation is increasingly desired by payers, referral sources, providers, patients, and other consumers of health care services. In response to this need, the FOTO musculoskeletal outcomes measurement system initially started with the Medical Outcomes Study SF-36™ health status survey (Medical Outcomes Trust, Boston, MA). The SF-36 (Short Form-36) health status survey has been previously tested for reliability and validity[5–9] and has become a preferred and accepted method in the measurement of patient-reported health status in ambulatory health care services.

In early piloting and implementation of the FOTO musculoskeletal outcomes measurement system (1993–1994), in addition to the SF-36, the original design included disease specific measures for orthopedic conditions. These included the Oswestry Low Back Pain Disability Questionnaire,[10] the Neck Disability Index,[11] and the Lysholm scale[12] for low back, neck, and knee patients respectively. FOTO was able to demonstrate the responsiveness and utility of some of the domains of the SF-36 in outpatient musculoskeletal rehabilitation (unpublished work, personal communication, Alan Jette, PhD, PT, New England Research Institute, Watertown, MA). Later, correlation was found[13,14] between the domains of bodily pain, physical functioning (an example of this domain is displayed in the box), and role limitations-physical and the disease specific measures. Our analyses determined that we would not lose much power in the instrument if we did not collect the disease specific questions. As a result, FOTO deleted a limited number of questions of the SF-36; however, all items of the physical domain were retained. FOTO deleted entirely the disease specific questionnaires, which reduced respondent burden.

Outcomes Index

FOTO reports the change in patient health status as the Outcomes Index (OI).[15] The FOTO OI is calculated as a functional score of the six domains (bodily pain, physical, role limitations-physical, social function, energy/fatigue, and health perceptions). Using the functional scores of each of the six domains calculated at both admission to and discharge from rehabilitation, we can compute an effect size change score.[16,17] The OI is defined as:

$$\frac{\text{Health status score at discharge} - \text{health status score at admission}}{\text{Standard deviation of health status score at admission}}$$

The OI is calculated as an average of the effect sizes. For simplification in reporting, the OI is then multiplied by 100. A greater gain in health status is reflected by a higher OI.

The OI documents the magnitude of the effect size, and represents the change in health status over the time of the rehabilitation episode. A typical OI is interpreted as a standardized unit of functional improvement. For example, an OI of "56" means that the patient improved from admission to discharge .56 standard deviation units.

SF-36: Physical Functioning Domain

The following items are about activities you might do during a typical day. Does your health now limit you in these activities? If so, how much? (Responses are: yes, limited a lot; yes, limited a little; no, not limited at all)

- Vigorous activities, such as running, lifting heavy objects, participating in strenuous sports
- Moderate activities, such as moving a table, pushing a vacuum cleaner, bowling, or playing golf
- Lifting or carrying groceries
- Climbing several flights of stairs
- Climbing one flight of stairs
- Bending, kneeling, or stooping
- Walking more than a mile
- Walking several blocks
- Walking one block
- Bathing or dressing yourself

Courtesy of Medical Outcomes Trust, Boston, Massachusetts.

The value of timing of rehabilitation onset on the OI will be evaluated in patients with musculoskeletal dysfunction.

Value Index

The effectiveness of rehabilitation must be balanced with the cost of the provision of services. FOTO reports an index on the value of the health status change achieved for the costs of the rehabilitation incurred over an episode of care, known as the Value Index (VI).[17] The FOTO VI is calculated as:

$$\frac{\text{Outcome Index}}{\text{Episode Cost}}$$

Episode is defined in days from the initiation until the conclusion of rehabilitation. The cost is defined as the net cost incurred following any initial adjustment for provisions in payer contracts.

The effect of timing of rehabilitation on the VI will be evaluated in patients with musculoskeletal dysfunction.

Patient Satisfaction

Patient satisfaction has been utilized for several years as an essential indicator of outcome. The FOTO system includes nine items pertaining to patient satisfaction (see box). A patient satisfaction index (PSI) has been developed to report on a rating of overall patient satisfaction result in the facility. PSI is calculated and reported as a percentage, with a range possible from 0 to 100 percent, with higher percentages representing greater levels of patient satisfaction. An examination will be made of the database to evaluate the effect of rehabilitation timing on PSI in patients with musculoskeletal dysfunction.

RESULTS

The efficiency and effectiveness of rehabilitation in 24,196 patient episodes, collected during 1995–1996 by FOTO, were evaluated. There were 14,033 females (58 percent) and 10,163 males (42 percent). The age of the sample population ranged from 18 to 93 years, with a mean of 44.8 years.

The timing of rehabilitation onset was evaluated against the mean of each of the following: the number of visits, cost, OI, VI, and PSI. The results of the analysis are displayed in Tables 1–3. Visits, cost, OI, VI, and PSI are evaluated in categories of: all patients; patients less than 45 years of age; and patients equal to or greater than 45 years of age, respectively.

VISITS

The mean number of visits for all patients was 7.5 visits at 0–7 days postinjury, increased to a peak of 8.7 visits at 31–60

Patient Satisfaction Items

Over the course of treatment for this primary injury/condition, how satisfied were you with: (responses are very satisfied; somewhat satisfied; neither satisfied nor dissatisfied; somewhat dissatisfied; very dissatisfied)
- The information you were given about your condition?
- The treatments for your condition?
- Your overall therapy care?
- Your primary clinician?
- Your ability to schedule a convenient appointment time?
- Length of time in the waiting room?
- Getting through to the office by phone?
- Convenience of the location?
- Based on my experience at this facility, I would tell a friend that I was?

Courtesy of Focus On Therapeutic Outcomes, Inc., Knoxville, Tennessee.

days, and declined to 7.8 visits for over 121 days. In patients less than 45 years of age, the mean number of visits was 7.0 visits at 0–7 days postinjury, increased to a peak of 8.4 visits at 31–60 days, and declined to 7.6 visits for over 121 days. In patients 45 years of age or older, the mean number of visits was 8.3 visits at 0–7 days postinjury, increased to a peak of 9.1 visits at 16–30 days, then declined to 8.0 visits for over 121 days.

The overall mean for all patients is approximately 8.0 visits. Fewer visits tend to occur if rehabilitation is initiated within the first 30 days after onset of the condition. In this preliminary review, there does not appear to be a relationship demonstrated between the number of visits and the acuity level of the condition.

COST

The mean cost for all patients generally increased as the length of elapsed time increased from the onset of the injury to the initiation of rehabilitation. For all patients, the mean cost was least at $748, 0–7 days postinjury, and peaked at

$869, 91–120 days postinjury. In patients less than 45 years of age, the mean cost was least at $692, 0–7 days postinjury, and peaked at $890, 91–120 days postinjury. With patients 45 years of age or older, the mean cost was least at $761, 121+ days postinjury, and peaked at $872, 16–30 days postinjury.

In this preliminary review there does not appear to be a correlation of cost and the acuity of the patient's injury, although patients 45 years of age or greater tend to exhibit higher cost for rehabilitation services.

OUTCOMES INDEX

When patients of all ages and diagnoses are evaluated, the mean outcomes index (69.0) peaks at a high of 8–15 days after onset of injury, then declines steadily as the elapsed time increases since onset of injury. A similar pattern emerges for the group of patients less than 45 years of age, and the group of patients 45 years of age or greater.

VALUE INDEX

The mean value index (61.8) for patients of all ages and diagnoses peaks at 0–7 days after onset of injury, then declines steadily as the elapsed time increases since onset of injury. A similar pattern is evident for patients less than 45 years of age. In the age group of patients 45 years of age or greater, the mean value index (69.3) peaks at 8–15 days after onset of injury, then declines steadily as the elapsed time increases since onset of injury.

PATIENT SATISFACTION INDEX

The mean patient satisfaction index for all patients peaked at 96.1 for the groups of 8–15 days and 16–30 days after onset of injury until initiation of rehabilitation. In patients less than 45 years of age, the patient satisfaction index peaks at 96.2 for the groups of 0–7 days and 8–15 days after onset of injury. In patients 45 years of age or greater, the patient satisfaction index peaks at 96.5, 16–30 days postinjury. Patient satisfaction was higher in the patient age group of 45 years and older.

Table 1. Total Elapsed Days From Injury Until Onset of Rehabilitation: All Patients

Days	0–7	8–15	16–30	31–60	61–90	91–120	121+
Visits	7.5	8.4	8.5	8.7	8.5	8.5	7.8
Cost	$748	$840	$844	$859	$842	$869	$761
OI	61.8	69.0	57.1	48.2	39.4	36.0	32.6
VI	82.6	82.1	67.6	56.1	46.8	41.4	42.9
PSI	95.9	96.1	96.1	95.3	95.4	95.3	94.3

Table 2. Total Elapsed Days From Injury Until Onset of Rehabilitation: Patients under 45 Years of Age

Days	0–7	8–15	16–30	31–60	61–90	91–120	121+
Visits	7.0	8.1	8.0	8.4	8.0	8.3	7.6
Cost	$692	$828	$821	$862	$814	$890	$761
OI	70.8	76.6	62.2	50.7	39.6	40.1	35.3
VI	102.4	92.6	75.7	58.9	48.6	45.1	46.3
PSI	96.2	96.2	95.7	95.0	94.2	94.5	93.4

• • •

The timely onset of outpatient orthopedic rehabilitation services following a musculoskeletal impairment has been recommended by both physicians and rehabilitation professionals for a variety of reasons. The rationale for early intervention stems from a desire to manage the inflammatory process of the injury, to provide education for the patient on appropriate body mechanics and protection for the injury, and to facilitate the necessary healing through controlled movement and exercise while minimizing the potential detrimental effects of immobilization. As a patient's injury becomes more chronic in nature, particularly in workers' compensation and litigated cases, the potential influence and effect upon outcome from secondary gain factors should be considered.

In an attempt to explore the potential effect of elapsed time from injury until the initiation of rehabilitation upon outcome, a sample of patients with orthopedic dysfunction contained in the FOTO database were assessed. The outcome measures selected included the number of visits, cost, patient HRQL (OI and VI), and patient satisfaction (PSI). The database sample was explored in total, as well as in two age ranges: those patients less than 45 years of age, and those patients 45 years of age and greater.

There were no apparent consistent trends in the number of visits or cost in the seven categories of acuity evaluated: 0–7 days, 8–15 days, 16–30 days, 31–60 days, 61–90 days, 91–120 days, and 121+ days elapsed from injury until onset of rehabilitation, or for patients in all age ranges. The similarity in utilization (visit) levels among patients with acuity levels 0–121+ days suggests that there are factors other than acuity level that are driving the utilization level. These factors can include the type of payer, influence of managed care, and increased cost shifting directly to patients.

Both the OI and VI showed positive gain, on an average, with the patients sampled. The magnitude of the gains were higher in patients less than 45 years of age. Patients treated within the first 15 days postinjury had greater improvement in HRQL. The magnitude of gain declined as the number of total elapsed days increased from the time of injury until onset of rehabilitation.

There were no apparent differences in PSI across all patient ages. Patients at least 45 years of age tend to rate their satisfaction levels higher than patients less than 45 years of age.

The measurement and achievement of patient outcome is complex. Outcome effectiveness and efficiency may be influenced by a number of confounding factors, including many that are beyond the control of the rehabilitation service provider. In an attempt to evaluate the potential effect upon outcome by the timing of onset for rehabilitation, the FOTO orthopedic database was examined. In this preliminary review, there was no apparent trend toward fewer visits or less cost with earlier rehabilitation intervention. There was a tendency toward a greater gain in HRQL with earlier rehabilitation intervention. This study and its results suggest the need to further evaluate outcomes of rehabilitation in outpatient orthopedic practice with statistical control of potential confounding variables, and by specific diagnosis classifications.

Table 3. Total Elapsed Days From Injury Until Onset of Rehabilitation: Patients 45 Years of Age or Older

Days	0–7	8–15	16–30	31–60	61–90	91–120	121+
Visits	8.3	8.8	9.1	9.0	9.0	8.65	8.0
Cost	$827	$858	$872	$856	$866	$850	$761
OI	50.7	59.5	52.1	45.8	39.5	32.5	30.5
VI	61.3	69.3	59.7	53.5	45.6	38.2	40.1
PSI	95.6	96.0	96.5	95.7	96.3	96.1	95.1

REFERENCES

1. Von Korff, M. "Studying the National History of Back Pain." *Spine* 30, no. 185 (1994): 2041S–46S.

2. Deyo, R. "Practice Variations, Treatment Fads, Rising Disability. Do We Need a New Clinical Research Paradigm?" *Spine* 18, no. 15 (1993): 2153–62.

3. Dobrzykowski, E. "Risk Adjustment in Rehabilitation." *Journal of Rehabilitation Outcomes Measurement* 1, no. 2 (April 1997): 11–15.

4. Wadell, G. "A New Clinical Model for the Treatment of Low Back Pain." *Spine* 12 (1987): 632–44.

5. McHorney, C.A., Ware, J.E., Rogers, W.H., Razek, A., and Lu, J.F.R. "The Validity and Relative Precision of MOS Short- and Long-form Health Status Scales and Dartmouth COOP Charts: Results from the Medical Outcomes Study." *Medical Care* 30(suppl. 5) 1992: MS253–MS265.

6. Ware, J.E., Kosinski, M., and Keller, S.D. "A 12-Item Short-Form Health Survey; Construction of Scales and Preliminary Tests of Reliability and Validity." *Medical Care* 34, no. 3 (1996): 220–33.

7. Jenkinson, C., Wright, L., and Coulter, A. "Criterion Validity and Reliability of the SF-36 in a Population Sample." *Quality Life Research* 3, no. 1 (1994): 7–12.

8. Lyons, R.A., Perry, H.M., and Littlepage, B.N. "Evidence for the Validity of the Short-Form 36 Questionnaire (SF-36) in an Elderly Population." *Aging* 23, no. 3 (1994): 182–84.

9. Ruta, D.A., Abdalla, M.I., Garratt, A.M., Coutts, A., and Russell, I.T. "The SF-36 Health Survey Questionnaire: I. Reliability in Two Patient-based Studies." *Quality in Health Care* 32, no. 3 (1994): 180–85.

10. Fairbank, J.C.T. "The Oswestry Low Back Pain Disability Questionnaire." *Physiotherapy* 66, no. 8 (1980): 271–73.

11. Vernon, H., and Mior, S. "The Neck Disability Index: A Study of Reliability and Validity." *Journal of Manipulative and Physiological Therapeutics* 14 (1991): 409–15.

12. Tegner, Y., and Lysholm, J. "Rating Systems in the Evaluation of Knee Ligament Injuries." *Clinical Orthopaedics and Related Research* 198 (1985): 43–48.

13. Jette, D.U., and Jette, A.M. "Physical Therapy and Health Outcomes in Patients with Spinal Impairments." *Physical Therapy* 76, no. 9 (1996): 930–41.

14. Jette, D.U., and Jette, A.M. "Physical Therapy and Health Outcomes in Patients with Knee Impairments." *Physical Therapy* 76, no. 11 (Nov. 1996): 1178–87.

15. Dobrzykowski, E., and Nance, T. "The Focus On Therapeutic Outcomes (FOTO) Outpatient Orthopedic Rehabilitation Database: Results of 1994–1996." *Journal of Rehabilitation Outcomes Measurement* 1, no. 1 (Feb. 1997): 56–60.

16. Stratford, P.W., Binkley, J.M., and Riddle, D.L. "Health Status Measures: Strategies and Analytic Methods for Assessing Change Scores." *Physical Therapy* 76, no. 10 (1996): 1109–23.

17. Kazis, L.E., Anderson, J.J., and Meenan, R.F. "Effect Sizes for Interpreting Changes in Health Status." *Medical Care* 27, no. 3 (1989, suppl.): S178–89.

21

Hip Fracture and Subacute Service Utilization of Medicare Beneficiaries: Trends and Patterns

Thomas T.H. Wan, Meri Beth Stegall, and Scott Stegall

INTRODUCTION

Care following that received in an acute care hospital has been variously described as subacute, postacute, or posthospital. According to the International Subacute Healthcare Association and the Joint Commission on Accreditation of Healthcare Organizations, subacute care is defined as "comprehensive services rendered immediately after, or instead of, acute hospitalization to treat one or more specific, active complex medical conditions or to administer one or more technically complex treatments in the context of a person's underlying long-term conditions and overall situation."[1] Relatively little literature exists on the changes in the relationship between the use of hospital services and subsequent use of rehabilitation services.

Hip fractures cause considerable morbidity, mortality, and expense for the elderly. The annual incidence of hip fracture is 8.2 per 1,000 population aged 65 and older in the United States. Every year there are, on average, 250,000 hip fracture patients, costing an estimate of $10–20 billion in direct medical care.[2–5] The objective of this study is to examine the relationship between the use of acute hospital services to treat hip fracture and the destination at discharge.

After implementation of Medicare's prospective payment System (PPS), concomitant changes in services utilization were observed in the elderly population: increase in use of rehabilitation services and decrease in the average length of their hospital stays. Rehabilitation and long-term care facilities are excluded from PPS reimbursement; Medicare pays them on a reasonable cost basis. Evidence in recent years has illustrated that PPS has increased the likelihood that patients will be discharged home in an unstable condition; the studies have empirically validated the widely held perception that under PPS Medicare patients were being released "sicker and quicker."[6–9] Length of stay reductions in acute care hospitals have created an increased use of rehabilitation services in subacute settings; in effect, care in these settings is being substituted for care in the acute care setting.[10,11] A serious concern for Medicare beneficiaries needing rehabilitative care is that care across all subacute settings is not equivalent. It follows that comparable rehabilitative outcomes are not ensured. Although the combined short-term costs of acute care and rehabilitation may be lower when rehabilitation care takes place outside the acute care setting, that is, in a rehabilitation hospital or unit, an implication is that the long-term cost may be more, because hip fracture patients may remain in nursing homes over the long term; costs are being shifted from the acute care sector to the long-term care sector.

This study examined whether care in subacute settings is being substituted for that in acute care settings, for patients with hip fractures. The primary proposition of the study was that subacute care is being used as a substitute for acute care services, for patients with continued care needs. Two hypotheses were formulated, using the discharge destinations from hospital data for Medicare patients to identify utilization patterns, as follows:

Hypothesis 1: The average proportion of patients discharged to subacute care settings is positively related to the average length of stay (ALOS) in the acute care hospital, after controlling for the differences in patient and hospital characteristics.

Hypothesis 2: The average proportion of patients discharged to subacute care settings is inversely related to the average deflated total inpatient charge, after controlling for the differences in patient and hospital characteristics.

J Rehabil Outcomes Meas, 1997, 1(4), 23–34

RELATED RESEARCH

Medicare is the single largest payer for rehabilitative services, covering over 50 percent of all discharges from such facilities, which account for, on average, 40 percent of revenues in rehabilitation hospitals and more than 50 percent in distinct-part units.[12,13] Since the implementation of the PPS for acute care hospitals, Medicare expenditures for rehabilitation services have increased. Expenditures for care rendered in rehabilitation hospitals and units increased from 0.6 percent of Medicare total inpatient hospital payments in 1984, to 1.1 percent in 1985, 1.4 percent in 1986, and 1.5 percent in 1987.[13] Table 1 presents the growth of rehabilitation hospitals and distinct-part units from 1984 to 1994.

Medicare regulations exclude the following five types of hospitals from PPS reimbursement: psychiatric hospitals, rehabilitation hospitals, children's hospitals, long-term care hospitals, and cancer hospitals. In addition, rehabilitation distinct-part units within a hospital are also exempt from PPS reimbursement. Medicare will reimburse these hospitals and units on a reasonable cost basis, subject to an annual target ceiling or target amount.[1,14,15]

The target ceiling is a cap on the operating costs per case for which Medicare will reimburse the specialty hospital or units.[14] Each provider's target amount equals the provider's allowable operating costs per case for the base period, increased by a statutorily prescribed inflation factor. For specialty hospitals, the primary reimbursement issue has concerned costs that exceed the provider's target amount. A Prospective Payment Assessment Commission analysis based on 1989 cost data is shown in Table 2.[16]

Subacute care sites for hip fracture patients reimbursed under the Medicare Part A benefit include home services provided by a home health agency, skilled nursing facilities, rehabilitation hospitals, and distinct-part rehabilitation units of acute care hospitals. The purposes of providing services by varying service settings are noted in Table 3.

Factors Associated with Postacute Care Utilization

A few studies have examined the combined effect of patient, hospital, and community attributes on the use of postacute care services.[17–19] Neu and Harrison[20] used personal attributes and medical market area characteristics to explain variations in Medicare postacute care utilization. They found that skilled nursing facility services and home health care appear to be substitutes for each other (*substitution* was defined as a substitution in practice; the study did not assess whether these two services are medical substitutes). Neu and Harrison[20] also suggested that the availability of skilled nursing facility (SNF) beds in metropolitan areas only has a negligible effect on the variation in use of postacute care. In analyzing the use of postacute care services by Medicare patients, Kane et al.[10] found that the variables significantly associated with the discharge location vary with the diagnosis-related group (DRG) and geographic location examined. However, functional status and living situation of Medicare patients were better predictor variables than the DRG and geographic location for the choice of a care modality (e.g., no formal care at home, home health care, nursing home care, or rehabilitation).

Hip Fracture Studies

In a study of elderly persons admitted to a large community hospital from 1981 to 1986, Fitzgerald, Moore, and

Table 2. ProPAC Analysis of Costs That Exceed Provider's Target Amount

Type of facility	Percentage over target amount
Rehabilitation facilities	53
Hospital	43
Distinct-part units	55
Psychiatric facilities	66
Hospital	61
Distinct-part units	68
Long-term hospitals	72
Children's hospitals	58
Cancer hospitals	57

Source: Reprinted from ProPac, Interim Report on Payment Reform for PPS-Excluded Facilities, Congressional Report C-92-05, October 1992.

Table 1. Number of Rehabilitation Hospitals and Distinct-Part Units Excluded from the Medicare Prospective Payment System: Fiscal Years 1984–1994

	1984	1985	1986	1987	1988	1990	1992	1993	1994
Hospital	49	68	79	84	100	135	166	184	187
Units	308	386	473	535	565	687	—	—	804

Note: — Data not available.

Table 3. Definition of Health Facility Purpose

Health benefit	Purpose
Home health agency	To provide a less intensive and less expensive alternative to short-stay hospital inpatient care.
Skilled nursing facility	To reduce the length of stay in acute-care hospitals for patients who need daily skilled nursing or rehabilitative services, but who no longer require the constant availability of physician services in the hospital setting.
Distinct-part rehabilitation	To provide rehabilitation services within the units established by acute-care hospitals.
Rehabilitation hospital	To provide rehabilitation services in a rehabilitation hospital.

Dittus[7] found: (1) the mean length of hospitalization for hip fracture decreased; (2) patients were discharged more often to the nursing home; and (3) after one year, patients were more likely to still be in nursing homes. The findings of this study also illustrate that patients having surgery for hip fracture after the implementation of PPS have 50 percent fewer in-hospital therapy sessions than before. Additionally, more of the PPS patients are discharged to a nursing home for rehabilitation; 33 percent of hip fracture patients, compared to 9 percent before PPS, transferred to the nursing home. These types of responses to PPS may have significant implications for changes in utilization patterns as the cost of care for Medicare beneficiaries increases, as long-term care providers exercise their option to admit lighter care, as private-pay patients need less services, and as more patients are discharged to rehabilitation hospitals and units.

Palmer and his colleagues[21] replicated the study design of Fitzgerald et al. by analyzing the experience of 386 Medicare beneficiaries with hip fractures in a private, suburban teaching hospital between the years 1981 and 1987. They found: (1) a decrease in mean acute length of stay, from 17 to 12.9 days; (2) a decrease in the mean number of physical therapy sessions, from 11.1 to 9.8; (3) an increase in the number of physical therapy treatments per day, from 1.2 to 1.4; (4) no change in the proportion of patients discharged to nursing homes, 52.9 percent before PPS compared to 54.6 percent after PPS; (5) no significant difference between the proportions of patients institutionalized at six months, 22.6 percent versus 19.9 percent; (6) no difference in total adjusted average hospital charges before and after PPS; and (7) no difference in the six-month ambulation status.

In a study of changes in medical stability upon admission to a free-standing rehabilitation facility, Marciniak, Heinemann, and Monga[22] found that readmission patterns differed by diagnosis: stroke, brain injury, and hip fracture patients were infrequently readmitted, and spinal cord injury and amputation patients were more likely to be readmitted. Thus, a focus on the utilization patterns of patients with infrequent readmissions is more appropriate when examining the substitution of rehabilitation services for hospital acute care.

In a report prepared by the Prospective Payment Assessment Commission, an exploratory analysis of Medicare data on episodes of illness in 1988 showed that only 8.2 percent of Medicare patients with hip fractures were discharged to rehabilitation facilities for postacute care, whereas 35 percent of patients used SNF services and 31 percent used home health services. Forty-one percent of these patients did not use any postacute care. The demographic and insurance characteristics of users of postacute care services are detailed in Table 4.

From multivariate statistical analysis of the Medicare data on episodes of illness (Prospective Payment Assessment Commission, 1992), sicker patients with hip fractures—measured by length of hospital stay, number of secondary diagnoses during hospitalization, prior SNF use, and prior home health use—were more likely to use SNFs and less likely to use home health services. Several nondemographic and health status characteristics, such as reimbursement rates and supplies of SNF beds, were associated with use of SNFs and home health services. These findings shed some light on the inequitable use of postacute care services by hip fracture patients. However, the substitutability between acute and subacute care services is not apparent from the analysis of Medicare data on episodes of illness.

METHODS

This study examines the relationship between acute care hospitalization and use of subacute care services to discover if a substitution of rehabilitation services for acute care hospital services is occurring. Therefore, a diagnosis (e.g., hip fracture) that does not require frequent rehospitalization but does require subsequent rehabilitative services in a subacute care setting is selected for examination.

Diagnosis

DRG 210 includes the following operating room procedures:

7705	Femoral sequestrectomy	7835	Femur length change
7725	Femoral wedge ostectomy	7845	Oth femur repair/plastic
7735	Femoral division NEC	7855	Internal fixation—femur
7785	Partial ostectomy—femur	7875	Osteoclasis—femur
7795	Total ostectomy—femur	7895	Insert bone stim—femur
7805	Bone graft to femur	7915	Closed red—int fix femur

Table 4. Use of Post–Acute Care by Hip Fracture Patients in 1988

Demographics	None	Rehabilitation	Skilled nursing facility	Home health agency
Age				
< 65	7.9%	13.9%	21.8%	56.4%
65–74	8.6	21.7	27.0	42.7
75–84	8.8	34.4	22.5	34.3
85+	6.9	40.8	14.6	37.6
Sex				
Male	7.9	30.7	20.1	41.3
Female	8.1	35.3	20.2	36.5
Race				
White	8.0	35.1	19.9	37.0
African American	7.8	17.3	28.1	46.7
Other	7.7	21.7	25.9	44.8
Unknown	8.4	31.9	17.1	42.6
Medicare eligible				
Disabled	8.1	13.8	23.1	55.1
Aged	8.0	34.1	20.2	37.1
Medicaid				
Dual-eligible	4.5	34.0	15.6	46.0
Non–Medicaid	8.5	34.3	20.8	36.4

Source: Reprinted from Prospective Payment Assessment Commission, *Interim Report on Payment Reform for PPS-Excluded Facilities.* Washington, DC: Prospective Payment Assessment Commission, Congressional Rep C-92-05, 1992.

7925	Open reduction—femur fx	8015	Oth arthrotomy—hip
7935	Open reduc—int fix femur	8045	Hip structure division
7945	Close reduc—femur ephiphy	8075	Hip synovectomy
7955	Opn red—sep ephiphy—femur	8095	Excision of hip NEC
7965	Debrid opn fx—femur	8121	Arthrodesis of hip
7985	Open reduc—hip dislocat	8140	Repair of hip, NEC
7995	Femur injury op NOS	8310	Adductor tenotomy of hip
8005	Arthrot/prs remov—hip		

Sample and Data Sources

The population chosen for this study consisted of all short-term, general, acute care hospitals in urban areas. In the present study only survivors of hospitalization are included. Hospitals in states with Medicare waivers (Maryland, New York, Massachusetts, and New Jersey) were excluded. Only urban hospitals were included, in order to control for differences in trends due to the availability of rehabilitation services. In addition, the exclusion criteria included: hospitals not under the PPS, hospitals with fewer than 15 discharges in DRG 210, and patients under 70 years of age.

The study focused on the following three subgroups of hospitals over a period of seven years (1984–1990): (1) those with a rehabilitation unit for all seven years of the study; (2) those that began and continued such a unit in 1986 or 1987; and (3) those that did not have a unit any time during the seven-year study period. After excluding missing and problematic data, a total of 7,456 hospital-years were analyzed. The unit of analy-sis is the hospital-year. Hospitals without a rehab unit during the entire period represent 5,764 hospital-years. Hospitals with a unit throughout the period represent 1,098 hospital-years. Those that began a rehabilitation unit in either 1986 or 1987 represent the remaining 594 hospital-years.

Data were compiled from the Medicare Provider Analysis and Review (MEDPAR) files collected by the Health Care Financing Administration. Data from the annual surveys of the American Hospital Association were merged with MEDPAR files. The patient level data from these files were aggregated to the hospital level, in order to perform an organizational level analysis of substitution effects of subacute care services on hospital acute patient care.

Measurement

The patient and hospital characteristics are operationally defined and used as risk adjustment factors (see Appendix). The utilization variables reflecting patient discharge destinations are measured by the percentages of discharges to specific categories of destination, per year: percent discharged home, percent discharged to SNF, percent discharged to rehab hospitals or units, percent discharged to a home health agency, and percent discharged to other facilities. Furthermore, two additional utilization variables, average length of hospital stay and total deflated hospital charges, reflecting the inpatient service intensity, are also included.

Analyses

Descriptive analysis was performed to present the overall trends or changes in the percentage distribution of each discharge destination category over seven years. A pooled cross-sectional regression analysis was conducted in order to adjust for the differences in patient and hospital characteristics, so that the substitutability of subacute care for hospital acute care services could be properly examined. Each utilization variable (e.g., percent discharged to a specific destination) regressed on a series of patient and hospital characteristics. A residual variable (the difference between predicted and observed) from each regression equation was computed. This variable is used as an adjusted measure of the probability of being discharged to a given setting after controlling for the effects of 22 patient and hospital factors. Six residual variables were generated: (1) discharged home, (2) discharged to SNF, (3) discharged to home health agency, (4) discharged to rehabilitation units, (5) average total deflated charges, and (6) average length of stay.

A causal model was developed to examine the substitutive or complementary relationship between inpatient care and subacute care services (Figure 1).

The analysis of residual variables derived from the six regression equations was conducted to determine the substitutive (a negative path coefficient between two residual variables) and the complementary (a positive path coefficient between two residual variables) relationships of the service indicators. More specifically, the interrelationships of varying types of subacute care services were explored by using a structural equation modeling technique. Finally, the goodness of fit statistics of the path analytic model were calculated, using LISREL 8W programs.

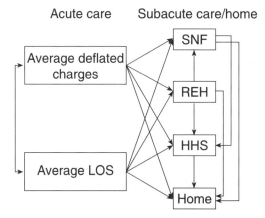

Figure 1. A causal relationship between acute care and subacute care services used.

FINDINGS

Trend Analysis

Discharge Destination

Figure 2 shows several remarkable trends in hospital patient discharges for hip fractures in the United States. An opposite direction of patient discharges was observed for the proportions discharged to home (dsthome) and to skilled nursing facilities (dstsnf). The average proportion discharged home declined rapidly, from 49.6 percent in 1984 to 21.8 percent in 1990. The average proportion discharged to a skilled nursing facility increased substantially, from 29.4 percent in 1984 to 44.5 percent in 1990. A steady increase was also observed in the average proportion of patients discharged to rehabilitation service units (dstreh) and to home health care agencies (dsthhs). When the trend for patient discharges to home was further examined in three different groups of hospitals (hospitals with no rehabilitation units, hospitals with rehabilitation units in the period of 1987–1990, and hospitals with rehabilitation units since 1984), a consistent downward trend in the average proportion discharged to home was found.

Average Length of Stay (ALOS) Trends

A sharp declining trend in the average length of hospital stay for hip fracture patients was found, irrespective of the hospital having or not having a rehabilitation unit (see Figure 3). The ALOS in all hospitals in the study ranged from 15.32 days in 1984 to 12.65 days in 1990. The ALOS in hospitals without rehabilitation units was always shorter than in the other two groups of hospitals with rehabilitation units. The analysis of ALOS by discharge destination and year shows a distinct pattern: 1) those who were discharged to rehabilitation units had a much shorter ALOS in acute care hospitals; and 2) for this group, the ALOS in hospitals increased from 5.5 days in 1984 to 8.5 days in 1990.

Trends in Deflated Total Charges

Figure 4 presents trends in deflated total charges for all the study hospitals, as well as hospitals with and those without rehabilitation units. Hospitals with rehabilitation units consistently showed higher deflated total charges: in 1990, an average of $9,733 per discharge in rehabilitation units; the average was $8,941 in hospitals with no rehabilitation units. The average deflated costs per hospital discharge increased from $8,108.6 in 1984 to $9,109 in 1990.

Patterns of Patient Discharge: Substitutive Versus Complementary Relationship

The analysis reveals that a large proportion of hip fracture patients, who in previous years had been discharged to home

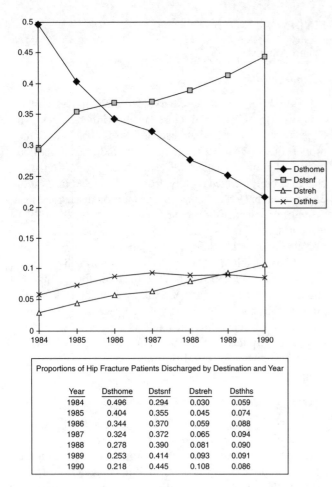

Figure 2. Proportions of hip fracture patients discharged by destination and year. Standard deviations for Figures 2–4 can be obtained from the authors on request.

and hospital characteristics were simultaneously controlled. A substitutive relationship is established between the two service types (e.g., residual variables) if a negative association is found, whereas a complementary relationship is established if a positive association is found.

Multivariate analysis of six residual variables was performed, using adjusted-average deflated charges (RCHG) and adjusted average length of stay (RLOS) as exogenous variables, and adjusted percent discharged to a skilled nursing facility (RSNF), adjusted percent discharged to a rehabilitation unit (RREH), adjusted percent discharged to a home health agency (RHHS), and adjusted percent discharged to home (RHOME) as endogenous variables. This analytic strategy was applied independently to the total study sample (number of observations = 3,428), to the hospitals

after a stay in an acute care hospital, are increasingly being transferred to other settings instead. In essence, alternative care settings may substitute for some part of the care which used to be complemented in an acute care hospital. Multivariate analysis of residual variables regarding patient discharge destinations for a pooled cross-sectional data set (1984–1990) of the study hospitals was undertaken to examine whether or not subacute care services were substituting for acute care services. The residual variable for each discharge destination can be interpreted as the adjusted percentage of patients discharged to the specific destination. Similarly, the residual variables for ALOS and average total hospital deflated charges can be interpreted as the adjusted average hospital length of stay and the adjusted total charges for acute care. The risk adjustment methodology was based on regression analysis of each subacute care service type (percent discharged to a given destination), or of each of the two acute care service indicators when the effects of patient

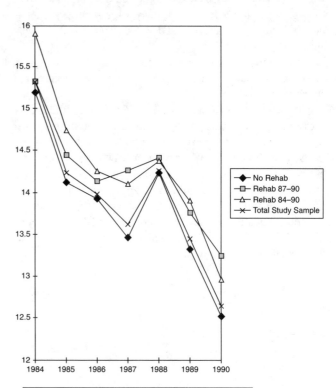

Figure 3. Mean average length of stay (ALOS) for those discharged to all destinations.

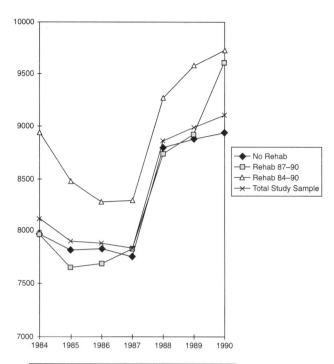

Trend in Deflated Total Charges for DRG 210 Patients			
Group=	A	B	C	D
		Rehab	Rehab	Total Study
Year	No Rehab	87–90	84–90	Sample
1984	7956.62	7968.84	8939.57	8108.63
1985	7821.47	7654.74	8478.27	7905.64
1986	7836.32	7694.27	8275.88	7889.89
1987	7761.81	7833.51	8294.60	7843.13
1988	8792.12	8736.23	9270.62	8860.55
1989	8879.54	8922.37	9584.33	8988.80
1990	8941.46	9612.31	9733.16	9109.04

Figure 4. Trend in deflated total charges for DRG 210 patients.

---

without rehabilitation units ($N = 2,404$), and to the hospitals with rehabilitation units ($N = 708$) for a period of seven consecutive years (1984–1990).

The Total Study Sample

Figure 5 shows a path diagram of the relationship between exogenous and endogenous variables, as well as the relationship between endogenous variables. Statistically significant relationships ($p < 0.05$) are noted in Figure 5. Key findings can be summarized as follows:

1. The adjusted ALOS is positively associated with the subsequent use of subacute services (nursing home care, rehabilitation care, and home health care). Thus, a complementary rather than a substitutive relationship exists between acute care services and subacute care services.

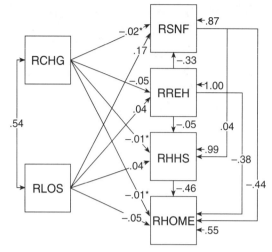

*Not statistically significant at 0.05 level.

Figure 5. Causal analysis of subacute care services in the total study hospitals.

---

2. An inverse relationship is present between RLOS and RHOME. It suggests that a shorter length of stay in an acute care hospital is associated with a higher proportion of hip fracture patients discharged to home.

3. Lower deflated charges are associated with a higher percentage of patients discharged to rehab units for subacute care. Thus, rehab units are being used to substitute for costly acute care.

4. The adjusted average deflated charges are not associated with subsequent use of SNF and home health services.

5. A moderate negative relationship exists between SNF and rehabilitation unit use (beta = −0.33). It suggests that nursing home care is being used to substitute for hospital rehabilitation services.

6. Hospitals that are more likely to discharge their patients home are those who do not require skilled nursing care (beta = −0.44), home health care (beta = −0.46), or rehabilitation (beta = −0.38).

7. A summary of the goodness of fit statistics is presented in Table 5. Two acute-care utilization variables account for 13 percent of the variance in the subsequent use of SNF, and 45 percent of the variation in the discharge to home; and their effect on subsequent use of rehabilitation units and home health agencies is negligible.

Hospitals without Rehabilitation Units

Figure 6 shows the results of path analysis. Key findings include:

1. The adjusted ALOS is not statistically significantly related to subsequent use of rehabilitation units and home

Table 5. Summary Statistics of Path Analysis: Total Study Sample; Hospitals With No Rehab Units; and Hospitals with Rehab Units

Endogenous variable*	Total variance explained by two exogenous variables (RCHG and RLOS)	X²	P	RMSR	NNFI
Total study sample: (with 2 degrees of freedom)		0.003	0.96	0.0004	1.01
Skilled nursing facility	0.13				
Rehab units	0.00				
Home health agency	0.01				
Home	0.45				
Hospitals with no rehab units: (with 2 D.F.)		0.002	1.00	0.0004	1.01
Skilled nursing facility	0.12				
Rehab units	0.00				
Home health agency	0.01				
Home	0.46				
Hospitals with rehab units: (with 2 D.F.)		0.001	1.00	0.0000	1.00
Skilled nursing facility	0.20				
Rehab units	0.03				
Home health agency	0.02				
Home	0.50				

*The residual variable is used.
RCHG: the adjusted average deflated charges.
RLOS: the adjusted average length of hospital stay.
RMSR: Root mean square residual.
NNFI: Non norm fit index.

---

health care. The adjusted proportion of patients discharged to home is not influenced by either of the two acute care indicators.

2. A positive association (gamma = 0.19) exists between the adjusted LOS and the proportion discharged to a skilled nursing facility.

3. Use of rehabilitation units is inversely related to use of SNF and home health care. This result suggests that care rendered by rehabilitation units is being used to substitute for other subacute care services.

4. A moderately strong negative association (–0.46) is present between SNF use and patients discharged to home.

5. No statistically significant relationship exists between adjusted hospital charges and subacute care services.

Hospitals with Rehabilitation Units

The analysis of six utilization (residual) variables illustrates that a complementary relationship exists between the adjusted ALOS and two subacute care services (RSNF and RREH). A substitutive relationship exists between the adjusted hospital charges and the proportion of patients discharged to other settings for subacute care (Figure 7). An inverse relationship between RSNF and RREH was identified: skilled nursing facilities substitute for hospital rehabili-

tation services. The discharge to a home setting is a logical, workable alternative to subacute care, as indicated by a moderately strong negative association between the percentage of patients discharged to home and the percentages of patients discharged to other alternative settings.

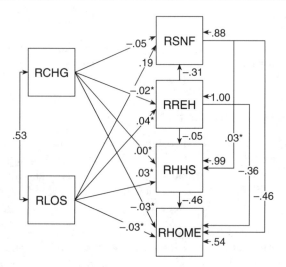

*Not statistically significant at 0.05 level.

Figure 6. Causal analysis of subacute care services in hospitals with no rehab units.

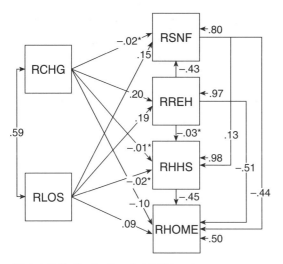

Not statistically significant at 0.05 level.

Figure 7. Causal analysis of subacute care services in hospitals with rehab units.

• • •

This study examined whether care in subacute care settings is being substituted for that in an acute care setting, for patients with hip fractures. Reductions in LOS have been observed. Whether these reductions have resulted in more use of rehabilitation in subacute care settings, in effect substituting care in those settings for that previously received in acute care settings, is an empirical question.

In this examination of the patterns of urban hospital discharge destinations and hospital utilization of older hip fracture patients during the period 1984 through 1990, it was found that the percentage of discharges to home has declined, and that patients with hip fractures are more likely to be transferred to other settings for subacute care. The analysis shows that a rapid change has occurred in the use of subacute care and provides a clear picture of hospital discharge patterns to either a subacute care setting or a home setting.

The ALOS for hip fracture patients shows a steady decline over the study period. Different discharge patterns emerged from the inspection of data collected from hospitals with and without rehabilitation units. Hospitals are more likely to discharge their longer-stay patients to subacute care settings rather than to home. Hospitals with higher average charges and shorter-stay patients are more likely to discharge patients to rehabilitation units for subacute care. These findings reinforce current concerns about the appropriateness of the timing of discharges from an acute care hospital into a rehabilitation setting.

The existing administrative database of MEDPAR files offers little information about the medical necessity for discharging patients to any alternative setting for subacute care.

Furthermore, no information is available for assessing whether or not the substitutions are inappropriate. In order to examine the relationship between rehabilitation services and acute care, it is essential to identify the supply-side information about the number of SNF beds, rehabilitation service providers, and home care agencies in the communities where hospitals are located.

This study was unable to separate the types of rehabilitation units (orthopedic versus any other type). Therefore, it is impossible to sort out the effect of having an orthopedic rehabilitation unit for hip fracture patients. Future studies should also establish a relational database that will integrate data measuring both the administrative and the functional outcomes of treating hip fracture patients in different subacute care settings.

REFERENCES

1. Griffin, K.M. *Handbook of Subacute Health Care.* Gaithersburg, MD: Aspen Publishers, Inc., 1995.
2. Institute of Medicine. "Hip Fracture: Setting Priorities for Effectiveness Research." Report of a study by a committee of the Institute of Medicine, Division of Health Care Services, eds. K.A. Heithoff and K.N. Lohr. Washington, DC: National Academy Press, 1990.
3. Lindsay, R. "The Burden of Osteoporosis: Cost." *The American Journal of Medicine* 98 (Suppl 2A) (1995): 9S–11S.
4. Schroder, H.M. "The Cost of Hospitalization Hip Fracture Patients Has Increased Despite Shorter Hospitalization Time." *Injury* 22, no. 2 (1991): 135–38.
5. Riggs, B.L., and Melton, L.J. "The Worldwide Problem of Osteoporosis: Insights Afforded by Epidemiology." *Bone* 17, no. 5 (1995): 505S–511S.
6. Fitzgerald, J.F., et al. "Changing Patterns of Hip Fracture Care Before and After Implementation of the Prospective Payment System." *Journal of the American Medical Association* 258, no. 2 (1987): 218–21.
7. Fitzgerald, J.F., Moore, P.S., and Dittus, R.S. "The Care of Elderly Patients with Hip Fracture: Changes Since the Implementation of the Prospective Payment System." *New England Journal of Medicine* 319, no. 21 (1988): 1,392–97.
8. Gaumer, G.L., and Stavins, J. "Medicare Use in the Last Ninety Days of Life." *Health Services Research* 26, no. 6 (1992): 725–42.
9. Manton, K.G., et al. "Use of Medicare Services Before and After Introduction of the Prospective Payment System." *Health Services Research* 28, no. 3 (1993): 269–92.
10. Kane, R.L., et al. "Use of Post-hospital Care By Medicare Patients." *Journal of the American Geriatric Society* 44, no. 3 (1996): 242–50.
11. Katz, B.P., et al. "Demographic Variation in the Rate of Knee Replacement: A Multi-Year Analysis." *Health Services Research* 31, no. 2 (1996): 125–40.
12. Hosek, S., et al. "Expanded Access to Rehabilitation Services for Older People: An Urgent Need." *Journal of the American Geriatric Society* 38 (1990): 1,055–56.
13. Langenbrunner, J., et al. "Developing Payment Refinements and Reforms under Medicare for Excluded Hospitals." *Health Care Financing Review* 10, no. 3 (1989): 91–107.

14. Department of Health and Human Services. *Subacute Care: Policy Synthesis and Market Area Analysis.* Washington, DC: DHHS, 1995.

15. Traxler, H., and Dunaye, T. "Emerging Patterns in Transitional Care." *Health Affairs* 6 (1987): 57–68.

16. Prospective Payment Assessment Commission. *Interim Report on Payment Reform for PPS-Excluded Facilities.* Washington, DC: Prospective Payment Assessment Commission, Congressional Rep C-92-05, 1992.

17. Morrisey, M., Sloan, F., and Valvona, J. "Shifting Medicare Patients Out of the Hospital." *Health Affairs* 7, no. 5 (1988): 52–64.

18. Morrisey, M., Sloan, F., and Valvona, J. "Medicare Prospective Payment and Posthospital Transfers to Subacute Care." *Medical Care* 26 (1988): 685–98.

19. Harrington, C., and Swan, J. "The Impact of State Medicaid Nursing Home Policies on Utilization and Expenditures." *Inquiry* 24 (1987): 157–72.

20. Neu, C., and Harrison, S. *Medicare Patients and Postacute Care.* Santa Monica, CA: RAND Corporation (R-3780-MN), 1989.

21. Palmer, R., et al. "The Impact of the Prospective Payment System on the Treatment of Hip Fractures in the Elderly." *Archives of Internal Medicine* 149 (1989): 2,237–41.

22. Marciniak, C., Heinemann, A., and Monga, T. "Changes in Medical Instability Upon Admission to a Rehabilitation Unit." *Archives of Physical Medicine and Rehabilitation* 74 (1993): 1,157–60.

PART **IV**

Stroke and Brain, Spinal Cord, and Head Injury
Rehabilitation Outcomes

22

Outcome Measures and a Program Evaluation Model for Postacute Brain Injury Rehabilitation

Daniel P. Harris

Rapid social and economic change is now the norm for U.S. health care providers. Rehabilitation professionals are under increasing pressure to produce meaningful measures of treatment outcome in an environment of shifting trends in service models and reimbursement constraints. The enormous difficulty of this task is underscored by the fact that no universally accepted outcome measures have been developed in the 30 years since a framework for doing so was described.[1] Heroic efforts have been made, but the results can be likened to the fable of the blind men who tried to describe an elephant while touching different parts of its body. Rehabilitation outcome often is viewed differently by different people. This fundamental reality may be the greatest challenge that providers face today in trying to develop representative outcome measures for patients with differing needs and levels of function.

MANAGED CARE: THE "M" WORD

In the late 1980s and early 1990s, a marked increase in the number of facilities providing postacute brain injury treatment coincided with the emergence of managed care concepts in rehabilitation. Hundreds of facilities arose rather suddenly, offering the public a dizzying array of services. However, consumers and third-party payers did not have any means of differentiating quality and value among programs.[2] Many rehabilitation professionals perceived the resulting unfocused competition between providers and the disorganized cost-cutting strategies of payers as a destructive process, fueled by the lack of outcome measures. Managed care became the "M" word in professional circles, not to be mentioned in polite conversation. However, providers with fore-

sight realized that it was imperative to develop models of care based on outcome, in order to satisfy the external demands of competition and cost containment, while developing useful internal measures of treatment effectiveness and efficiency.

OUTCOME MEASUREMENT AND TREATMENT PROGRAM MODELS

In 1992, we (Healthcare Rehabilitation Center) began developing rehabilitation outcome measures by creating treatment programs based on patients grouped according to cognitive levels and rehabilitation needs. We hoped to track improvement in cognitive status and reduction of dependence as universal outcome indicators for patients at various levels of function. This seemed like a simple idea, but we immediately ran into several problems in selecting criteria to form program populations, estimate prognosis for individual patients, assess treatment progress, and track outcome. For example, the Rancho Los Amigos Levels of Cognitive Functioning Scale[3] (RLAS) was one of the few instruments available at the time for classifying cognitive status in postacute brain-injured individuals. However, in applying the Rancho Scale we found that patients could be classified according to cognitive level upon admission for rehabilitation, but as treatment progressed they might make substantial progress without meeting any of the criteria for advancing up the broad steps of the scale.

We considered using other instruments, such as the Functional Independence Measure[4] and the Disability Rating Scale,[5] to rate performance in activities of daily living, but many of our patients had problems in daily living skills because of psychological and behavioral deficits, rather than physical inability to perform specific tasks. These individuals were typically admitted to our facility many months, or

J Rehabil Outcomes Meas, 1997, 1(2), 23–30
© 1997 Aspen Publishers, Inc.

even years, after their injury. As a result, extensive improvement in cognitive and/or physical function was not likely, and therefore not usually the main goal of rehabilitation. Often, the precipitating factors for referring a patient to our treatment center had to do with social and emotional problems, such as physical aggression, chemical dependency, family dysfunction, or sexual misconduct. Admitting diagnoses for any particular individual frequently included both medical and psychiatric conditions. Many rehabilitation settings have not focused on providing services for such patients, but the need to treat them and the consequences of failing to do so have been documented.[6–11] Unfortunately, we found that no single cognitive or daily living scale seemed to provide the range of indicators necessary to address their complex needs.

We subsequently attempted to devise a combination of outcome assessments, including some scales created by our staff to track patient behavior, but in trying to provide for the infinite permutations of possible symptoms, treatments, and results, these systems quickly grew to unmanageable size. Seasoned clinicians became bogged down in a swamp of instruments and indicators. When we tried to measure postdischarge outcome with some of these complicated approaches, patients, their family members, and external professionals also were dragged into the mire. Extensive questionnaires sent out by mail to these individuals had a low rate of return, and telephone contact follow-ups often proved to be arduous, unproductive experiences on both ends of the line.

It soon became apparent that patients and their family members often had a different perspective from us and even from each other on treatment outcome. Furthermore, they were not motivated to visualize outcome as some pattern of functional levels within a scaling system. They found it more important to discuss at length the reasons why an individual had succeeded or failed at remaining in a particular postdischarge placement. Also, regardless of the type of placement, those we contacted often spontaneously reported whether a patient was now doing worse, the same, or better on specific personal needs and objectives, compared to the way they were before treatment. Because the postdischarge placement and personal objectives of the patient were universally important to our consumers, we decided to include these two dimensions of outcome in our program evaluation model as key indicators for the quality of care. Many other measures were required in addition to outcome criteria as the model developed. The time and resources necessary to administer an elaborate outcome scaling system were not available, and the rewards were not apparent, so we abandoned that approach.

A PROGRAM EVALUATION MODEL

By 1993, our efforts to design services according to patient levels of cognitive function and rehabilitation needs had evolved into three treatment programs. Table 1 lists these programs and provides descriptions of their respective patient populations and treatment goals. Once the programs were organized, the necessity to provide evidence of quality monitoring for certification by CARF . . . The Rehabilitation Accreditation Commission and the Joint Commission on Accreditation of Healthcare Organizations (Joint Commission) led to the development of program evaluation indicators. Figure 1 shows a diagram of the program evaluation model implemented to measure quality and efficiency for each of the three treatment programs. The model was developed by the facility's Quality Improvement Committee, which was made up of a cross-section of personnel, including physicians, program directors, therapy managers, nurse managers, and support staff. According to the committee's specifications, outcome measures are integrated into one of five general areas of indicators: treatment models, treatment plans, progress and outcome, consumer satisfaction, and resource utilization. Measurement instruments for each of the five areas are derived from standing quality improvement indicators, or created specifically to assess important processes within each area. For example, an existing database of treatment plan objectives has been modified to measure progress made by patients in each program toward meeting objectives on schedules established by their treatment teams. On the other hand, a patient/family satisfaction survey had to be originated by interviewing consumers and recording the most frequent criticisms and compliments about the facility's admission process, daily care, living environment, treatment programs, and discharge planning. Survey questions then were formulated from the interview responses.

OUTCOME MEASURES WITHIN THE MODEL

Outcome measures within the program evaluation model are based on our experience that two themes consistently seem important to rehabilitation consumers: the patient's ability to succeed across time in the postdischarge placement and to pursue constructive personal objectives. By definition, individuals are often admitted to our facility because they cannot perform acceptably in some other environment (community, home, school, work, outpatient therapy, etc.). It is a logical approach, then, for our treatment teams to measure outcome by predicting at admission the most appropriate discharge placement for each patient, monitoring the accuracy of predictions, and tracking the ability of each patient to maintain the actual postdischarge placement, whether or not it ends up being the one predicted. Patient progress toward significant personal objectives can also be tracked in the context of determining important skills and activities that may contribute to success in a particular discharge placement. For example, an adult individual discharged to independent living in the community may benefit from joining a

Table 1. Treatment programs, patient Rancho Los Amigos Scale Levels, and therapeutic goals for a postacute brain injury rehabilitation facility

Program	RLAS levels	Therapeutic goals
Medical rehabilitation	II—Generalized response: inconsistent, nonspecific responses to stimuli. III—Localized response: inconsistent, but specific responses to stimuli. May follow simple commands.	Increase arousal, reduce spasticity and improve mobility, manage feeding and swallowing disorders, improve medical condition, control seizures, discontinue any tracheostomy tube, start continence training.
Neurobehavioral rehabilitation	IV—Confused-agitated: bizarre and nonpurposeful behavior, incoherent speech, lacks attention and memory. V—Confused-inappropriate: responds to simple commands, coherent automatic speech, unable to learn new skills or information. VI—Confused-appropriate: has goal-oriented behavior, follows simple directions, relearns old skills, new skills affected by memory loss.	Improve orientation, increase independence in activities of daily living(ADLs) and basic vocational activities, improve emotional self-control and adjustment to disability, compensate for memory loss, increase communication skills.
Community reentry	VII—Automatic-appropriate: independence in and oriented in routine activities, slowed cognitive processing, shallow recall, impaired judgment.	Improve home and personal management skills, attain job readiness, reduce risk of substance abuse, establish a community support system.

support group, seeking realistic levels of vocational training, and assuming responsibility for his or her own finances. Conversely, an adolescent discharged to the family home may need to comply with school programming, behave appropriately at home, find a positive peer group, and develop constructive recreational activities in order to function acceptably for any length of time. No existing scaling system appears flexible enough to classify postdischarge objectives that could vary widely from patient to patient, but we now recognize 11 general descriptive categories (Table 2) that can capture almost all combinations.

For the purposes of program evaluation, it is necessary to generate quality monitoring data for each treatment program across all five areas of indicators in the program evaluation model. To enable data comparisons between programs, the Quality Improvement Committee has created a single set of program evaluation goals and measures that can be applied uniformly for all three programs. Goals for treatment outcome center on the "effectiveness" of each patient's discharge placement, and on the patient's ability to make progress after discharge toward objectives developed at the time of discharge from the facility. Measurement criteria for outcome goals within programs are expressed simply as percentages of patients who are able to maintain their initial discharge placements and progress toward postdischarge objec-

tives during specific periods of time (1 month, 6 months, and 12 months postdischarge). Two definitions have been developed to classify the effectiveness of discharge placements and patient progress toward postdischarge objectives:

1. A discharge placement is considered effective if either of two criteria is met at the time of any postdischarge follow-up contact.
   a. The level of clinical care, supervision, or financial support required by the patient in his or her current placement has not increased, compared to the level required in the initial discharge placement.
   b. The patient has progressed to a less restrictive, more appropriate level of care since the initial discharge placement, even though increased resources may be required.
2. A patient is considered to be progressing toward his or her postdischarge objectives at the time of any follow-up if the individual contacted reports that more than 50 percent of the patient's objectives are being "maintained" or "advancing."

Two criteria are required for judging the effectiveness of discharge placements because some individuals may need to be discharged to inappropriately restrictive environments until more suitable placements can be obtained (no. 1b

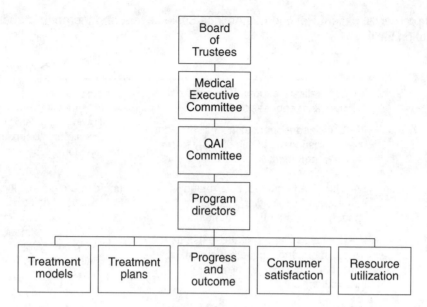

Figure 1. A program evaluation model implemented to measure quality and efficiency for postacute brain injury rehabilitation treatment programs.

above). For example, an adult initially might be placed in the home of his or her parents until a supervised apartment becomes available. An apartment is a much more appropriate living situation for the adult offspring, but the cost of supervision and rent is greater than expenses incurred if he or she remains in the parents' home. In such a scenario, a super-

vised apartment placement would be classified as effective, even though added resources would be required to support the individual in that setting. For program evaluation, group data on the effectiveness of placements is obtained by categorizing types of placements that patients may have before and after treatment at our facility (Table 3). Outcome mea-

Table 2. Categories of objectives after discharge for postacute brain injury rehabilitation patients

Objective type	Category criteria
Behavior	Personal conduct related to social and emotional function, may focus on reducing negative actions or increasing positive behaviors.
Community living skills	Skills required to use community services such as transportation systems, libraries, restaurants, theaters, parks, etc.
Community resources	Support to be obtained through community service agencies (i.e., support groups, clubs, charity, governmental agencies).
Family counseling	Psychiatric or psychological services for individual family members or the family group (patient may be included).
Patient counseling	Psychiatric or psychological services for the patient, apart from the family.
Education (school)	Placement in public or private school for academic development (excludes vocational training).
Medical	Physician, nursing, or rehabilitation services necessary after discharge, may include patient and/ or family training in medical management.
Peer group	Development of age-appropriate leisure skills.
Personal living (ADLs)	Basic skills to be applied during daily routines (i.e., dressing, hygiene, meal preparation).
Substance abuse	Participation in public or private substance treatment programs, may have personal objectives to remain free of substance abuse and attend a support group.
Vocational (work/training)	Enrollment in public or private vocational programs, seeking employment or returning to the pre-injury job, participating in paid or volunteer work for community service agencies.

Table 3. Types of placements before and after treatment for patients in a postacute brain injury rehabilitation facility

Placement type	Category criteria
Community independent	Adult (18 years old or more), head of own household, does not require supervision to manage home, finances, or job duties.
Community supervised	Adult, not living with family members or other caregivers (i.e., has own apartment), does not require direct assistance but needs supervision to consistently manage home, finances, or job duties.
Home with family	Adult or child, lives with family members in the family home, requires assistance or supervision to complete daily routines, job duties, or school work, may be in outpatient treatment.
Group home	Non–hospital-licensed facility, staffed by professionals or trained paraprofessionals, communal living environment, assisted or supervised activities provided for all residents.
Inpatient rehabilitation	Hospital-licensed facility, freestanding or part of general medical hospital system, patients are housed and treated on premises by rehabilitation professionals.
Psychiatric facility	Psychiatric-licensed facility, freestanding, or part of hospital/institutional system, patients are housed and treated on premises by psychiatric treatment professionals.
Nursing facility	Skilled nursing or long-term nursing care facility, residents require ADL assistance and regular nursing care.
Correctional facility	Adult or juvenile incarceration unit operated by governmental authority.

sures are based on percentages of patients who are able to maintain or improve the effectiveness of placements within each category at 1 month, 6 months, and 12 months postdischarge.

Only one simple set of criteria is required to obtain ratings of patient progress toward postdischarge objectives (no. 2 above). Follow-up contacts are asked to report whether the patient is "regressing," "maintaining," or "advancing" on each objective. These objectives are written by the treatment team (with patient cooperation, if possible) at the time of discharge to address the patient's future needs. In designing each patient's objectives, the team also assigns a staff member to make follow-up contacts and identifies the appropriate individual or agency to contact regarding the patient after discharge. All contacts are made by telephone, and the sample to be contacted includes every patient who has been treated at the facility for at least four weeks before discharge. Group data for program evaluation is obtained by assigning each objective as it is written to one of 11 possible categories (Table 2). Outcome measures are based on percentages of patients who are rated as maintaining or advancing on objectives within each category.

RESULTS

Because our outcome measures are tracked by a database system, it is relatively easy to display data in many different forms. Program evaluation goals for each treatment team and the facility as a whole require quarterly reports on percentages of effective discharge placements and patient progress toward postdischarge objectives for groups at 1 month, 6

months, and 12 months postdischarge. Figure 2 provides a global example of data on the effectiveness of discharge placements for patients in the database to date who have been followed for at least 6 months after discharge. The sample includes 112 patients (85 males, 27 females; mean age 28.6 years) admitted between 1993 and 1996 for postacute rehabilitation following traumatic brain injuries. Data for the five most common placements before and after treatment are shown. The figure presents four measures for each type of placement across all treatment programs:

1. Number of patients in the specific type of placement immediately before admission to our facility.
2. Number of patients at the time of admission predicted for discharge to the specific type of placement.
3. Number of patients actually discharged to the specific type of placement.
4. Number of patients at 6 months postdischarge in the specific type of placement.

Several points of information useful for program evaluation are available in the data. For example, only 36 of the 112 patients in the sample were admitted to the facility from independent living, supervised living in the community, or the family home. Data for those three placements were combined to provide an overall "community living" sample. In Figure 2, it can be seen that a total of 70 patients were predicted for discharge to that setting. However, 79 patients actually were discharged to community living, and 65 of those individuals maintained effective placements until at least 6 months after discharge. Treatment teams in each program

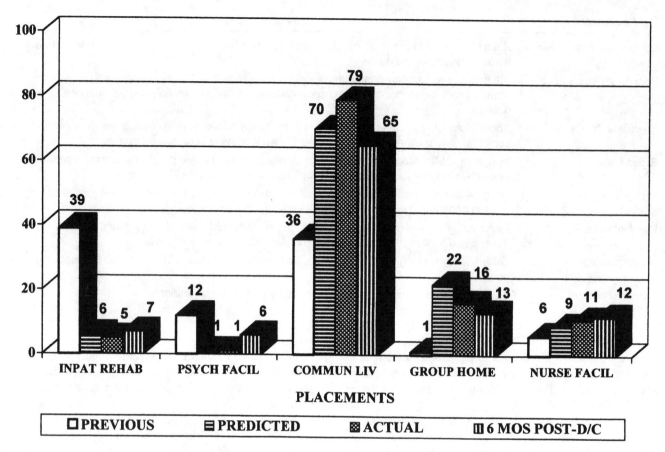

Figure 2. Example data on the effectiveness of discharge placements for postacute brain injury rehabilitation patients at 6 months after discharge.

have used this kind of information as justification for developing more therapies focused on preparing patients and families to cope with specific problems in community living, particularly for those individuals who previously have not succeeded in that environment. To the extent that these therapies might influence outcome, the percentage of effective placements in the family home or independent living may increase across time. Table 4 presents evidence from

program evaluation reports supporting this concept. The data in the table show that between 1993 and 1996 the percentage of effective placements for community living increased from 76 to 91, when measured at 6 months postdischarge.

It would be very naive to propose that there is a straightforward relationship between the specific therapies provided for any particular patient and the outcome of his or her rehabilitation measured at various points in time. Many variables that

Table 4. Percentage of effective community living placements and patients advancing on postdischarge objectives (1993–1996) for brain injury rehabilitation patients at 6 months postdischarge

	1993		1994		1995		1996	
Community living	*N*	*(%)*	*N*	*(%)*	*N*	*(%)*	*N*	*(%)*
Total placements	29		20		19		11	
Effective placements	22	(76)	17	(85)	16	(84)	10	(91)
Objectives advancing	18	(62)	11	(55)	10	(63)	6	(55)

can influence a patient's chance of success or failure in a given discharge placement are beyond the control of the treatment team and outside its scope of responsibilities. The data in Table 4 agree with such an observation, in that the smallest percentages of patients reported to be advancing toward postdischarge goals (55 percent in 1994 and 1996) coincide with the greatest percentages of effective placements (85 percent in 1994 and 91 percent in 1996).

•　　•　　•

A great deal of work still remains to determine the relationships between variables that can shape rehabilitation outcome within the larger context of forces that mold a patient's life. Hopefully, the experiences, methods, and example data described in this brief article will provide some indication of how this complex task may be addressed. Database management of outcome measures, and the integration of outcomes data into program evaluation models, appears to be a promising approach for two basic reasons. First, the potential number of variables to be investigated is so large, even within individual treatment facilities, that database systems currently are the only information tools powerful enough to accomplish comprehensive data analyses. Fortunately, attempts are also presently being made to form rehabilitation outcomes databases at state and national levels.[12] Second, outcomes data can have a greater impact on the quality of care when integrated into the process of program evaluation, rather than being viewed solely as an end product of treatment. The best way to maximize treatment planning and therapy skills in brain injury rehabilitation programs is to provide regular, meaningful feedback to professionals on the outcomes of their own patients. In doing so, we can progress toward truly describing the "elephant," even though our sight is yet limited.

REFERENCES

1. Donabedian, A. "Evaluating the Quality of Medical Care." *Milbank Memorial Fund Quarterly* 44 (1966): 166–206.
2. Evans, R.W., and Ruff, R.M. "Outcome and Value: A Perspective on Rehabilitation Outcomes Achieved in Acquired Brain Injury." *Journal of Head Trauma Rehabilitation* 7, no. 4 (1992): 24–36.
3. Hagen, C. "Language Cognitive Disorganization Following Closed Head Injury: A Conceptualization." In *Cognitive Rehabilitation: Conceptualization and Intervention,* ed. L.E. Trexler. New York: Plenum Press, 1982.
4. Granger, C.V., and Hamilton, B.B. "UDS Report—The Uniform Data System for Medical Rehabilitation." *American Journal of Physical Medicine and Rehabilitation* 73 (1992): 108–13.
5. Rappaport, M., et al. "Disability Rating Scale for Severe Head Trauma: Coma to Community." *Archives of Physical Medicine and Rehabilitation* 63 (1982): 118–23.
6. Barin, J.J., et al. "Counseling the Head Injured Patient." In *Head Injury Rehabilitation: Children and Adolescents,* ed. M. Ylvisaker. San Diego: College Hill Press, 1985, 361–82.
7. Hackler, E., and Tobis, J.M. "Reintegration into the Community." In *Rehabilitation of the Head Injured Adult,* eds. M. Rosenthal, E.R. Griffith, M.S. Bond, and J.D. Miller. Philadelphia: F.A. Davis Company, 1984, 421–34.
8. Jones, M.L., and Evans, R.W. "Outcome Validation in Post-acute Rehabilitation: Trends and Correlates in Treatment and Outcome." *Journal of Insurance Medicine* 24, no. 3 (1992): 186–92.
9. Malec, J.F., et al. "Outcome Evaluation and Prediction in a Comprehensive-integrated Post-acute Outpatient Brain Injury Rehabilitation Programme." *Brain Injury* 7, no. 1 (1993): 15–29.
10. Rosen, C.D., and Gerring, J.P. *Head Trauma: Educational Reintegration.* San Diego: College Hill Press, 1986.
11. Willer, B., et al. "Assessment of Community Integration Following Rehabilitation for Traumatic Brain Injury." *Journal of Head Trauma Rehabilitation* 8, no. 2 (1993): 75–87.
12. Dahmer, E.R., et al. "A Model Systems Database for Traumatic Brain Injury." *Journal of Head Trauma Rehabilitation* 8, no. 2 (1993): 12–25.

A Seven- to Fourteen-Year Follow-Up Study of Adults with Very Severe Intellectual Impairment following a Neurological Insult

Barbara A. Wilson and Janet Cockburn

The natural history of change following brain injury is an important element in understanding the likely long-term outcome of people with neurological conditions. Follow-up studies have been reported on certain diagnostic groups such as severe head injury[1-4] or stroke.[5,6] Other studies have focused on particular cognitive deficits such as acquired disorders of memory,[7] language,[8] or reading.[9] Little is known of the long-term outcome of people with very severe intellectual impairment following acquired, nonprogressive brain injury other than on broad, very general measures such as the Glasgow Outcome Scale.[10] Although we know that severity of injury, duration of coma, length of posttraumatic amnesia, and reduced mobility affect outcome in general,[4,11-14] few details are provided of the social, vocational, and cognitive outcome of people with profound intellectual deficits. The present study has concentrated on a series of patients admitted for rehabilitation after acquired neurological damage, whose intellectual status at the time rendered them untestable on standard neuropsychological tests for adults. Twenty-four of the 30 patients were traced 7 to 14 years later and 15 survivors were reassessed.

SUBJECTS

The sample comprised all severely impaired patients referred to the first author for neuropsychological assessment between 1979 and 1986 (17 men and 13 women, approximately 8 percent of all referrals). Although varying considerably in etiology and age at insult, all had intellectual impairments severe enough to preclude them from assessment on standardized neuropsychological tests for adults. Assessment of their abilities was made using tests designed for children with special needs, including the Vineland social maturity scale,[15] the Portage developmental checklists,[16] the British Ability Scales (BAS),[17] and the Leiter International Performance Scale.[18]

The mean age of the sample at initial assessment was 32.1 years (sd 13.5, range 15–65 years). The majority (17) had sustained a very severe head injury with mean coma duration 9.27 weeks (sd 7.46), range 4–32 weeks. Six patients had sustained a cerebral vascular accident, three had been treated for cerebral tumor, three had suffered an anoxic episode, and one was thought to have had a viral infection (Table 1). Twelve of the subjects had severe physical problems, defined as "confined to a wheelchair and needing help with transfers," in addition to their intellectual handicaps. Eighteen had less severe or no physical problems.

At follow-up, eight patients had died. Although, on average, older than those still alive, they covered the full age range of the original sample (Table 1). Three stroke patients had died of a further stroke; two cerebral tumor patients died as a consequence of the tumor; and three head-injury patients died, one from a seizure, one an embolus, and one, aged 59, of "natural causes." Six had both severe physical and intellectual problems and two (one head-injury, one stroke) had severe intellectual problems without severe physical defects. One patient, a young head-injured man, refused follow-up, and six could not be traced. The remaining 15 subjects, four of whom had severe physical as well as intellectual problems when first seen, consented to reassessment and were seen in the most convenient setting for them, usually their place of residence or regular day center.

REASSESSMENTS

Subjects were seen for three to six hours on one to three occasions. A carer, usually a relative, was also interviewed

J Rehabil Outcomes Meas, 1997, 1(2), 60–66
© 1997 Aspen Publishers, Inc.

Table 1. Ages at insult and diagnoses of the 30 subjects

	Age (years)			Diagnostic group					
	Mean	sd	Range	Head injury	Stroke	Tumor	Anoxia	Undiagnosed	Total
Those seen	28.73	9.96	17–52	10	2	1	2	—	15
Those who died	41.87	19.43	15–65	3	3	2	—	—	8
Those uncontacted	29.16	5.74	22–34	3	1	0	1	1	6
Refused	22	—	—	1	—	—	—	—	1
Total	32.10	13.50	15–65	17	6	3	3	1	30

to verify factual information or to provide information for subjects unable to communicate.

The interviews took the following format:

1. A reminder about the purpose of the visit and a recollection of when we last met.
2. The administration of a social and vocational questionnaire.[7]
3. Reassessment on as many of the original tests or scales as possible. Standard tests from the Wechsler Adult Intelligence Scale (WAIS-R)[19] were also administered to those participants now able to attempt them.

RESULTS

Social and Vocational Questionnaire

Domestic Circumstances

Ten subjects were living at home with relatives or a spouse, and one man (anoxic brain damage) was living in his own home with support from a rota of volunteer carers. The remaining four, three men and one woman, all of whom had suffered a severe head injury, lived in long-term residential accommodation. The woman (LO), who had spent several years in private care until her parents could no longer afford the fees, was in a National Health Service (NHS) hospital. One man lived in an NHS residence for profoundly disabled people and one young man (VU) lived in a hostel for people with severe learning difficulties. Despite having considerable freedom, sheltered employment, and regular contact with his family, he was unhappy about his circumstances. Having sustained his head injury at the age of 17 years, he could remember being without cognitive and physical problems, and was able to articulate the differences, as he saw them, between himself and other residents, who had developmental disorders. The third man was in a Cheshire Home, run by a charity for people with physical and intellectual handicaps. His wife felt very guilty that, after 11 years, she could no longer cope with him at home, saying: "I ought to

be able to cope but . . . I can't go out and I can't have any life. He gets jealous of me and of (daughter). He does things for attention. . . ."

Five subjects had been married before the neurological insult, four of whom were still married. One (in residential care) was separated from his wife but still in contact with her. Nine were unmarried with no sexual partner. The remaining subject, a man in his early forties (TK), had a current sexual partner who was also one of his carers.

Vocational and Employment Status

None of the participants were in paid employment, although one woman worked as a volunteer and one man attended a sheltered workshop each day. A further person, who had been involved in an industrial accident in 1976 when a piece of metal tubing had penetrated his skull, kept up his premorbid interest in antique clock repair and restoration. When assessed in 1979 he was unable to read, write, or count, had severe expressive and receptive language impairments, and performed in the subnormal range on tests of nonverbal reasoning. In 1993, despite still being unable to read, write, or count and with naming ability at a seven-year-old level, he maintained an impressive collection of clocks and a sophisticated clock repair workshop. His skills were sought after in the clock restoration field, although his relatives had to deal with all the financial transactions.

Most of the remaining subjects who were living at home attended day centers or special education classes. Only two had no regular commitments. One had declined the opportunity to attend a special club for people with aphasia. The other (ED) maintained his premorbid interests in motorcycles and watching football.

Table 2 summarizes the residential, marital, and cognitive status at follow-up.

Cognitive Assessments

Most people (12, i.e., 80 percent) had improved on the cognitive assessments, two had deteriorated, and one man (the surviving tumor patient) had not changed.

Table 2. Current status of the 15 subjects seen at follow-up

	Living with relatives/ spouse	Living in hospital/ residential home	Living in hostel	Living alone	Married before and still married	Married before and now separated	Unmarried before and current sexual partner	Unmarried before and no current sexual partner	Cognitively improved	Cognitively unchanged	Cognitively deteriorated
Severe physical and intellectual impairment	2	2	—	—	2	—	—	2	2	—	2
Severe intellectual impairment only	8	1	1	1*	2	1	1	7	10	1	0
TOTAL	10	3	1	1	4	1	1	9	12	1	2

*With support.

Three illustrations of patients who improved are provided below:

ED

This man sustained a severe head injury in a motorcycle accident when he was 26 years old and was in a coma for several weeks. A psychological assessment was carried out in February 1985, 10 months postinjury. He passed 7 of the 17 Vineland social maturity scale items at the nought- to one-year-old level and one item at the one- to two-year-old level. No further items were passed. These items included:

Item	Therapist's comments
2. Balances head	He can only do this for short periods—e.g., during a meal.
11. Drinks from a cup assisted	Yes, can do this.
13. Grasps with thumb and forefinger	Yes, can do this.
17. Follows simple instructions	If he is shown a picture of a toothbrush and asked "Show me what you do with this," he will pretend to brush his teeth.

On the Portage developmental checklists, ED failed many items at the nought- to one-year-old level and *all* the items on the motor scale.

The report said, "There is little doubt that ED is severely physically and intellectually handicapped. It is impossible to assess his 'true' level of cognitive ability because a) his motor skills are so limited he cannot carry out many of the tasks used to assess cognitive function, b) he has no adequate means of communicating, c) some of the tasks on the checklists are inappropriate for a man of his age, and d) he may be unwilling to cooperate with some of the activities requested. . . . Whatever his real inner cognitive strengths are, he is currently *functioning* at a level well below that of the average one-year-old."

When reassessed in 1992, ED was living with his wife and baby son in a converted bungalow. He used a computer to write letters and keep a diary. Although dysarthric, his speech was mostly intelligible. He could write in large print, was at ceiling on all Portage scales except the motor scale, and was testable on standardized neuropsychological tests.

On the Raven's standard progressive matrices,[20] ED scored 44 points (IQ equivalent 108). His age-scaled scores on three subtests of the WAIS-R[19] were in the average range, as were scores on tests of memory and the modified Wisconsin Card Sorting Test.[21] He was still very physically impaired, using an electric wheelchair.

MI

This woman sustained a severe head injury at the age of 17 years in a road traffic accident and was unconscious for several weeks. At that time she was head girl of her school and expected to go on to university. When first assessed eight months postinjury, she was severely intellectually impaired, being unable to recognize any letters or words and at chance on a lexical decision task (selecting real from nonsense words). She could name only four items on the Oldfield-Wingfield test of naming[22] (a score in the severely impaired range) and her mental age scores on the BAS[17] ranged from five years (digits) to eight years (matrices—a nonverbal reasoning test). She could copy accurately, count the number of items on a page, and match shapes and colors.

When reassessed 10 years later, MI's reading age on the Schonell graded word reading test[23] was 11.5 years. She could name 13 items on the Oldfield-Wingfield test.[22] As a result of her general improvement it became possible to establish that MI had a semantic memory disorder,[24] that is, she had lost much of her general knowledge particularly for living things,[25] a relatively rare and specific neuropsychological syndrome previously difficult to detect among a host of other cognitive deficits.

MI has a right hemiplegia but has taught herself to write neatly with her left hand. Her favorite occupation is to do the family ironing, which she does impeccably with her left hand. She spends two days a week as a volunteer helper in a nursery school.

TK

At the age of 29 years, TK, an engineer, attempted suicide with carbon monoxide. No details about coma were available. He was psychologically assessed four months later. On the Vineland social maturity scale, his overall social age was estimated to be at the two- to three-year-old level with his first failure at nought-one years ("reaches for nearby objects"), and his highest success seven-eight years ("combs hair"). He could not draw or write but could make a few scribbles on a piece of paper. He could count forwards from one through 20, but not backwards from 20 through one, and could say the alphabet from A through M before making errors. He could spell six words correctly (*cat, see, red, big, eat, him*), but was unable to read any printed words or letters. He named six out of 15 words from description, but could not name any pictures to confrontation.

The report at the time said 1) he was profoundly intellectually handicapped in all areas of functioning, and 2) it was impossible to assess how far his problems were confounded by sensory visual deficits and how far they were due to more central difficulties. For example, he might have visual object agnosia, but it was not possible to exclude poor acuity as an explanation for his failure to recognize objects. He also appeared to have both expressive and receptive language problems.

In 1993, TK was still unable to name to confrontation, scoring 0 out of 24 on a difficult naming test.[26] However, his naming to description was good, and he scored 21 out of 24 when the same 24 items were described to him. His three errors were *snowplough* for *sledge, moorhen* for *swan,* and *car* for *motorcycle.*

TK appeared to have an apperceptive agnosia.[27] He could not reliably tell me how many pens were held in front of him, nor whether two pictures were the same, yet he could point out particular flowers in the garden and does not consider himself visually impaired. Patients with apperceptive agnosia are often considered blind until they report seeing something or are noticed avoiding obstacles in their path.[28]

Both patients who deteriorated had encountered further medical problems since leaving rehabilitation:

LO was involved in a horse-riding accident when she was 28 years old, sustaining a compound fracture of the right parietal bone with left temporal contre-coup injury and subdural haematoma, which was surgically removed. She was referred for neuropsychological assessment six months later, at which time she could speak three words (*yes, no,* and *today*). On the Leiter international performance scale, LO passed all the tests at the two-year-old level; three out of four tests at the three-year-old level; two out of four tests at the four-year-old level; and one out of four tests at the five-year-old level, giving an overall score of 3.5 years. On the Portage checklists LO scored below a one-year-old level on the language scales; between a one- to two-year-old level on the motor scales; between a two- to three-year-old level on the socialization scales; and between a three- to four-year-old level on the self-help scales. In 1985, almost two years after her head injury, LO had a plate fitted in her head to repair the fracture. About a year later an infection set in and she deteriorated. On reassessment she was no longer able to say any words, had changed little on the Portage scales, and was physically less able than before.

HD was a laborer who was involved in a motorcycle accident in 1984, aged 22 years, and was in coma for six weeks. When assessed seven months later, he failed all the two-year-old items on the Leiter international performance scale and made some failures at the one- to two-year-old level on the Portage cognitive checklist. Nevertheless, his digit span was five forwards and four backwards, he showed evidence of learning on a six-piece formboard (becoming faster with successive trials) and could draw a barely recognizable man and attempt some writing to dictation (Figure 1).

When seen in 1993, HD was living in a home for people with profound handicaps and could do none of the tasks administered in 1985. His parents said that HD started having seizures soon after discharge from the rehabilitation center, had two or three periods of status epilepticus, and continued to suffer from severe epilepsy.

• • •

The patients reported in this study suffered very severe brain damage as a consequence of neurological insult. As they were too impaired to be assessed on standardized neuropsychological tests for adults, they were given tests for children. Using such developmental tests to assess brain-damaged adults is not new[29] and items are not always appropriate. Nevertheless, they provide an objective, quantifiable measure that is preferable to claims that the patient is untestable.

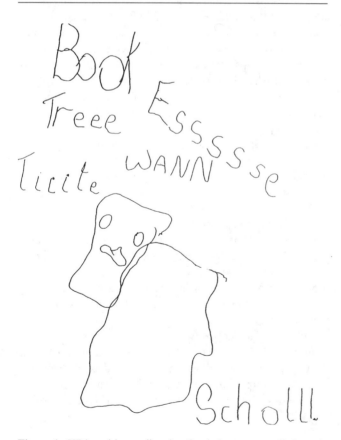

Figure 1. HD's writing to dictation (book, is, tree, man, little, and school) and drawing of a man in 1985.

There are, perhaps, four major messages from the results of this study.

1. Most people, even those with extremely severe intellectual impairment, continue to improve over time. ED, whose first assessment took place 10 months postinjury, after the generally accepted period of optimum recovery, made substantial improvement during the next eight years. The few who deteriorate may well have encountered further medical complications.

2. The majority of severely intellectually impaired people live outside of hospital care. Only three (20 percent) of the present sample were in long-term residential care and this includes two patients who had deteriorated. A further patient was living in a hostel for people with learning difficulties, apparently because his large family found it difficult to provide him with the consistent day-to-day environment he needed.

3. More subjects had died than might have been expected from this age group. Although one person was 70 when he died, the remaining seven ranged from 16 to 63 years at death. Whereas the death rate among stroke patients was similar to that found over a five-year period in a community study,[6] with 50 percent of the sample dying (aged 48, 63, and 70 years), three (21 percent) of the 14 head-injured people traced had died, aged 32, 36, and 59 years. It is a commonly held belief that, after the acute stage, head-injured people have a normal, or nearly normal, life span. Although firm evidence is sparse, Field,[30] whose subjects were survivors from World War I, suggested head-injured survivors only have a 3 to 5 year reduction in life span. More recently, Gilchrist and Wilkinson[4] reported that only 4 (6 percent) of 72 patients followed up 9 months to 15 years after rehabilitation had died. Jennett and McMillan,[31] also indicated little reduction in life span, a finding substantiated by a report from the Medical Disability Society[32] that better management in the immediate postinjury stage has contributed to increased numbers of patients with brain injury having normal life expectancy. Whatever the truth for head-injured people in general, the present results do not suggest normal life expectancy for those with very severe impairments and those with both severe intellectual and physical handicaps are more likely to die than those with only severe intellectual handicap. In the former group, six (50 percent) were known to have died at follow-up, compared with only two (11 percent) of the latter.

4. A number of patients had resolved into having more clear-cut neuropsychological syndromes that were originally obscured by widespread cognitive deficits. MI had a classic semantic memory disorder with a particularly severe loss of semantic information about liv-

ing creatures. VU demonstrated a specific semantic memory disorder over and above general cognitive deficits. TK, thought to have visual agnosia in 1982, showed a picture typical of apperceptive agnosia when reassessed 10 years later.

Despite increasing evidence about the effectiveness of rehabilitation in returning people to work or to a more independent lifestyle,[33] it is not possible to tell from this study whether, or to what extent, rehabilitation affected the outcome of these subjects. All had received rehabilitation, most for many months. Some now expressed a wish for further rehabilitation and, given that most subjects showed improvements in their cognitive functioning, they may now be in a better position, even at such a late stage postinjury, to benefit from more structured cognitive rehabilitation programs.

REFERENCES

1. Brooks, D.N., et al. "The Effects of Severe Head Injury on Patient and Relative within Seven Years of Injury." *Journal of Head Trauma Rehabilitation* 2 (1987): 1–13.

2. Oddy, M., et al. "Social Adjustment After Closed Head Injury: A Further Follow-Up Seven Years After Injury." *Journal of Neurology, Neurosurgery, and Psychiatry* 48 (1985): 564–68.

3. Thomsen, I.V. "Late Psychosocial Outcome in Severe Blunt Head Trauma: A Review." *Brain Injury* 1 (1987): 131–43.

4. Gilchrist, E., and Wilkinson, M. "Some Factors Determining Prognosis in Young People with Severe Head Injuries." *Archives of Neurology* 36 (1979): 355–59.

5. Bamford, J., et al. "A Prospective Study of Acute Cerebro-Vascular Disease in the Community: The Oxfordshire Stroke Project 1981–1986." *Journal of Neurology, Neurosurgery, and Psychiatry* 53 (1990): 16–22.

6. Burn, J., et al. "Long-Term Risk of Recurrent Stroke After a First-Ever Stroke: The Oxfordshire Community Stroke Project." *Stroke* 25 (1994): 333–37.

7. Wilson, B.A. "Long Term Prognosis of Patients with Severe Memory Disorders." *Neuropsychological Rehabilitation* 1 (1991): 117–134.

8. Wade, D., and Hewer, R.L. "Functional Abilities After Stroke: Measurement, Natural History and Prognosis." *Journal of Neurology, Neurosurgery, and Psychiatry* 50 (1987): 177–82.

9. Wilson, B.A. "Remediation of Acquired Dyslexia: A 6–10 Year Follow-Up Study of Seven Brain Injured People." *Journal of Clinical and Experimental Neuropsychology* 16 (1994): 354–71.

10. Jennett, B., and Bond, M. "Assessment of Outcome After Severe Brain Damage: A Practical Scale." *Lancet* 1 (1975): 480–84.

11. Smith, A. "Duration of Impaired Consciousness as an Index of Severity in Closed Head Injuries: A Review." *Diseases of the Nervous System* 22 (1961): 69–74.

12. Levin, H.S., O'Donnell, V.M., and Grossman, R.G. "The Galveston Orientation and Amnesia Test: A Practical Scale to Assess Cognition After Head Injury." *Journal of Nervous and Mental Disease* 167 (1979): 675–84.

13. Eyman, R.K., et al. "The Life Expectancy of Profoundly Handicapped People with Mental Retardation." *New England Journal of Medicine* 323 (1990): 584–89.

14. Vogenthaler, D.R., Smith, K.R., and Goldfader, P. "Head Injury, A Multivariate Study: Predicting Long-Term Productivity and Independent Living Outcome." *Brain Injury* 3 (1989): 369–85.

15. Doll, E.A. *The Measurement of Social Competence*. Minneapolis: Educational Publishers, 1953.

16. Wilson, B.A. "Adapting 'Portage' for Neurological Patients." *International Rehabilitation Medicine* 7 (1985): 6–8.

17. Elliot, C.D., Murray, D.J., and Pearson, L.S. *British Ability Scales*. Windsor: NFER-Nelson, 1977.

18. Leiter, R.R. *Examiner's Manual for the Leiter International Performance Scale*. Chicago: Stoelting, 1969.

19. Wechsler, D. *Wechsler Adult Intelligence Scale*. New York: The Psychological Corporation, 1981.

20. Raven, J.C. *Guide to the Standard Progressive Matrices*. London: Lewis & Co, 1960.

21. Nelson, H.E. "A Modified Card Sorting Test Sensitive to Frontal Lobe Defects." *Cortex* 12 (1976): 313–24.

22. Oldfield, R.C., and Wingfield, A. "Response Latencies in Naming Objects." *Quarterly Journal of Experimental Psychology* 17 (1965): 273–81.

23. Schonell, F.J., and Schonell, F.E. *Diagnostic Attainment Testing*. Edinburgh: Oliver & Boyd, 1963.

24. Patterson, K., and Hodges, J. "Disorders of Semantic Memory," in *Handbook of Memory Disorders*, eds. A.D. Baddeley, B.A. Wilson, and F.N. Watts. Chichester: Wiley, 1995.

25. Warrington, E.K., and Shallice, T. "Category Specific Semantic Impairments." *Brain* 107 (1984): 829–54.

26. Hodges, J., Salmon, D.P., and Butters, N. "Semantic Memory Impairment in Alzheimer's Disease: Failure of Access or Degraded Knowledge?" *Neuropsychologia* 30 (1992): 301–14.

27. Lissauer, H. "Ein Fall Von Seelenblindheit Nebst Einem Beitrage Zur Theorie Derselben." *Archives für Psychiatrie und Nervenkrankheiten* 21 (1890): 222–70.

28. Rubens, A.B. "Agnosia," in *Clinical Neuropsychology*, eds. K.M. Heilman and E. Valenstein. New York: Oxford University Press, 1979.

29. Eson, M.E., Yen, J.K., and Bourke, R.S. "Assessment of Recovery from Serious Head Injury." *Journal of Neurology, Neurosurgery, and Psychiatry* 41 (1978): 1036–42.

30. Field, J.H. *Epidemiology of Head Injuries in England and Wales*. London: HMSO, 1976.

31. Jennett, B., and McMillan, R. "Epidemiology of Head Injury." *British Medical Journal* 282 (1981): 101.

32. Medical Disability Society. *Report of the Working Party on the Management of Traumatic Brain Injury*. London: Royal College of Physicians, 1988.

33. McMillan, T.M., and Greenwood, R.J. "Model of Rehabilitation Programmes for the Brain-Injured Adult. II: Model Services and Suggestions for Change in the United Kingdom." *Clinical Rehabilitation* 7 (1993): 346–55.

24

A Protocol for Multidisciplinary Assessment of the Outcome of Traumatic Brain Injury in Adults after Two Years or More

Rolland S. Parker, Hussein Abdel-Dayem, Sidney I. Silverman, Michael Hutchinson, Daniel Luciano, and Alireza Minagar

Precise assessment of adaptive outcome two or more years after traumatic brain injury (TBI) caused by an accident is a multidisciplinary task, since the head injuries and the consequent dysfunctions can be both neurobehavioral and somatic. Outcome is defined as current level and style of adaptation, compared with a known or estimated pre-injury baseline. When TBI outcome is assessed imprecisely or incorrectly, treatment is inappropriate or neglected. The focus is upon TBI caused by mechanical forces, often accompanied by other injuries. To illustrate the complexity of outcome assessment, and its multidisciplinary requirements, in one group of head-injured patients one third of motor sequelae were not related to the head injury.[1] Our guiding assumptions are: (1) TBI interferes with *adaptation,* defined as the integrated way in which a person copes with his environment; (2) accurate assessment involves multidisciplinary study of a wide range of functions.

Two years is selected as a reasonable postinjury interval since most recovery will have occurred, and one must assess the patient's status for compensation, further treatment, and need for rehabilitation. Orderly information gathering is particularly needed for concussion or minor head injury since their effects are denied by such phrases as "self-limiting . . . (inviting) exaggeration . . . 'ambulance chasing' . . . deliberate inflation . . . disproportionate to the consequences of injury."[2] When a large group of impaired TBI victims are not counted, the safety issues and social costs are not reflected in official statistics and policy. Further, one cannot agree with Stuss,[3] who exaggerates our precision in understanding TBI at different phases: "The severity of TBI must be defined by the acute injury . . . not by severity . . . at random points after

trauma . . . symptoms of mild TBI gradually improve." Some authors question whether mild concussion is really a cerebral dysfunction, that is, subtle brain damage.[4] Clinical experience with paradoxically large dysfunctions, and experimental neuropathological data concerning whiplash (inertial or nonimpact loading) associated with lesser level of disturbed consciousness,[5,6,7] certainly support the position that significant impairment can occur when a set of physical conditions occur either without involving impact at all, or after high acceleration/deceleration of the skull and enclosed brain.

Errors occur at information gathering of both acute and chronic phases. The presence of TBI may not be recognized: lack of diagnosis by an examining doctor; incorrect statements in the record about loss or altered consciousness, post-traumatic or retrograde amnesia; lack of examination after an accident; nonattention to head injury due to attention to other systems; discrepancy between emergency and hospital records and what the patient remembers. The patient had recovered consciousness by the time the emergency personnel arrived, seemed alert in the emergency room, when in fact prior loss of consciousness was not known or the patient remained confused, or still in posttraumatic amnesia. Further, examiner and research errors can exaggerate recovery after TBI.[8,9] Too narrow a range of functions may be studied. Assessment procedures may be less precise than the current standard of psychometric assessment. "Good" or "complete" recovery may be reported without precise or wide-range examination (in contrast, a major head injury research study of outcome utilized 40 hours, including 16 hours of neuropsychological testing[10]). The very existence of TBI may not be recognized: A detailed study of major injuries determined an increase of 74 percent compared to the official statistics, while minor injuries exceeded official statistics by 384 percent.[11] Finally, the patient's vulnerability to further injury or late-developing disorders may go unrecognized.

J Rehabil Outcomes Meas, 1997, 1(3), 1–22
© 1997 Aspen Publishers, Inc.

Outcome studies of TBI have faced technical obstacles, particularly for mild TBI or concussion:

- There may be no common diagnostic category, conceptual schema, or formal rating system.[6,12,13,14,15]
- *Criteria are arbitrary* for specifying the level of impairment.
- *Criteria vary* with the procedures.
- *Insensitive procedures* ignore subtle deficits and may not take into consideration the difference between patients with and without persistent postconcussional symptoms (PCS) or a history of head injury.[16]
- A "whole person impairment"[14] is imprecise insofar as it does not consider compensatory strategies or loss of actual functions within a particular environment.
- *Somatic injury, pain, and headaches* synergistically enhance TBI effects that interfere with work, community living, and autonomic and immune functions.
- *Symptoms of the PCS and mild TBI occur without head injury* so that the diagnosis of TBI becomes more difficult.[17,18,19]

Accurate assessment of outcome will be enhanced by our information-gathering protocol, which includes comparison of the estimated pre-injury baseline with current performance; multidisciplinary study of a wide range of functions; alertness to noncerebral medical conditions consequent to head trauma; differentiating positive and negative symptoms; considering the maladaptive consequences of "distractors" that reduce effectiveness; and offering recommendations and prognosis. TBI in children may require a longer period of deferred judgment to determine the developmental trajectory.[20]

CHANGES OVER A LONG INTERVAL

The process of TBI can continue after an injury.[21,22,23] This accounts in part for symptom persistence and late-developing medical and neurobehavioral conditions (see below). Although it has been asserted that MTBI effects are resolved after three months,[24] this does not reflect clinical experience with persistent, documented postconcussion syndrome. One group of patients, selected on the basis of apparent whiplash injury, offered not only an estimated mean cognitive loss of nearly one standard deviation (SD) (14 points) of Wechsler Intelligence Scale Revised (WAIS-R) Full Scale IQ,[25] but numerous previously undetected head impacts.[26] For another subset of patients (three or more PCS symptoms), approximately one quarter with uncomplicated mild head injury had increased numbers of cognitive and emotional/vegetative symptoms, were more intolerant to intense sound and light, and had higher interference scores on the Stroop procedure. Both cognitive and emotional vegetative symptoms were associated with other dysfunctions.[16]

The phases of TBI may be conceptualized:

1. *Preexisting TBI.* The extent of traumatic brain injury and impairment can be increased by a preexisting condition (prior brain injury or fragile adaption). A seemingly mild impact or deceleration may synergize the prior dysfunctions, rendering the new condition major. A large proportion of college students reported prior head injury (23–34 percent of males and 12–16 percent of females). Thus the cumulative proportion of people having a prior head injury increases with age, explaining one source of paradoxically grave level of impairment after apparently minor head injury.[27]
2. *Primary.* Mechanical forces (head impact, neck movement, skull deformation, brain movement in the skull) create brain shearing relative to the skull and between parts with or without torn blood vessels, but with damaged axons and contusions or lacerations. Since the full extent of axonal damage requires 12 hours to develop, outcome may be contingent upon the immediate availability of treatment.[7] Primary phase TBI alone ("concussion" or "mild head injury") does not preclude occult injuries that are expressed later as tertiary or quaternary symptoms.
3. *Secondary.* This phase may include pathophysiological processes initiated by primary trauma (hemorrhage and mass effects; interference with blood brain barrier and brain autoregulation, including perfusion; ischemia and anoxia; cytotoxic effects).[7]
4. *Tertiary.* Here occur disorders of physiological dysfunctioning. Early disorders are endocrine dysfunctioning, such as diabetes insipidus. Late disorders are endocrine-related developmental dysfunctions.
5. *Quaternary.* Occurring in this phase are neurological conditions that develop after the acute phase of trauma (dementing conditions; posttraumatic epilepsy).

It has been asserted that the majority of recovery occurs in the first six months, with improvement occurring at a reduced rate up to several years postinjury.[28] Actually, changes in both directions occur for a long period, with the trajectory of recovery varying between functions. When assessment was performed during the two- to five-year interval after injury (primarily after moderate and severe TBI), positive and status changes occurred.[23] There was an increase in the number of problems (visual; headaches; word-finding; memory; slowed thinking; concentration; easy fatigability; irritability and aggression; reduced social life; self-centered and socially inappropriate behavior). Of those employed at the time of the accident, 50 percent were employed at two years, and only 40 percent at 5 years. Only 4 percent of the unemployed group at two years had gained employment at five years. Some patients improved in activities of daily living, including domestic tasks, community activities, and return to driving. In the more seriously in-jured requiring inpatient rehabilitation, older individuals (55 and older) stayed twice as long as younger persons, owing to decreased physical reserve, preexisting medical conditions, and higher incidence of medical complications.[29] Consistency of performance improves more than five years after a TBI.[28]

MEDICAL DISORDERS CONTRIBUTING TO IMPAIRMENT

After serious trauma, the damaged systems may not re-cover fully, adding to the stress of the posttraumatic period and impairing adaptive functioning. Somatic damage signifi-cantly impairs ability to work.[30]

Systems Injured During Accidents

Gastrointestinal, genitourinary, respiratory, cardiovascu-lar, skin, musculoskeletal, endocrinologic, and orthopedic systems may suffer from impact.[31] Orthopedic trauma may incur joint contractures, heterotopic ossifications, and cra-nial or craniofacial defects. Respiratory failure, pneumonia, tracheostomy, gastrostomy, and jejunostomy were associ-ated with longer length of stay in acute care and rehabilita-tion. Particular bodily functions to be assessed include swal-lowing and feeding, recovery from pelvic fractures, upper and lower extremity strength, and coordination[32]; autonomy of the thermoregulatory system is also important.[33]

The Immune System and General Health

Changes of health and bodily functioning may occur early, or later, because of impaired immune functions and physiologic disruptions. Severe head injury (hypoxia, is-chemia, hypotension, etc.) creates widespread brain dam-age,[7] impairing structures that maintain health functions. One mechanism is an exchange between the neural, immune, and hormonal systems (neuroimmunomodulation), through neural and blood cells (lymphocytes), and neurohormonal and endocrine substances. Feedback control of the hypo-thalamus by adrenal cortical glucocorticoids and other chemicals is changed during posttraumatic stress disorder (PTSD).[34] Excess glucocorticoids (such as cortisol), secreted by the adrenal cortex in stress, suppress immunological and inflammatory responses.[35] Psychological stress, depression, and particular lesions also affect the immune function, al-though the precise neuroendocrine pathway is unknown.[36]

Neck Injury

The neck is the most injured body region in noncontact crashes as a result of tension, shear, bending, rotation, and com-pression by muscles.[37] Vulnerable structures include the ca-rotid artery; ligaments; trigeminal sensory vascular network; sympathetic cervical chain; vertebral artery; bone fracture damaging soft tissues and spinal cord; vertebrobasilar occlu-sion; dysfunction of spinal afferents; radicular injury; mid-cer-vical fractures at C3-4 level which may compress the cord. Damage can have neurobehavioral effects through pain, im-paired sensory and motor nerve supply, interference with auto-nomic nervous system reflexes, interference with cerebral blood supply, and restricted range of motion. Neck injury im-plies that rotational and angular momentum was probably transmitted to the head and the contained brain. Dysfunctions attributed to neck injury include headache; referred pain; myofascial pain or fibromyalgia; sensory loss and hypersen-sitivity (including vision, audition and tinnitus, balance, touch, pain, unstable temperature); dystonia; Horner's syn-drome; muscular weakness based upon cranial nerve dys-function; dysarthria; nausea; vomiting; syncope; confusion; and transient ischemic attacks.[37-44] Patients selected on the basis of whiplash exhibit loss of mental ability, comorbid psychiatric syndromes,[26] and deficits of information process-ing and concentration.[45]

CHRONIC POSTTRAUMATIC STRESS DISORDER (PTSD)

The complex physiological, anatomical, and behavioral ba-sis of PTSD interacts with TBI effects, somatic trauma, the re-covery process, the hypothalamic-pituitary adrenocortical axis (HPA), the sympathetic nervous system (SNS), and the im-mune system. The proportion of individuals who suffer from PTSD after accidents is controversial, with estimates varying from common[46] to low after minor head injury.[8] In one sample[47] there were 10 cases from a sample of 300 with moder-ate to severe head injury with intracranial injury and uncon-sciousness up to 14 days. It was noted that symptoms of these conditions overlap. It was documented in 16 of 31 patients in one sample with persistent symptoms after a whiplash acci-dent.[26] Chronic PTSD has numerous neurobehavioral effects: restriction of the range of activity due to hyperarousal and dys-phoric symptoms; alterations in regulatory physiology[48]; in-creased arousal and autonomic hyperactivity[49]; decreased nore-pinephrine secretion, increased cortisol, and inhibited immune reaction.[50] The stress response, with its antigrowth, antireproductive, catabolic, and immunosuppressive effects, is designed to be time limited.

In contrast, chronic PTSD (hyperactivation of the hypo-thalamic-pituitary adrenal axis) potentiates psychosocial and physiological symptoms: the Selye stress syndrome (behav-ioral, neuroendocrine, autonomic, and immunological fea-tures; reduced pain threshold; weight gain). Chronic PTSD terminating in hypoarousal (reduced corticotropin releasing hormone secretion) is associated with fatigue and depres-sion.[34] Stress inhibits the reproductive axis, the growth axis, thyroid axis, and growth hormone production, and decreases some mood disorders (anxiety; melancholic depression). Stress-related gluconeogenesis with excess glucocorticoids, leads to insulin resistance, resulting in poor control of diabetes and adiposity.[34,51–56]

Cognitive loss has been documented after PTSD. A group of patients with PTSD alone had WAIS-R IQ scores below estimated baseline. Their deficits were less severe than those in a demographically similar group with TBI.[57] Such loss may be consequent to altered information processing,[58] impaired monitoring, regulation of memory, and processing bias for disaster-specific information. Cognitive loss is greater when there is a concurrent comorbid diagnosis.[59] For older accident victims, the mechanism for dementia may be moderate stress adding to aging of the hippocampus.[60] The enhanced incidence after TBI of Alzheimer's Disease is to be considered as a possible outcome.

Physiological and Health Dysfunctions

Catecholamines, particularly dopamine, inhibit gonadotropin release, possibly attributable to adrenergic release by the SNS.[51] The conflict between adaptive response to stress (increased energy mobilization and analgesia) and the immune response (reduced activity to spare energy consumption for repair) may partially account for the frequent complaint of low stamina in traumatized patients. Further, the immune system seems to stimulate hyperalgesia, which reduces work efficiency.[61] There is increased vulnerability to medical conditions, including viral diseases.[62]

Cumulative lifelong exposure to stress (hyperarousal), suggested by increased cortisol levels in older people, may cause sleep disorders and cognitive deficits.[63] Partial and full PTSD at three months predicted dissociative consciousness changes at 12 months after emotional trauma alone.[64] To differentiate psychologically motivated dissociation from TBI-related altered consciousness is an unresolved technical question.

PTSD Contributes to Psychiatric Disorders

An endocrine pattern seen in TBI, such as adrenocorticoid hypersecretion of cortisol (accompanying PTSD) and hypothyroidism, is also found in psychiatric depression.[65] While the proportion of TBI patients described as *depressed* is high, *depression* is an ambiguous term including many disparate dysfunctions (psychodynamic, anatomical, chemical). A study of Alzheimer's disease indicated that HPA axis deregulation is associated with depressive symptoms and hippocampal atrophy. HPA axis dysregulation was increased in both depressed patients and controls.[66] This is consistent with an age-related effect of stress upon the hippocampus.

HYPOTHALAMICO-PITUITARY AXIS (HPA) AND TARGET ENDOCRINES

The hypothalamic-pituitary endocrine axis contributes to development and homeostasis. Normal development is the outcome of integrated physiological functioning. Growth, for example, is contingent upon thyroid secretions, growth hormone, insulin, glucocorticoids, catecholamines, CNS biogenic amines, inhibitory effects of the CNS independent of sex steroids, and reduced sensitivity of the hypothalamus to inhibitory effects of sex steroids and CNS inhibition.[67] Homeostasis is controlled through feedback loops from the endocrine glands that maintain hormone levels rather precisely by feeding back to the hypothalamus and the pituitary. Hypothalamic influence is positive in all instances except secretion of prolactin (PRL), so that damage causes a release of PRL.[68] Hypothalamic damage interferes with maintenance of body homeostasis.[33] Hypothalamic-pituitary damage is caused by blunt trauma, mass effects causing compression of the hypothalamo-hypophyseal portal vessels,[183] shearing movements of the brain tearing the pituitary stalk,[69] and bullet wounds outside the brain.[70] Basilar skull fractures that tear the pituitary stalk, rupturing the neural connections to neurohypophysis and vascular connections to the adenohypophysis, disrupt delivery of releasing or inhibiting factors to the pituitary. A severe enough lesion of any part of the HPA leads to loss of endocrine homeostasis, by disturbing excitatory and inhibitory stages of endocrine signaling to the hypothalamus and pituitary gland.[63] Damage to the hypothalamic-pituitary axis commonly causes secondary hypopituitarism, expressed as somatic, sexual, and developmental problems. The degree of hormonal reduction reflects the severity of the trauma.[64]

SEXUAL PROBLEMS POST TBI

Sexual dysfunctions may be present or absent, and drive can be reduced or increased. The range of reported complaints has varied from 4 to 71 percent. Varied etiology of sexual dysfunction, and procedures for study of particular aspects of physiological functioning, have been reviewed.[71] Sexual problems exacerbate other psychosocial effects of head injury: capacity for intimacy; mood; physical abilities; self-esteem.[72] A majority of marriages where one partner has incurred TBI result in divorce. PCS was followed by sexual dysfunction in 58 percent of one group, including reduced libido and erective dysfunction. Changes in cognitive level and personality are more distressing than changes in physical ability. The history of pre-injury marital stability and coping skills can aid in overcoming such problems as reduced affection, and reduced income. Roles within the family change. Sexuality is interfered with by cognitive factors, and physical problems such as headache and fatigue.[73]

Sexual outcome varies with location (patients with frontal and right hemisphere lesions reporting more satisfaction than others), and interval since injury (arousal levels decreasing with time). Amenorrhea[74–76] may signal hypopituitarism. Marital and sexual problems may result from pain; damage to neural circuits and cerebral areas (frontal, frontotemporal, septal); deficits of neurotransmitters, endocrines; functions such as sensorimotor, neuroorthopedic, cognitive-behavioral, bowel, bladder, libido, and genital; mood disorders (depression, stress, fatigue).[71,72,77] Epileptic seizures trigger changes in hormones involved in reproductive function, further affecting excitability of CNS neurons and the seizure threshold. Antiepileptic drugs in turn affect reproductive hormones and behavior, creating risks for women of reproductive age or currently pregnant.[78] A protocol for assessing endocrine and sexual performance is available.[18]

BEHAVIORAL AND EMOTIONAL CHANGES

Outcome can include a variety of diagnostic categories: cerebral personality syndromes and symptoms (e.g., the frontal lobe disorder and aprosodia; reduced motivation; catastrophic reaction[79]; inflexibility and perseveration; irritability; disinhibition (sexuality, violence); inappropriate mood and affect (laughing, crying); social insensitivity; endogenous depression; aprosodia; difficulties in initiation and completion of activities; behavior not modified by experience[80]; psychiatric conditions (in remission and initially expressed); posttraumatic stress disorder (see above); mood changes (psychodynamic, cerebral personality disorder, and brain damage, including anger, depression, sexuality, anxiety); loss of social skills and interest; change of identity (feels unattractive, damaged, and vulnerable); changed body schema as a neurological disorder.[57,81]

TAXONOMY OF NEUROBEHAVIORAL FUNCTIONS: ORGANIZING DATA

Organizing neurobehavioral findings through the Taxonomy of Neurobehavioral Functions[57,82] described elsewhere enables the examiner to detect informational gaps in the record and to plan an examination without redundancy. Findings can be presented in an orderly way, and comparison made with baseline and examinations at different postinjury intervals. See representative symptoms by Taxa in Table 1.

I. Basic Systems

A. Awareness, perception, and arousal. Arousal, consciousness, and experience of self, activities, and the external world, with capacity for memory.

B. Information processing. Encoding external stimuli and mental contents, foresight, error monitoring, focused attention, concentration, sequencing, manipulating information.

C. Integrated sensorimotor functions and body schema. Reception and utilization of external and internal stimuli, integrating them with motor output, and body schema.

D. Neurophysiological and health. Vegetative, endocrine, and immune systems.

E. Cerebral personality functions. Permanent changes in behavior, experience, and expression of affect directly caused by brain trauma.

II. Cognitive Functions

A. General intelligence and cognitive processing. The range, level, and complexity of information that can be manipulated, and applied to problems ("crystallized"), or new and abstract tasks ("fluid"), in structured or unstructured situations.

Table 1. Samples of Positive and Negative Symptoms

Taxon	Type I (new)	Type II (reduced)
Awareness	Arousal; altered consciousness	Numbing; reduced vigilance
Information processing	Perseveration; concrete thinking	Mental slowness; poor error monitoring
Sensorimotor	Movement disorders; hypersensitivity	Weakness; incoordination
Neurophysiological	Dysregulation; diabetes insipidus	Reduced development; sexual deficits
Cerebral personality	Frontal lobe syndrome; dyscontrol	Endogenous depression; aprosodia; adynamia
Intelligence	(None)	Dementia; factors
Memory	Confabulation; denial	Working memory; long-term storage; amnesia
Language	Jargon; dysarthria	Anomia; aphasia
Pain behavior	Social role; somatic orientation	Pessimism; impaired concentration
Posttraumatic stress	Intrusive anxiety; avoidance; dissociation	Fatigability
Psychodynamic	Dysphoria; defenses; embarrassment	Hypoarousal; hopeless; numbing
Identity; Weltanschauung	Reduced self-esteem; sees world as dangerous	Withdrawal; loss of social interest
Adaptive functions	Somatization	Reduced effectiveness in work, education, community

B. Memory. The storage of sensations, events, information, mental contents, and action patterns, and meanings with retrieval after varying intervals.

C. Language. Receiving, comprehending, communicating information and instructions, using grammatical rules with verbal, symbolic, or nonverbal representation, and motor speech, in order to achieve goals and social needs. Aphasia is a generic term for loss of speech.

III. Adaptive Functions

A. Posttraumatic stress. An unusual frightening experience leads to a pattern of anxiety and hyperarousal that varies in intensity from the "acute" stage (attempt to return to homeostasis) to "chronic" state (hypoarousal and exhaustion). Positive symptoms: Anxiety; arousal and autonomic hyperactivity; anger; preoccupation; dissociative states (depersonalization, derealization). Negative symptoms (chronic PTSD): hopelessness; deficient coping and motivation; hypoarousal (numbing; depression; asexuality; social withdrawal).

B. Pain behavior. Postaccident pain (headaches, neck, shoulder, back, upper and lower limb) has been reported in varying proportions of patients with TBI (18–95 percent). Lesser levels in severe cases is perhaps attributable to inadequate self-monitoring, but data may be biased by the information gathering procedure.[83] Pain increases after chronic stress, depression, anger, and tension reduce adaptive efficiency through impairing attention and memory.[83-89]

C. Psychodynamic. Emotional reactions to our experiences, unconscious processes, the meaning we give to life, and neurotic defenses.

D. Attitude towards oneself and the world (altered identity).[90] Reduced self-confidence; reduced self-esteem (less attractive, damaged, vulnerable to further injury, victimized); the world outlook (Weltanschauung) is dangerous, bleak, and unsupportive.

E. Complex adaptive functions. Combinations of injury, dysphoria, brain damage, and discouragement contribute to disability due to persistence of symptoms, evidenced by such problems as inability to perform integrated daily tasks.[91]

INDICATIONS FOR SELECTED PROCEDURES AFTER TWO YEARS

Indications for a Dental Examination

Oro-dental problems associated with brain damage include functional disorders characterized by faulty oral and pharyngeal phases of swallowing, by speech and language disorders associated with breathing, voice production, articulation of vowels and consonants, and by syntactical and other cognitive disorders. Direct injury to the orofacial and dental structures during head trauma may present immediate injury to the teeth

and dento-alveolar structures, and to the lingual, oral, and facial musculature. If the injuries induce fracture of teeth, or of the maxilla or mandible, dental care problems may persist for two or more years. Avulsed or mobile teeth may require splinting to retain them. The occluding surfaces of teeth may not be in a stable interdigitation relationship and can thus induce speech, swallowing, and esthetic disorders with associated prosthetic, psychological, and emotional problems. If the temporomandibular joint is injured, it may require several years of treatment to reduce the pain and muscle spasm associated with injury to the joint.

After a two-year postinjury interval, injury to the brain (cortex, basal ganglia, brainstem, and cranial nerves) can be manifested in the disturbed orificial sensorimotor function, expressed as aberrant jaw motion and deviant motor activity of the tongue, lips, and masticatory muscles.

Simple effective clinical tests of these symptoms may suggest referral. Testing is suggested for the tongue motoric activity required in speech, chewing, and swallowing. To stabilize head and neck posture the patient is requested to sit in the upright position with the eyes focused on a target five feet away at eye level for the following procedures:

First, the patient is asked to furl, curl, point, and blade the tongue tip. The mobility of the tongue during any *one* of these tasks when asked to do them three times at two- to three-second intervals may not be significant if not within the normal range. However, when they can't do several of the motor movements, these inabilities coupled with the following tests may be evidence of peripheral and/or central brain changes to the hypoglossal (XII) nerve. The patient is asked to say the K, G, KG sounds. If nasality exists where it did not before the head injury, the IX, X, and XI cranial nerves may be damaged.

Second, the patient is asked to distend cheeks with impounded air, first both the cheeks and then alternately. The patient is asked to retrude the lips and protrude them, to perform bilateral and unilateral nasal grimacing. The inability to do these tasks appropriately may be a form of relative hypodyskinesia or hyperdyskinesia, perhaps indicating a central brain disorder.

Finally, the patient is asked to perform some mandibular jaw motion patterns. If patient has no overt orthodontic or prosthodontic occlusion reasons for limited mobility patterns, the patient should receive the following tests:

1. Open and close the jaw without pain to a distance of two or three finger digits wide, 30–45 mm.
2. The patient should be able to tap upper and lower incisor teeth tip to tip at least three times in three seconds.
3. The patient is asked to tap the upper left cuspid tooth to the lower left cuspid tooth and conversely on the right side. The cuspid should be tapped two or three times without pain, and again within two to three seconds.

If they can not open the jaws easily, reach the opposing incisor or cuspid teeth, one should heed the deficiency carefully. It may be because of dental problems and a dentist should be consulted to rule out orthodontic or prosthodontic tooth disorders. However, patients with central brain or peripheral cranial nerve disorders may not be able to achieve these movements because of peripheral nerve sensory loss or central brain disorder. In all instances where faulty movement and function of the oral facial and dental structures are not clearly associated with neurologic deficit, a dental consultation should be obtained for clarification of movement disorders or sensory deficiencies.

Indications for a General Medical Examination

Major advances in our understanding of the neurophysiology and pathologic mechanism of traumatic brain injury, and innovations in neurological scanning procedures, and delivery of services, have markedly decreased the mortality and morbidity of head injury. Consequently, more patients survive several years posttrauma, and will be examined with residual medical conditions whose traumatic origin at one time would have been more patent. The medical examination of TBI outcome is part of a continuum that begins in the first hours of insult and may last for years.

Due to immune system deficits, and continuing traumatic stress effects, victims of head trauma should be regarded as compromised hosts and therefore at risk for infection. Additional infectious conditions requiring attention, with alertness to possible attribution to a head injury, are posttraumatic meningitis, subdural empyema, and brain abscesses, which may be detected after a delay. Any patient with recurrent meningitis should activate alarms in the mind of examiners about history of head injury, particularly skull fractures.

Consequent to damage to the hypothalamus and brain stem from severe head trauma, there are hyperdynamic cardiovascular responses that may be encountered in the rehabilitation phases. Unexplained hypertension and ST-T changes in the electrocardiogram (ECG) may be related to the long-term effects of head trauma, and alert an examiner to other somatic and neurobehavioral dysfunctions.

Respiratory complications are common after severe injuries, and may require a tracheostomy. Therefore, that head trauma patient remains at risk for pulmonary complications such as an embolism or deep vein thrombosis, even after a considerable interval.

It is noteworthy that coagulopathy is a common complication of severe head injury.[92]

Indications for an Adult Endocrinological Examination

Head trauma can cause defects ranging from isolated ACTH deficiency to panhypopituitarism with diabetes insipidus.[68] Any suggestion of damage to the sella turcica should initiate study of pituitary function, which may take years to deteriorate.

Symptoms of hypopituitarism may be total or partial.[70,74] Panhypopituitarism is rare, and is associated with alterations in arousal and awareness. Hypopituitarism is clinically evident after 70–75 percent destruction of the adenohypophysis. Total loss of pituitary secretion requires 90 percent glandular destruction and may accompany prolonged coma. Recovery of pituitary function usually parallels neurological improvement. Residual impairment is not uncommon.[93] Prompt treatment is essential after suspicion of a pituitary injury.

The integrity of the pituitary end-organ axis is investigated by studying pituitary and organ hormone levels, and pituitary response to hypothalamic releasing hormones. Endocrine evaluation includes MRI exploration of hypothalamic-pituitary structures, and integrity of the pituitary end-organ axis (pituitary and organ hormone levels; pituitary response to hypothalamic releasing hormones).[51]

Alerting endocrine symptoms: polyuria, polydipsia, thirst (diabetes insipidus[94] is associated with reduced levels of vasopressin after severe head trauma, but may occur after minor head trauma), hypothalamus, hypophysectomy, retrograde degeneration of axons into the supraoptic and paraventricular hypothalamic nuclei.[95,96] With delayed onset,[97] permanent antidiuretic hormone insufficiency is expected.[7,36,74,75,76,98] Other symptoms are excessive and inappropriate secretion of antidiuretic hormone (SIADH)[99] and thyroid dysfunction. Galactorrhea, amenorrhea, and hirsutism,[100] and inhibition of gonadotropin secretion resulting in secondary hypogonadism in boys,[101] may indicate hypothalamic damage with hyperprolactinemia. Further symptoms might be loss of axillary and pubic hair[51]; growth failure; acquired gonadotropin deficiency[98]; hypothyroidism; ACTH deficiency[70]; transient hypogonadotrophic hypogonadism[52] or permanent hypogonadotrophic hypogonadism[98]; reduced thyroid function, possibly associated with a stress-related sympathetic discharge of catecholamines[53]; hyponatremia (cerebral salt wasting, or natriuresis, a syndrome of inappropriate antidiuretic hormone secretion characterized by vasopressin or ADH [SIADH])[102,103]; myxedema; dwarfism; obesity; hypothermia; bradycardia[33]; dermatological (waxy or dry skin; wrinkling around eyes and ears); anemia; psychiatric disturbance (mental slowing; apathy; delusions; paranoid psychosis); hypoglycemia; weakness; lethargy; cold intolerance; decreased libido; constipation; bradycardia; hoarseness; myxedema; increased, decreased menstrual flow and amenorrhea; delayed resumption of menstruation.[99]

Indications for a Child or Adolescent Endocrinological Examination

Indications for an endocrinological exam in nonadults include growth retardation[104,105]; lack of achievement of puberty; precocious puberty (defined as the onset of secondary sexual characteristics before age 8 in girls and 9 in boys[106]), with growth acceleration and skeletal maturation, or dilation of the third ventricle[51] consequent to a tear of the hypothalamus[75] which may commence within a few months of injury[76]; gonadotropin releasing hormone (GnRH) release in girls due to hypothalamic damage[107]; interference with inhibition of gonadotropin secretion by the mass effects of head trauma due to hypothalamus damage[108]; growth hormone deficiency[75] that may commence within a few months of injury[76]; absent secondary sexual development consequent to hypopituitary insufficiency[13,45,109,110]; and gonadal failure with loss of libido, impotence, amenorrhea,[111] amenorrhea and sexual infantilism consequent to hypothalamic insufficiency.[74]

Single Photon Emitted Computerized Tomography (SPECT)

Single photon emission computer tomography (SPECT) brain perfusion imaging is achieved by the intravenous injection of technetium Tc 99m–labelled lipophilic compounds that are able to cross the normal blood brain barrier. The patients are imaged two hours after the intravenous injection, using multihead detector gamma cameras, which have better resolution and decrease image acquisition time. In traumatic brain injury, SPECT brain perfusion imaging plays an important role in defining areas of perfusion abnormalities in the absence of morphological abnormalities on the X-ray, computed tomography (CT), or magnetic resonance imaging (MRI). Morphological changes on the CT or MRI imply decreased brain perfusion below critical levels for a prolonged period of time. Mild changes in cerebral brain perfusion, on the other hand, can be detected easily with SPECT brain perfusion imaging.

Indications for a SPECT study:

1. Moderate and minor traumatic brain injury with or without history of loss of consciousness, with neurobehavioral changes such as lack of concentration, attention, amnesia, and so on. It should be noted that presence of positive findings on X-ray CT or MRI does not limit the use of SPECT because the sensitivity to dysfunction is higher.
2. Early imaging within one week following the accident is more sensitive than delayed imaging.
3. Delayed SPECT imaging in traumatic brain injury is indicated only in symptomatic patients with abnormal neuropsychological testing, regardless of whether the X-ray CT or MRI are positive or negative.

Indications for a Neurological Examination

The role of the neurological consultation is to synthesize an ordered vision of the extent to which the brain trauma or organic disease contributes to the clinical presentation. Closed head injury may be associated with epidural hematoma, subdural hematoma, subarachnoid hemorrhage, frontal and temporal lobe contusions, shearing injury, and carotid or vertebral artery dissection. Knowledge of a head trauma is a cue to the need for later study. Hematoma causes headaches, loss of mental acuity, drowsiness, weakness, seizures, or coma. Shearing injuries are associated with loss of mental function, seizures, and damage to the pituitary. A history of hydrocephalus (usually after brain contusion) is associated with gait abnormalities (a sliding or "magnetic" gait), urinary incontinence, and progressive dementia. Carotid or vertebra dissection can lead to stroke and transient ischemic attack, with their characteristic syndromes an example of cerebral effects consequent to neck injury.

The long-term neurologic sequelae of closed head injury can include headache, imbalance, fainting, loss of consciousness, urinary incontinence, gait disorder, loss of mental functions, depression masquerading as dementia, episodic behavioral changes, convulsions, vertigo, polydipsia. A patient presenting with these symptoms should prompt a neurological consultation and exploration of possible head trauma. Some, but by no means all, of these symptoms may correlate with abnormalities on brain MRI or CT. Some abnormalities may appear on the MRI but not on the clinical exam and vice versa. Therefore, an MRI should never be regarded as the final answer. A normal MRI does not rule out brain trauma, nor does an abnormal scan necessarily pinpoint the cause of the presenting complaint. Moreover, the standards of interpretation of the MRI are variable, and it remains an unfortunate fact that scans are frequently misinterpreted. Furthermore, a given complaint may suggest a particular kind of imaging study. For example, the complaint of constant urination could represent either psychiatric disease or damage to the pituitary stalk in a shearing injury, perhaps prompting a detailed imaging study of the pituitary, rather than an image of the whole brain.

Negative focal neurological examination findings are sometimes found in PCS, but positive findings encourage investigation of other functional areas. The following neurological symptoms have a high incidence: vertigo, dizziness, distorted stance and gait[112]; headaches[113]; visual, pupillary, and oculomotor dysfunction[114]; paroxysmal alterations of consciousness[115]; hearing loss,[116] articulation problems, and laryngeal dysfunction[117,118]; seizures; motor, sensory, visual field, other cranial nerve deficits[10]; movement disorders.[119]

Some Cranial Nerve Dysfunctions Sometimes Ignored

Nerve I: Olfactory

Chemosensation is a generic term involving olfaction (smell), gustation (taste), and chemical sense (irritation or pungency). All three contribute to flavor. Olfaction and the chemical sense contribute to detection of vaporous molecules. Trigeminal and vagal nerves contribute to sensations of feel, warmth, cold, irritation, and pungency in the perception of chili peppers and mint, crisp versus soft, and so on.[120] The complaint of inability to "taste" may really mean inability to distinguish flavors. Patients may attribute trigeminal cues to olfactory cues, that is, pungent odorants such as ammonia are detected by a common chemical sense. The olfactory nerve is vulnerable to shearing tears in the cribriform plate. Odor loss may not be reported if not inquired into, and the patient may be unaware if it is unilateral. Dysfunction may be temporary or permanent, peripheral (loss of sensitivity), or central (loss of ability to identify odors). Deficits of taste (ageusia) (Nerve V) may occur with damage to chemoreceptive areas of the medial frontal and anterior temporal lobes,[121] or bilateral shearing.[122] Testing with noxious stimulants such as ammonia should be avoided since they may excite pain afferents.[123]

Nerve II: Optic N

The long course of Nerve II, its radiations, and branches to the midbrain, is vulnerable to TBI, and thus invites visual field study. When found, the visual defects are often not related to TBI if there is "no damage to the globe." Specification of postorbital or retro-chiasmal deficits is vital. Visual problems associated with head trauma include diplopia, fourth nerve palsy, abduction defects, loss of color vision.[114,124]

Nerve V: Trigeminal

Taste alteration (dysgeusia) is stated to be more common than taste loss or decrement.[125] There may be a dissociation between loss of olfactory and loss of chemical sensation; what is termed *odor* is really a chemical sensation received in the mouth. Cerebral lesions rarely impair taste, though it may be lost together with the sense of smell as a result of head injury.[126] Dysfunctions may be consequent to unilateral thalamic and parietal lobe lesions. A gustatory aura is occasionally experienced at the beginning of a frontoparietal seizure.[127]

Late Developing Neurological Conditions

Functionally significant abnormalities may be detected only by late MRI.[128] Neurodegenerative diseases: premature senility or dementia, dystonia, and posttraumatic epilepsy (see also PTSD).[129–134] Dystonia: hemidystonia, bilateral dystonia, and torticollis.[135] Guillain-Barre Syndrome may be an immunological dysfunction.[136] Head trauma has been directly implicated in deposition of β amyloid protein,[134] leading to increased incidence of senile dementia (Alzheimer's disease)[131,137–139] and Parkinson's disease.[140–142]

Indications for a Partial Seizure Study

Posttraumatic epilepsy is a well recognized late consequence of TBI.[143–148] Epileptic seizures affect reproductive function (see section on sexuality, above). Apparent partial seizures can accompany the persistent postconcussion syndrome, and should be actively sought (interview; checklist). Partial seizures have a risk of recurrence.[149] Posttraumatic tumors[150] can cause alterations of affect and consciousness that resemble partial seizures.[151]

Posttraumatic epilepsy is, by definition, a partial epilepsy with seizures beginning in a restricted area of cortex. If there is no alteration of awareness during such seizures, they are defined as simple partial, while complex partial seizures do include such an alteration. It is crucial that clinicians be aware of the delay in development of epilepsy following head trauma, as well as the sometimes bizarre manifestations of seizures arising in cortical areas most likely to be effected. It is important to realize that seizures may develop after even relatively mild loss of consciousness.[152] Other sources of confusion resulting in the failure to diagnose delayed posttraumatic seizure disorders are the limited diagnostic value of many routine EEG studies, as well as a lack of understanding of the varied and at times bizarre manifestations of seizures.

The areas frequently injured by deceleration injuries include the orbitofrontal cortex and polar regions of the temporal and frontal lobes. Since most of these regions lie deep, and may be relatively electrically shielded from detection by standard EEG electrodes, EEGs in such patients can be normal even during an actual seizure. Sometimes this results in the diagnosis of pseudoseizures.[153] Thus, in such patients, the use of special electrodes (sphenoidal, supra/infraorbital) may be necessary to detect epileptiform activity.

Seizures may take the form of staring or generalized shaking, but also manifest themselves in milder or more unusual seizures arising from such areas as the mesial or inferior frontal lobes. It is in this group of patients that misdiagnosis is most likely to occur, particularly since even ictal EEGs may be normal. The initial or sole phenomena experienced ictally can indicate to the physician the region of ictal onset, such as simple visual hallucinations arising in the occipital lobe.[154] In the case of the mesial temporal lobe, neuropsychiatric ictal phenomena can occur, at times leading to confusion with psychiatric disorders. In fact, patients may not report such experiences to their physicians for fear of being thought insane. Panic attacks may occur, as well as episodes of déja or jamais vu, derealization, depersonalization, autoscopy (out-of-body perception), depression, and paranoia.[156] Isolated autonomic changes may also occur, such as flushing or piloerection. When such seizures remain partial, the majority will have no associated ictal EEG changes.[155] Frontal lobe epilepsy may also present with bizarre seizures, which may at times be felt to be functional, particularly since even the ictal EEG may be normal in approximately 20 percent of cases.[153] Seizures arising in the deep frontal cortex may involve bizarre episodes, often occurring daily and in sleep, with unusual behavior such as screaming, cursing, boxing, or bicycling movements.[151]

It is crucial that the limitations of EEG as a diagnostic tool be appreciated. Physicians should consider a comprehensive seizure evaluation of any head trauma patient presenting with new paroxysmal symptoms. Seizures may occur at the time of, or shortly after, head trauma. However, there may be a lag of years or even decades before posttraumatic seizures occur. This lag represents the time necessary for the development of gliosis and functional reorganization resulting in an epileptogenic focus.

Indications for Neuropsychological Examination

The neuropsychologist is called upon to study sensorimotor functions of varying complexity, for example, coordination, strength, and sensory functions; cognitive level (IQ testing); information processing; academic and vocational capacity and potential; and emotional changes. Procedures include review of records, clinical observations, interview (see below) of patient and collaterals, formal testing using nationally standardized, special neuropsychological procedures, measures of academic achievement, memory, and information processing, computerized tests of concentration, vigilance, and attention,[157,158] and projective and questionnaire procedures for assessing personality, moods, and psychiatric disorders. Current functioning is compared to baseline, including possible preexisting conditions, and exaggeration or loss of pretraumatic personality characteristics. Referral questions include: the neurobehavioral diagnosis of traumatic brain injury in the "mild" or concussive range; capacity to return to a former vocation or receive vocational retraining; capacity for formal academic education; explanation for specific difficulties at work (fatigability); cognitive difficulties, problem solving, attention, concentration, and memory; study of clumsiness and complex sensorimotor deficits; personality, psychiatric, and mood changes; marital and social relationships; posttraumatic stress disorder. Detection of malingering may be the cause for referral, although the examiner is cautioned about lack of acceptable validity for detection procedures.[159,160]

OUTCOME ASSESSMENT

Estimating the Baseline

It is incorrectly presumed that the baseline cannot be estimated; an example is Faust's[161] contention concerning the executive function. Baseline components include lifestyle (use of free time); health (strength, stamina, coordination); development (emotional and physical); personality (sociability; level of dysphoria; sexuality; frustration tolerance); achievement (educational and vocational); and cognitive level (pre-injury IQ[170] and achievement tests).[162] Sources of baseline information include:

1. *Educational achievement scores.* Early school records offer percentiles from nationally standardized achievement tests that correlate well with IQ.[163] These are more objective than grades, and can be compared to current psychometric findings. School grades can be reduced by lack of motivation, disinterest, poverty, change of residence, and many other factors.

2. *Years of education.* The GED certificate is a 12-year education equivalent[164] or WAIS-R Scales, tables by age and education offer an estimated mean pre-injury IQ,[165,166] or percentile ranks.[167] A poorly representative estimate of pre-injury IQ could be obtained from records that reflect low education if motivation or circumstances acted to reduce given educational potential.

3. *Current test patterns.* Estimation of pre-injury learning ability through use of scores believed to be stable is called "hold" versus "nonhold." Doubt has been expressed concerning its utility for premorbid ability.[168] However, sparing of Verbal IQ relative to Performance IQ has been frequently found. It was demonstrated in 161 consecutive patients with diffuse TBI tested at a postinjury interval up to 10 years: Verbal IQ 91.7; Performance IQ 85.9; Full Scale Intelligence Quotient (FSIQ) 88.2.[57] However, a score could underestimate the baseline because of unreliability, poor education, lateralization effects, sensory processing deficits, loss of long-term memory, or aphasia. Published formulas that estimate pre-injury IQ demographically (race, education, geographic region, and occupation) use vague categories, restrict the range of IQ, and underestimate a bright, undereducated person's ability.[169]

4. *Military record.* This extreme environment can demand sensorimotor capacity, intelligence, stress resistance, personality traits of hardiness and leadership, physical strength and stamina, responsibility, leadership, verbal and nonverbal skills, and ability to learn a wide range of skills and concepts. Determine the military occupational specialty, training and highest rank, duties, combat experience, and so on as examples of baseline level.

5. *Vocational record.* Obtain work samples, employment reviews, skill level, training, job requirements, job stability, promotions, and temperament and personality.[170]

6. *Clinical observation.* Pre-injury development can be estimated through verbal usage, and through nonverbal aspects of behavior such as demeanor and expressed frustration at not performing particular activities (in conjunction with problem-solving style such as use of preplanning versus trial-and-error).

7. *Interview with collaterals.* Interview family, friends, and work associates to inquire about work, independence, re-

sponsibility, personality and temperament, social inter-est, frustration tolerance, and use of leisure time.

A Wide Range of Data Gathering

To assess outcome or status several years or more after an accident, the examiner should conduct a wide range examina-tion within his or her own specialty, and be alert to disorders outside his or her own area. The range of potential dysfunctions is so great that it is necessary to *customize the examination* to some extent for each patient, taking into consideration the ap-parent level of function, obvious impairment, demographic characteristics (education, employment, and facility with En-glish), and the specific concern of the referring source. Re-quired information is multidisciplinary: a wide range neurop-sychological examination (WRNE); record review (medical, dental, mental health, educational, employment); intensive in-terviewing of patient and collaterals (family, friend, employ-ers); and record review. Substantial study of personality and emotions are indicated, since disorders of these can interfere with interpersonal skills, family and other relationships, or positive attitudes can enhance the level of outcome. In the light of the tendency by some practitioners (clinical, legal, insur-ance) to assume exaggeration of effects after TBI, systematic information gathering and presentation (the wide range, multi-disciplinary examination) can contribute to overcoming the prejudice, assuming that litigation is a marker for malingering. The validity of procedures to establish the presence of malin-gering has been questioned.[159]

The Interview and Clinical Observation

The interview is essential to obtain social, subjective, and historical information. If a prior history of TBI is not known,[81] major complaints may appear incredible. A patient may forget or not know that a TBI-causing accident occurred in childhood.[9] The examiner should determine whether there is a credible accident that accounts for some complaints or documented dysfunctioning: how the head and body were injured; altered consciousness, retrograde and anterograde amnesia; emotional stress; somatic injuries to head, neck, torso, and extremities. Head injury can be elicited through queries concerning: head swelling, scratches, and dirt; decel-eration; loss and alterations of consciousness, retrograde and posttraumatic amnesia; pain in head, neck, and torso; cervi-cal vertebrae damage, and so on[171]; postinjury recovery. The interview is needed to document subjective complaints, adaptive level, and covert dysfunctions such as partial sei-zures and subclinical aphasia. Sexual information may be difficult to elicit due to the embarrassment of the patient, spouse, or examiner, or lack of patient insight. It is important to interview the sexual partner.[172]

Patient statements cannot be taken as definitive concerning their status ("expressive deficits"). They may assert that they are fine, or minimize distress, because of embarrassment about their condition, or be evasive due to communication problems, aphasia, poor memory, lack of insight, or comprehension.[57,173] Error of functional capacity often occurs when patient re-sponses in the interview are used as data. Assessments of "in the normal range" or "good recovery" frequently miss dysfunc-tions detected by more precise neuropsychological examina-tion: reductions below baseline capacity, aphasic difficulties and reduced intelligence, memory, and academic achievement. The clinician should be alert to discrepancies between the patient's claims of distress and apparent demeanor. Apparent indifference should not be mistaken for faking. Rather, the dull mood, as observed by comparison with test information con-cerning moods obtained by the Rorschach[174] or other personal-ity test, may offer evidence for the cerebral personality symp-tom of aprosodia.

Suitability of Assessment Procedures

The measurement of many functions requires psychomet-ric adequacy (nationally standardized, validated, reliable, and measuring a wide range of performance). Some test ma-terials can be invalid for particular TBI patients. For ex-ample, the commonly utilized Minnesota Multiphasic Per-sonality Inventory (MMPI) is dependent upon the integrity of functions that themselves are commonly impaired after TBI (comprehension and verbal skills). Also, the MMPI is normed with a pathological bias. In contrast, the verbally expressed Rorschach Inkblot Test, in addition to data about self-esteem, moods, and changed sense of self (identity), can signal incapacity to self-describe (reduced cognitive and comprehension level, insight, and verbal ability). Complex functions are more sensitive to brain damage than simple ones, whether academic skills or sensorimotor measures such as coordination.[4] For example, if long-term memory is spared, the spelling score might be high, while measures of complex functions such as writing to command and reading comprehension might be impaired. (Since otherwise intelli-gent normals may be poor spellers, it is advisable to consider only particular *patterns* of spelling errors, such as reversed letters, as in *pervious* for *previous* or *form* for *from*.) Cogni-tive assessment (memory, mental ability, achievement) can-not be precisely performed with brief testing or observation, requiring instead psychometrically adequate tests. Brief tests[175] are useful for screening purposes alone, but they are too imprecise for assessment of TBI outcome. Simple as-sessment procedures without age standards or estimated baseline ("serial sevens," calculations, abstractions), often provide overestimated levels due to slight patient success, although they may be revelatory of arithmetic versus verbal skills. Qualitative data (clinical observations of task ap-proach) does permit assessment of problem-solving style and morale. The significance of individual measurements to measure a general function should not be emphasized. A single function such as "attention" has varied components (speed, task complexity, focused attention) with different speeds of recovery for aspects of a given function.[28]

Repeated examination with the same procedures leads to a large *practice effect*. This spurious impression of improvement exaggerates extent of recovery, thus interfering with treatment planning, and creates deleterious forensic implications.[176] This has been reported with neuropsychological procedures.[177-179] A practice effect has been documented for IQ gain for children,[180] adolescents,[181] and adults.[182] I reexamined one man post–head injury, after other psychologists reported a 20-point gain in WAIS-R IQ with repeated WAIS-R testing. When an alternative mental ability test was administered,[183] the standard score was almost exactly at the postinjury level. There is no evidence for recovery of (group) mean IQ when a practice effect is avoided.[26,57]

Ecological validity reflects measurement of tasks of daily living, such as adaptation in the light of social support, and environmental demands such as work. To predict performance, a criterion of success is useful such as pre-injury performance. It is better to predict capacity for particular jobs (for example, the pre-injury employment) than general employability. The examiner selects procedures that test the skills needed for a particular position.[184] Should the patient be required to perform different or more complex functions, on the same or a different job, reserves may be inadequate. Therefore, the battery should confront the patient with tasks that are complex, speeded, and ecologically relevant.[185] Procedures may vary according to TBI status: Those for concussion may overlap little with those used for the severely brain traumatized patient, that is, they may not measure difficulties in daily living.[186] Subjective functioning is largely ignored by Outcome Measures of the Subcommittee of the NIH/NINDS Head Injury Centers because it lacks formal personality testing, and minimizes behavioral and psychosocial assessment.[187]

Clinical observations are important. Direct observation of personality is needed for overt expression of mood, problem-solving style, motivation, and credibility. Subtle emotional cues can lead to more intensive study. Dull affect requires the differential diagnosis between aprosodia, reactive depression (sadness), and endogenous depression (structural lesions or neurotransmitter dysfunctions). Aprosodia is common and suggested by the contrast between verbally or test-expressed complaints and a bland mood, which offers a false appearance of lack of distress; it is characterized also by excessive denial and concern.

SIGNIFICANT CONTRIBUTORS TO IMPAIRMENT

Adaptive effectiveness represents an interaction between spared functions, motivation, the impairing effect of "distractors" (as discussed below), the social milieu with its level of support, the availability of treatment and diagnostic facilities, and any later developing conditions. Outcome can be reduced by doubt or opposition to the claim of disability, which renders diagnostic and treatment services unavailable. Adaptive level fluctuates because of the complex play of forces and the patient's reaction to them.[188] TBI effects are cumulative, but prior injuries can be occult (for example, in children[20]), or revealed only under conditions of stress.[189] The effects of somatic trauma can reduce adaptive effectiveness regardless of the level of cerebral injury. Increased age reduces the level of outcome, perhaps lowering speed of information processing.[28] Vulnerability may be due to comorbidity and susceptibility to mechanical injury caused by predisposition to subdural hemorrhage, and reduced elasticity of the cerebral vessels and the brain.[92] Personality difficulties become more intense with chronicity, and interfere with work ability.[190,191] The effect of subjective complaints (headaches, dizziness, fatigability, feeling of impairment, anxiety, etc.) varies from reducing the quality of life[1] to impairing ability to work.[84] Particular symptoms can be directly impairing and associated with unemployed status or difficulty in finding work[10] (as observed in a military population of generally low velocity penetrating brain trauma): global aphasia; extensive paralysis; posttraumatic epilepsy; sensory loss including visual field loss, verbal memory deficit, reasoning loss, visual memory impairment, violent behavior, and isolation. Single symptoms did not affect relative employability, being compensated for, but the number of symptoms (disability score) predicted difficulty in finding work.[10]

Distractors

Adaptive capacity can be overestimated by considering test scores alone, without considering other symptoms (Mayberg comment[188]). Headaches, pain, hyperarousal, depression, posttraumatic stress, and partial seizures reduce efficiency for employability and ability to maintain independence. Distractors disturb consciousness, memory, identity, and perception of the environment,[64] synergizing with lesional effects to reduce ability, concentration, and motivation at work and home.[84] The physiological sequelae of whiplash, apart from shearing damage to the brain, create additional problems for the patients.[189] Pain can reduce treatment participation, while analgesics reduce mental ability. However, if the examiner's sole attention fixes on pain and injury, TBI may be ignored since TBI symptoms closely parallel those of chronic pain.[85] In contrast to pain, dissociation grants protection from the painful feelings of the trauma.

Considerations of Safety

Symptoms may create increased likelihood of accidents: sensorimotor dysfunction (poor balance, incoordination, motor weakness, dyskinesia, and other sensory loss); cognitive impairment (poor judgment creates inability to predict hazards); reduced ability to learn from experience; absence seizures and partial seizures of whose significance the patients may be unaware and may occur without warning.[149] There is danger from motor vehicle use, sports, ambulation, bicycling, the use of power and sharp tools. Accidents are reported before, during, and after anti-epileptic drug therapy.[190] Partial seizures may not interfere severely with capacity to attend school or work, but should the ordinary activity involve driving, swimming, or use of power tools, then jeopardy of safety implies a poor outcome.

Environmental Demands and Impairment

An exaggerated estimate of "recovery" can occur when the patient is examined while still unemployed, before the patient must confront demands for stamina, stress resistance, concentration under conditions of high noise and light, speeded output, emotional resources, and abrasive or nonsupportive social interactions. Such problems are not apparent in the quiet examiner's office or when the patient remains at home. The patient experiences stress when returning to work, school, or family.[192] If patient, doctors, and family are unaware of brain damage dysfunctions, distress might be attributed to an emotional disorder.[193] Distress over inability to cope (the catastrophic reaction) should be identified. Yet anxiety, anger, and depression, in the context of a good work history and supportive social milieu, is associated with a better rehabilitation outcome.[194] Even apparent success upon return to work, or continued work after injury, can be deceptive. Employment can be maintained through tolerance by management, or assistance by colleagues. Less domestic contribution may be condoned by a sympathetic family.

• • •

Outcome is the resolution of many factors: level of premorbid personality and development; recovery; family dynamics; community and social reaction to impairment; personal reaction to impairment; quality and timing of intervention; environmental demands (e.g., employment); situational stressors (financial obligations, response time of insurance companies to need for treatment); and subjective stressors (pain, guilt, reaction to litigation, and reduced income). Assessment of neurobehavioral outcome after TBI is a complex procedure that cannot be reduced to simple categories such as "good recovery" or "partially disabled." It is actually a complex, somewhat imprecise estimate, that represents a moment in time. It is judged relative to an estimated baseline, and utilizes a multidisciplinary study of the current range of neurobehavioral and medical deficits and dysfunctions. Its precision is enhanced by sampling a wide range of neurobehavioral systems, and study of possible traumatic, developmental, and degenerative processes that occur after TBI and related injuries. While a postinjury interval of at least two years is recommended before assessing outcome, there are numerous endocrinological and neurological conditions that may take a longer time to be expressed.

Outcome is more than level of functioning. It includes capacity to cope with the environment safely, maturely, and independently, including capacity for self-care, education, work, and social relationships.[194] Assessment of outcome takes into account associated conditions such as somatic injury, various emotional reactions, and the impairing effect of distracting symptoms such as pain, headaches, hyperarousal, partial seizures. The examiner considers the effects of social and community reactions to the injured person, the availability of treatment, and accommodations needed in the workplace, community, or home. The need for retraining, psychotherapy, medical treatment, and social support is a factor in assessment of outcome of TBI.

REFERENCES

1. Masson, F., et al. "Prevalence of Impairments 5 Years after a Head Injury, and Their Relationship with Disabilities and Outcome." *Brain Injury* 10 (1996): 487–97.

2. Pearce, J.M.S. "Polemics of Chronic Whiplash Injury." *Neurology* 44 (1994): 1993–97.

3. Stuss, D.T. "A Sensible Approach to Mild Traumatic Brain Injury." *Neurology* 45 (1995): 1251–52.

4. Greiffenstein, M.F., Baker, W.J., and Gola, T. "Motor Dysfunction Profiles in Traumatic Brain Injury and Postconcussion Syndrome." *Journal of the International Neuropsychological Society* 2 (1996): 477–85.

5. Ommaya, A.K. "Head Injury Mechanisms and the Concept of Preventive Management: A Review and Critical Synthesis." *Journal of Neurotrauma* 12 (1995): 527–46.

6. Francel, P., Alves, W.M., and Jane, J.A. "Mild Head Injury in Adults." In *Neurological Surgery*, 4th ed., ed. R. Youmans. Philadelphia: Saunders, 1996, pp. 1595–17.

7. Liau, L.M., Bergsneider, M., and Becker, D.P. "Pathology and Pathophysiology of Head Injury." In *Neurological Surgery*, 4th ed., ed. R. Youmans, pp. 1549–94.

8. Parker, R.S. "Reducing the Incidence of Unrecognized Traumatic Brain Injury in the Acute and Chronic Phases." *Journal of Neurological and Orthopaedic Surgery and Medicine* 16 (1995a): 118–25.

9. Parker, R.S. "Concussion: Not Always a 'Minor' Head Injury." *Journal of Neurological and Orthopaedic Medicine and Surgery* 15 (1994b): 123–26.

10. Schwab, K., et al. "Residual Impairments and Work Status 15 Years After Penetrating Head Injury: Report from the Vietnam Head Injury Study." *Neurology* 43 (1993): 95–103.

11. Haase, J. "Social-Economic Impact of Head Injury." *Acta Neurochirgica* 55(suppl), (1992): 75–79.

12. Brown, S.J., Fann, J.R., and Grant, I. "Postconcussional Disorder: Time to Acknowledge a Common Source of Neurobehavioral Morbidity." *Journal of Neuropsychiatry and Clinical Neurosciences* 6 (1994): 15–22.

13. Miller, L. "Neuropsychology and Pathophysiology of Mild Head Injury and the Postconcussion Syndrome: Clinical and Forensic Considerations." *Journal of Cognitive Rehabilitation* 14 (Jan./Feb. 1996): 8–23.

14. Evans, R.W. "The Postconcussion Syndrome and the Sequelae of Mild Head Injury." *Neurologic Clinics* 10, no. 4 (1992): 815–47.

15. Zasler, N.D. "Neurologic Impairment and Disability Evaluation." In *Head Injury and Postconcussive Syndrome,* eds. M. Rizzo and E. Tranel. New York: Churchill Livingstone, 1996, pp. 351–63.

16. Bohnen, N., Twijnstra, A., and Jolles, J. "Persistence of Postconcussional Symptoms in Uncomplicated, Mildly Head-Injured Patients: A Prospective Cohort Study." *Neuropsychiatry, Neuropsychology, and Behavioral Neurology* 6 (1993): 193–200.

17. Fox, D.D., et al. "Post-Concussive Symptoms: Base Rates and Etiology in Psychiatric Patients." *The Clinical Neuropsychologist* 9 (1995): 89–92.

18. Kosteljanetz, M., et al. "Sexual and Hypothalamic Dysfunction in the Postconcussional Syndrome." *Acta Neurologica Scandinavica* 63 (1981): 169–80.

19. Schrader, H., et al. "Natural Evolution of Late Whiplash Syndrome Outside the Medicolegal Context." *Lancet* 347 (1996): 1207–11.

20. Parker, R.S. "Neurobehavioral Outcome of Minor Head Injury in Children." *Seminars in Neurology* 14(1) (1994c): 67–73.

21. Bigler, E.S., et al. "Day of Injury CT Scan As An Index to Pre-Injury Brain Morphology." *Brain Injury* 8 (1994): 231–38.

22. Johnson, S.C., et al. "White Matter Atrophy, Ventricular Dilation, and Intellectual Functioning Following Traumatic Brain Injury." *Neuropsychology* 8 (1994): 307–315.

23. Olver, J.H., Ponsford, J.L., and Curran, C.A. "Outcome Following Traumatic Brain Injury: A Comparison Between 2 and 5 Years of Age." *Brain Injury* 10 (1996): 841–48.

24. Levin, H.S., et al. "Neurobehavioral Outcome Following Minor Head Injury: A Three-Center Study." *Journal of Neurosurgery* 66 (1987): 234–43.

25. Wechsler, D. *Wechsler Adult Intelligence Scale-Revised.* San Antonio, TX: Psychological Corporation, 1981.

26. Parker, R., and Rosenblum, R. "Intelligence and Emotional Dysfunctions After Mild Head Injury Incurred in a Car Accident." *Journal of Clinical Psychology* 52 (1996a): 32–43.

27. Crovitz, H.F., Diaco, D.S., and Apter, A. "Consistency in Recalling Features of Former Head Injuries: Retrospective Questionnaire vs. Interviews Retest." *Cortex* 28 (1962): 509–12.

28. Hetherington, C.R., Stuss, D.T., and Finlayson, M.A.J. "Reaction Time and Variability 5 and 10 Years After Traumatic Brain Injury." *Brain Injury* 10 (1996): 473–86.

29. Cifu, D.X., et al. "Functional Outcome of Older Adults with Traumatic Brain Injury: A Prospective, Multicenter Analysis." *Archives of Physical Medicine and Rehabilitation* 77 (1996): 883–86.

30. Dikmen, S.S., et al. "Employment Following Head Injuries." *Arch Neurol* 51 (1994): 177–86.

31. Kalisky, Z., et al. "Medical Problems Encountered During Rehabilitation of Patients With Head Injury." *Archives of Physical Medicine and Rehabilitation* 66 (1985): 25–29.

32. Englander, J.S., et al. "The Impact of Acute Complications, Fractures, and Motor Deficits on Functional Outcome and Length of Stay After Traumatic Brain Injury: A Multicenter Analysis." *Journal of Head Trauma Rehabilitation* 11, no. 5 (1996): 15–26.

33. Treip, C.S. "Hypothalamic and Pituitary Injury." *Journal of Clinical Pathology* 32(suppl. 4) (1970): 178–86.

34. Chrousos, G.P. "Organization and Integration of the Endocrine System." In *Pediatric Endocrinology,* ed. M.A. Sperling. Philadelphia: Saunders, 1996.

35. Miller, W.L., and Tyrrell, J.B. "The Adrenal Cortex." In *Endocrinology and Metabolism*, 3rd ed., eds. P. Felig, J.D. Baxter, and L.A. Frohman. New York: McGraw-Hill, 1995.

36. Reichlin, S. "Neuroendocrinology." In *Williams Textbook of Endocrinology*, 8th ed., eds. J.D. Wilson and D.W. Foster. Philadelphia: Saunders, 1992, pp. 135–219.

37. Nordhoff, L.S., Murphy, D., and Underhill, M.L. "Diagnosis of Common Crash Injuries." In *Motor Vehicle Collision Injuries: Mechanisms, Diagnosis, and Management,* ed. L.S. Nordhoff. Gaithersburg, MD: Aspen Publishers, 1996, pp. 1–69.

38. Davis, J.M., and Zimmerman, R.A. "Injury of the Carotid and Vertebral Arteries." *Neuroradiology* 25 (1983): 55–69.

39. Garrett, T.J., and Hubbard, S.A. "Vertebral Artery Thrombosis Due to Motor Vehicle Accident." *Annals of Emergency Medicine* 22 (1992): 141–43.

40. Chandler, W.F. "Trauma to the Carotid Artery and Other Cervical Vessels." In *Neurological Surgery,* 3rd ed., vol. 4, ed. R. Youmans. New York: Saunders, 1990, pp. 2367–76.

41. Auer, R.N., Krcek, J., and Butt, J.C. "Delayed Symptoms and Death After Minor Head Trauma With Occult Vertebral Artery Injury." *Journal of Neurology, Neurosurgery, and Psychiatry* 57 (1994): 500–502.

42. Binder, L.M. "Persisting Symptoms After Mild Head Injury: A Review of the Postconcussive Syndrome." *Journal of Clinical and Experimental Neuropsychology* 8 (1986): 323–46.

43. Sturzenegger, M., Radanov, B.P., and Di Stefano, G. "The Effect of Accident Mechanisms and Initial Findings on the Long-Term Course of Whiplash Injury." *Journal of Neurology* 242 (1994): 443–49.

44. Teman, A.J., Winterkorn, J.S., and Lowell, D.M. "Traumatic Thrombosis of a Vertebral Artery in a Hypoplastic Vertebrobasilar System: Protective Effect of Collateral Circulation." *New York State Journal of Medicine* 9 (1991): 314–15.

45. Radanov, B.P., Dvorak, J., and Valach, L. "Cognitive Deficits in Patients After Soft Tissue Injury of the Cervical Spine." *Spine* 17 (1992): 127–31.

46. Taylor, S., and Koch, W.J. "Anxiety Disorders Due to Motor Vehicle Accidents: Nature and Treatment." *Clinical Psychology Review* 15 (1995): 721–30.

47. McMillan, T.M. "Post-Traumatic Stress Disorder Following Minor and Severe Closed Head Injury: 10 Single Cases." *Brain Injury* 10 (1996): 749–58.

48. Putnam, F.W. "Traumatic Stress and Pathological Dissociation." In *Stress: Basic Mechanisms and Clinical Implications,* vol. 771 of *Annals of the New York Academy of Sciences.* ed. G.P. Chrousos. New York: New York Academy of Sciences, 1995, pp. 708–15.

49. Southwick, S.M., et al. "Psychobiologic Research in Post-Traumatic Stress Disorder." *Psychiatric Clinics of North America* 17(2) (1994): 251–64.

50. Haynes, S.N., et al. "Psychophysiological Assessment of Poststress Recovery." *Psychological Assessment* 3 (1991): 356–65.

51. Woolf, P.D. "Hormonal Responses to Trauma." *Critical Care Medicine* 20 (1992): 216–26.

52. Woolf, P.D., et al. "Transient Hypogonadotrophic Hypogonadism After Head Trauma: Effects on Steroid Precursors and Correlation With Sympathetic Nervous System Activity." *Clinical Endocrinology* 25 (1986): 265–74.

53. Woolf, P.D., et al. "Thyroid Test Abnormalities in Traumatic Brain Injury: Correlation With Neurologic Impairment and Sympathetic Nervous System Activation." *The American Journal of Medicine* 84 (1988): 201–208.

54. Dokas, L. A., Schlatter, L.K., and Barr, C.S. "Corticosteroid-Induced Proteins in Brain." *Brain Corticoid Receptors,* vol. 746 of *Annals of the New York Academy of Sciences.* New York: New York Academy of Sciences, 1994, pp. 157–65.

55. McEwen, B.S. "The Plasticity of the Hippocampus is the Reason for Its Vulnerability." *Seminars in Neuroscience* 6 (1994a): 239–46.

56. Eskay, R.L., et al. *Stress: Basic Mechanisms and Clinical Implications,* vol. 771 of *Annals of the New York Academy of Sciences,* ed. G.P. Chrousos. New York: New York Academy of Sciences, 1995, pp. 105–14.

57. Parker, R.S. *Traumatic Brain Injury and Neuropsychological Impairment.* New York: Springer-Verlag, 1990.

58. Gill, T., et al. "Cognitive Functioning in Post-Traumatic Stress Disorder." *Journal of Traumatic Stress* 3 (1990): 29–45.

59. Barrett, D.J.H., et al. "Cognitive Functioning and Posttraumatic Stress Disorder." *American Journal of Psychiatry* 153 (1996): 1492–94.

60. Kerr, D.S., et al. "Chronic Stress-Induced Acceleration of Electrophysiologic and Morphometric Biomarkers of Hippocampal Aging." *The Journal of Neuroscience* 5, no. 5 (1991): 1316–24.

61. Maier, S.F., Watkins, L.R., and Fleshner, M. "Psychoimmunology: The Interface Between Behavior, Brain, and Immunity." *American Psychologist* 49 (1994): 1004–1007.

62. McEwen, B.S. "Introduction: Stress and the Nervous System." *Seminars in Neuroscience* 6 (1994b): 195–96.

63. Van Cauter, E., Leproult, R., and Kupfer, D.J. "Effects of Gender and Age on the Levels and Circadian Rhymicity of Plasma Cortisol." *Journal of Clinical Endocrinology and Metabolism* 81 (1966): 2468–73.

64. Carlier, V.E., et al. "PTSD in Relation to Dissociation in Traumatized Police Officers." *American Journal of Psychiatry* 153 (1996): 1325–28.

65. Musselman, D.L., and Nemeroff, C.B. "Depression and Endocrine Disorders: Focus on the Thyroid and Adrenal System." *British Journal of Psychiatry* 168(suppl. 40) (1996): 123–28.

66. O'Brien, J.T., et al. "Clinical and Magnetic Resonance Imaging Correlates of Hypothalamic-Pituitary-Adrenal Axis Function in Depression and Alzheimer's Disease." *British Journal of Psychiatry* 168 (1966): 679–87.

67. MacGillivray, M.H. "Disorders of Growth and Development." In *Endocrinology and Metabolism,* 3rd ed., eds. P. Felig, J.D. Baxter, and L.A. Frohman. New York: McGraw-Hill, 1985, pp. 1619–73.

68. Molitch, M.E. (1995). "Neuroendocrinology." In *Endocrinology and Metabolism,* 3rd ed., eds. Felig, Baxter, and Frohman, pp. 221–28.

69. Graham, D.I. "Neuropathology of Head Injury." In *Neurotrauma,* eds. R.J. Narayan, J.E. Wilberger, and J.T. Povlishock. New York: McGraw-Hill, 1996, pp. 43–59.

70. D'Angelica, M., et al. "Hypopituitarism Secondary to Transfacial Gunshot Wound." *Journal of Trauma: Injury, Infection, and Critical Care* 39 (1995): 768–71.

71. Therapeutics and Technology Assessment Subcommittee of the American Academy of Neurology. "Assessment: Neurological Evaluation of Male Sexual Dysfunction." *Neurology* 45 (1995): 2287–92.

72. Elliott, M.L., and Biever, L.S. "Head Injury and Sexual Dysfunction." *Brain Injury* 10 (1996): 703–17.

73. Alison, M. "The Effect of Brain Injury on Marriage." *Headlines* (May/June 1993): 2–4.

74. Grossman, W.F., and Sanfield, J.A. "Hypothalamic Atrophy Presenting as Amenorrhea and Sexual Infantilism in a Female Adolescent: A Case Report." *Journal of Reproductive Medicine* 39 (1994): 738–40.

75. Attie, K.M., et al. "The Pubertal Growth Spurt in Eight Patients With True Precocious Puberty and Growth Hormone Deficiency: Evidence For a Direct Role of Sex Steroids." *Journal of Clinical Endocrinology and Metabolism* 71 (1990): 975–83.

76. Shaul, P.W., Towbin, R.B., and Chernausek, S.D. "Precocious Puberty Following Severe Head Trauma." *American Journal of the Diseases of Children* 139 (1985): 467–83.

77. Zasler, N.D., and Horn, L.J. "Rehabilitative Management of Sexual Dysfunction." *Journal of Head Trauma Rehabilitation* 5(2) (1990): 14–24.

78. Morrell, M.J. "Antiepileptic Drugs, Hormones, and Reproductive Health." In *Treatment of Epilepsy: Principles and Practice,* ed. E. Wyllie. Waverly Press, forthcoming.

79. Goldstein, K. "The Effect of Brain Damage on the Personality." *Psychiatry* 15 (1952): 235–59.

80. Kapp, B.S., et al. "Amygdaloid Contributions to Conditioned Arousal and Sensory Information Processing." In *The Amygdala: Neurobiological Aspects of Emotion, Memory, and Mental Dysfunction,* ed. J.P. Aggleton. New York: Wiley-Liss, 1992, pp. 229–54.

81. Parker, R.S. "The Spectrum of Emotional Distress and Personality Changes After Minor Head Injury: The Consequences of Motor Vehicle Accidents." *Brain Injury* 10 (1996b): 287–302.

82. Parker, R.S. "Neurobehavioral Approach to the Diagnosis and Assessment of Traumatic Brain Injury." In *A Guide to the Analysis, Understanding, and Presentation of Cases Involving Traumatic Brain Injury,* ed. C. Simkins. Washington, DC: National Head Injury Foundation, 1994d, pp. 79–89.

83. Lahz, S., and Bryant, R.A. "Incidence of Chronic Pain Following Traumatic Brain Injury." *Archives of Physical Medicine and Rehabilitation* 77 (1996): 889–91.

84. Parker, R. "The Distracting Effects of Pain, Headaches, and Hyper-Arousal Upon Employment After 'Minor' Head Injury." *Journal of Cognitive Rehabilitation* 13, no. 3 (1995b): 14–23.

85. Anderson, J.M., Kaplan, M.S., and Felsenthal, G. "Brain Injury Obscure by Chronic Pain: A Preliminary Report." *Archives of Physical Medicine and Rehabilitation* 71 (1990): 703–708.

86. Craig, K.D. "Emotional Aspects of Pain." In *Textbook of Pain,* eds. P.D. Wells and R. Melzack. New York: Churchill Livingstone, 1994, pp. 261–74.

87. Haas, D.C. "Acute Posttraumatic Headache." In *The Headaches,* eds. J. Olesen, P. Tfelt-Hansen, and K.M.A. Welch. New York: Raven, 1993a.

88. Haas, D.C. "Chronic Posttraumatic Headache." In *The Headaches,* eds. Olesen, Tfelt-Hansen, and Welch, pp. 629–37. New York: Raven, 1993b.

89. Perlman, S., and Kroening, R.J. "General Considerations of Pain and Its Treatment." In *Neurological Surgery,* 3rd ed., ed. R. Youmans. New York: Saunders, 1990, pp. 3803–12.

90. Parker, R.S. *Self-image Psychodynamics: Rewriting Your Life Script.* Englewood Cliffs, NJ: Prentice-Hall, 1983.

91. Ditunno, J.F., Jr. "Functional Assessment Measures in CNS Trauma." *Journal of Neurotrauma* 9(Supplement 1), 3/92 (1991): 301–305.

92. Vollmer, D.G. "Prognosis and Outcome of Severe Head Injury." In *Head Injury,* 3rd ed., ed. P.R. Cooper. Baltimore: Williams and Wilkins, 1993, pp. 553–81.

93. Frohman, L.A. "Diseases of the Anterior Pituitary." In *Endocrinology and Metabolism,* 3rd ed., eds. P. Felig, J.D. Baxter, L.A. Frohman. New York: McGraw-Hill, 1995, pp. 289–383.

94. Ganong, C.A., and Kappy, M.S. "Cerebral Salt Wasting in Children." *American Journal of Diseases of Children* 147 (1993): 167–69.

95. Kern, K.B., and Meislin, H.W. "Diabetes Insipidus: Occurrence After Minor Head Trauma." *Journal of Trauma* 24 (1984): 69–72 (abstract).

96. Robertson, G.O. "Posterior Pituitary." In *Endocrinology and Metabolism,* 3rd ed., eds. Felig, Baxter, and Frohman, pp. 385–432.

97. Hadani, M., et al. "Unusual Delayed Onset of Diabetes Insipidus Following Closed Head Trauma. Case Report." *Journal of Neurosurgery* 63 (1985): 456–58 (abstract).

98. Ferrari, S., and Crosignani, P.G. "Ovarian Failure without Gonadotropin Elevation in a Patient with Post-Traumatic Isolated Hypogonadotropic Hypogonadism." *European Journal of Gynecology and Reproductive Biology* 21 (1986): 241–44.

99. Bontke, C.F., Zasler, N.D., and Boake, C. "Rehabilitation of the Head-Injured Patient." In *Neurotrauma,* eds. R.J. Narayan, J.E. Wilberger, and J.T. Povlishock. New York: McGraw-Hill, 1996, pp. 841–58.

100. Rebar, R.W. "The Ovaries." In *Cecil Textbook of Medicine,* eds. J.C. Bennett and F. Plum. Philadelphia: Saunders, 1996, pp. 1293–1313.

101. Matsumoto, A.M. "The Testis." In *Cecil Textbook of Medicine,* eds. Bennett and Plum, pp. 1325–41.

102. Andrews, B.T. "Fluid and Electrolyte Management in the Head-Injured Patient." In *Neurotrauma,* eds. R.J. Narayan, J.E. Wilberger, and J.T. Povlishock. New York: McGraw-Hill, 1996, pp. 331–44.

103. Kokko, J.P. "Osmolality Disorders." In *Cecil Textbook of Medicine,* eds. Bennett and Plum, pp. 532–38.

104. Yamanaka, C., et al. "Acquired Growth Hormone Deficiency Due to Pituitary Stalk Transaction after Head Trauma in Childhood." *H.M. European Journal of Pediatrics* 152, no. 2 (1993): 99–101 (abstract).

105. Eichser, I., et al. "Isolated Growth Hormone Deficiency After Severe Head Trauma." *Journal of Endocrine Investigation* 11 (1988): 409–11 (abstract).

106. Towbin, R.B., Charron, M., and Meza, M.P. "Imaging in Pediatric Endocrine Disorders." In *Pediatric Endocrinology,* ed. M.A. Sperling. Philadelphia: Saunders, 1996, pp. 559–76.

107. Rosenfield, R.L. "The Ovary and Female Sexual Maturation." In *Pediatric Endocrinology,* ed. Sperling, pp. 331–85.

108. Styne, D.M. "The Testes: Disorders of Sexual Differentiation and Puberty." In *Pediatric Endocrinology,* ed. Sperling, pp. 423–76.

109. Pescovitz, O.H. "Pediatric Neuroendocrinology: Growth and Puberty." In *Neuroendocrinology,* ed. C.B. Memeroff. Boca Raton, FL: CRC, 1992, pp. 473–500.

110. Miller, W.L., Kaplan, S.L., and Grumbach, M.M. "Child Abuse As a Cause of Post-Traumatic Hypopituitarism." *New England Journal of Medicine* 302 (1980): 724–28.

111. Cytowic, R.E., Smith, A., and Stump, D. "Transient Amenorrhea after Closed Head Trauma" (letter). *New England Journal of Medicine* 314 (1986): 715.

112. Tusa, R.J., and Brown, S.B. "Neuro-otologic Trauma and Dizziness." In *Textbook of Head Injury,* eds. D.P. Becker and S.K. Gudeman. Philadelphia: Saunders, 1996, pp. 177–200.

113. Barcellos, C., and Rizzo, M. "Posttraumatic Headaches." In *Head Injury and Postconcussive Syndrome,* eds. Rizzo and Tranel, pp. 139–75.

114. Mishra, A.V., and Digre, K.B. "Neuro-Ophthalmologic Disturbances in Head Injury." In *Head Injury and Postconcussive Syndrome,* eds. Rizzo and Tranel, pp. 201–25.

115. Gates, J.R., and Granner, M.A. "Nonepileptic Events." In *Head Injury and Postconcussive Syndrome,* eds. Rizzo and Tranel, pp. 243–53.

116. Rovit, R.L., and Murali, R. "Injuries of the Cranial Nerves." In *Head Injury,* 3rd ed., ed. P.R. Cooper. Baltimore: Williams and Wilkins, 1993.

117. Aronson, A.E. "Editorial: Laryngealphonatory Dysfunction in Closed-Head Injury." *Brain Injury* 18 (1994): 663–65.

118. Theodoros, D.G., and Muirdoch, B.E. "Laryngeal Dysfunction in Dysarthric Speakers Following Severe Closed-Head Injury." *Brain Injury* 8 (1994): 667–84.

119. Krauss, J.K., Tränkle, and Kopp, K-H. "Post-traumatic Movement Disorders in Survivors of Severe Head Injury." *Neurology* 47 (1996): 1488–92.

120. Murphy, C., and Davidson, T.M. "Geriatric Issues: Special Considerations." *Journal of Head Trauma Rehabilitation* 7 (1992): 76–82.

121. Costanzo, R.M., and Zasler, N.D. "Epidemiology and Pathophysiology of Olfactory and Gustatory Dysfunction in Head Trauma." *Journal of Head Trauma Rehabilitation* 7 (1992): 15–24.

122. Joseph, R. *Neuropsychology, Neuropsychiatry, and Behavioral Neurology.* New York: Plenum, 1990.

123. Selhorst, J.B. "Neurological Examination of Head-Injured Patients." In *Textbook of Head Injury,* eds. D.P. Becker and S.K. Gudeman. Philadelphia: Saunders, 1989, pp. 82–101.

124. Lessell, S., Lessell, I.M., and Glaser, J.S. "Topical Diagnosis: Retrochiasmal Visual Pathways and Higher Cortical Function." In *Neuro-ophthalmology.* Philadelphia: Lippincott, 1990, pp. 213–38.

125. Doty, R. "Diagnostic Tests and Assessment." *Journal of Head Trauma Rehabilitation* 7 (1992): 47–65.

126. Walton, J. *Brain's Disease of the Nervous System,* 9th ed. New York: Oxford University Press, 1985.

127. Adams, R.D., and Victor, M. *Principles of Neurology,* 4th ed. New York: McGraw Hill, 1989.

128. Newberg, A.B., and Alavi, A. "Neuroimaging in Patients With Traumatic Brain Injury." *Journal of Head Trauma Rehabilitation* 11, no. 6 (1996): 65–79.

129. Gentleman, S., and Roberts, G. "Risk Factors in Alzheimer's Disease." *British Medical Journal* 304 (1992): 118–19.

130. Gedye, A., et al. "Severe Head Injury Hastens Age of Onset of Alzheimer's Disease." *Journal of the American Geriatric Society* 37 (1989): 970–73.

131. Graves, A.B., et al. "The Association Between Head Trauma and Alzheimer's Disease." *American Journal of Epidemiology* 131 (1990): 491–501.

132. Mortimer, J.A., et al. "Head Injury as a Risk Factor for Alzheimer's Disease." *Neurology* 35 (1985): 264–67.

133. Mortimer, J.A., et al. "Head Trauma as a Risk Factor for Alzheimer's Disease: A Collaborative Re-Analysis of Case-Control Studies." *International Journal of Epidemiology* 20, no. 2 (suppl. 2) (1991): S28–S35.

134. Roberts, G.W., et al. "Beta Amyloid Protein Deposition in the Brain After Severe Head Injury: Implications for the Pathogenesis of Alzheimer's Disease." *Journal of Neurology, Neurosurgery, and Psychiatry* 57 (1994): 419–25.

135. Krauss, J.K., et al. "Dystonia Following Head Trauma: A Report of Nine Patients and Review of the Literature." *Movement Disorders* 7 (1996): 263–72.

136. Duncan R., and Kennedy, P.G. "Guillain-Barre Syndrome Following Acute Head Trauma." *Postgraduate Medical Journal* 63 (June 1987): 479–80.

137. Van Duijn, C.M., et al. "Head Trauma and the Risk of Alzheimer's Disease." *American Journal of Epidemiology* 135 (1992): 775–82.

138. Nicoll, J.A.R., Roberts, G.W., and Graham, D.I. "The Neurobiology of Alzheimer's Disease." In *Annals of the New York Academy of Sciences,* vol. 777, eds. R.J. Wurtman et al. New York: New York Academy of Sciences, 1996, pp. 271–75.

139. Mayeux, R., et al. "Synergistic Effects of Traumatic Head Injury and Apolopoprotein-e4 in Patients with Alzheimer's Disease." *Neurology* 45 (1995): 555–57.

140. Stern, M., et al. "The Epidemiology of Parkinson's Disease." *Archives of Neurology* 48 (1991): 903–907.

141. Hubble, J.P., et al. "Risk Factors for Parkinson's Disease." *Neurology* 43 (1993): 1693–97.

142. Golbe, I. "Risk Factors in Young-Onset Parkinson's Disease." *Neurology* 43 (1993): 1641–43.

143. DeLorenzo, R.J. "The Epilepsies." In *Neurology in Clinical Practice,* eds. W.G. Bradley et al. Boston: Butterworth-Heinemann, 1991, pp. 1443–47.

144. Weiss, G.H., et al. "Predicting Posttraumatic Epilepsy in Penetrating Head Injury." *Archives of Neurology* 43 (1986): 771–73.

145. Devinsky, O. *Behavioral Neurology.* St. Louis: Mosby, 1992.

146. Willmore, L.J. "Posttraumatic Epilepsy." *Neurological Clinics* 10, no. 4 (1992): 869–78.

147. Walker, A.E., and Blumer, D. "Posttraumatic Seizures." *Archives of Neurology* 46 (1989): 23–26.

148. Lewis, R.J., et al. "Clinical Predictors of Post-Traumatic Seizures in Children With Head Trauma." *Annals of Emergency Medicine* 22 (1993): 1114–18.

149. Pedley, T.A., Scheuer, M.L., and Walczak, T.S. "Epilepsy." In *Merritt's Textbook of Neurology,* 9th ed. Baltimore: Williams and Wilkins, 1995, pp. 845–70.

150. Troost, D., and Tulleken, C.A. "Malignant Glioma After Bombshell Injury." *Clinical Neuropathology* 3, no. 4 (1984): 139–42.

151. Hochberg, H., and Pruitt, A. "Neoplastic Diseases of the Central Nervous System." In *Harrison's Principles of Internal Medicine,* 13th ed., vol. 2. eds. K.J. Isselbacher et al. New York: McGraw Hill, 1994, pp. 2256–69.

152. Devinsky, O. "Epilepsy After Minor Head Trauma." *Journal of Epilepsy* 9 (1996): 94–97.

153. Williamson, P.D., et al. "Complex Partial Seizures of Frontal Lobe Origin." *Annals of Neurology* 18 (1985): 497–504.

154. Palmini, A., and Gloor P. "The Localizing Value of Auras in Partial Seizures: A Prospective and Retrospective Study." *Neurology* 42 (1992): 801–808.

155. Devinsky, O., et al. "Clinical and Electroencephalographic Features of Simple Partial Seizures." *Neurology* 38 (1988): 1347–52.

156. Luciano, D. "Partial Seizures of Frontal and Temporal Origin." *Neurological Clinics* 11, no. 4 (1993): 805–22.

157. ForThought. *Vigil: Technical Reference Manual.* Nashua, NH., 1993.

158. Sandford, J.A., and Turner, A. *Intermediate Visual and Auditory Continuous Performance Test.* Richmond, VA: Braintrain, 1994.

159. Parker, R.S. "Documenting Malingering and Exaggerated Claims After Head Injury." In *A Guide to the Analysis, Understanding and Presentation of Cases Involving Traumatic Brain Injury,* ed. C. Simkins. Washington, DC: National Head Injury Foundation, 1994a, pp. 309–33.

160. Parker, R.S. "Enhancing Information-Gathering After Mild Head Injury in the Acute and Chronic Phases." *Journal of Neurological and Orthopaedic Medicine and Surgery* 16 (1996a): 118–25.

161. Faust, D. "Forensic Neuropsychology: The Art of Practicing a Science That Doesn't Exist." *Neuropsychology Review* 2 (1991): 205–31.

162. Hartlage, L.G. *Neuropsychological Evaluation of Head Injury.* Sarasota, FL: Professional Resource Exchange, 1990.

163. Anastasi, A. *Psychological Testing,* 6th ed. New York: Macmillan, 1988.

164. Dalton, J.E. "Neuropsychological Equivalence of the G.E.D." *International Journal of Clinical Neuropsychology* 12 (1990): 138–39.

165. Matarazzo, J.D., and Herman, D.O. "Relationship of Education and IQ in the WAIS-R Standardization Sample." *Journal of Consulting and Clinical Psychology* 52 (1984): 631–34.

166. Sattler, J.M. *Assessment of Children.* San Diego: Jerome M. Sattler, 1988.

167. Ryan, J.J., Paolo, A.M., and Findley, P.G. "Percentile Rank Conversion Tables for WAIS-R IQs at Six Educational Levels." *Journal of Clinical Psychology* 47 (1991): 104–107.

168. Larrabee, G.J., Largen, J.W., and Levin, H.S. "Sensitivity of Age-Decline Resistant ('hold') WAIS Subtests to Alzheimer's Disease." *Journal of Clinical and Experimental Neuropsychology* 7 (1985): 497–504.

169. Phay, A., Gainer, C., and Goldstein, G. "Clinical Interviewing of the Patient and History in Neuropsychological Assessment." In *Clinical Application of Neuropsychological Test Batteries,* eds. T. Incagnoli, G. Goldstein, and C.J. Golden. New York: Plenum, 1986, pp. 45–73.

170. Guilford, J.P. "The Structure-of-Intellect Model." In *Handbook of Intelligence,* ed. B.B. Wolman. New York: Wiley, 1985, pp. 225–66.

171. Teasdale, G., and Mathew, P. "Mechanisms of Cerebral Concussion, Contusion, and Other Effects of Head Injury." In *Neurological Surgery,* 4th ed., pp. 1553–58.

172. Sandel, M.E., et al. "Sexual Functioning Following Traumatic Brain Injury." *Brain Injury* 10 (1996): 719–28.

173. Prigatano, G.P., and Schachter, D.L., eds. *Awareness of Deficit After Brain Injury.* New York: Oxford University Press, 1991.

174. Piotrowski, Z.A. *Perceptanalysis.* New York: Macmillan, 1957.

175. Feher, E.P., et al. "Establishing the Limits of the Mini-Mental State: Examination of 'Subtests'." *Archives of Neurology* 49 (1992): 87–92.

176. Matarazzo, J.D. "Psychological Assessment Versus Psychological Testing: Validation from Binet to the School, Clinic and Courtroom." *American Psychologist* 45 (1990): 999–1017.

177. Collum, C.M., Heaton, R.K., and Grant, K. "Psychogenic Factors Influencing Neuropsychological Performance: Somatoform Disorders, Factitious Disorders, and Malingering." In *Forensic Neuropsychology: Legal and Scientific Bases,* eds. H.O. Doerr and A.S. Carlin. New York: The Guilford Press, 1991, pp. 141–71.

178. McCaffrey, R.J., et al. "Practice Effects in Repeated Neuropsychological Assessments." *The Clinical Neuropsychologist* 6 (1992): 32–42.

179. Galasko, D., et al. "Repeated Exposure to the Mini-Mental State Examination and the Information-Memory-Concentration Test Results in a Practice Effect in Alzheimer's Disease." *Neurology* 43 (1993): 1559–63.

180. Ruff, H.A., et al. "Declining Blood Lead Levels and Cognitive Changes in Moderately Lead-Poisoned Children." *Journal of the American Medical Association* 269 (1993): 1631–46.

181. Thompson, P.P., and Molly, K. "The Stability of WAIS-R for 16-Year-Old Students Retested After 3 and 8 Months." *Journal of Clinical Psychology* 49 (1993): 891–98.

182. Gregory, R.J. *Adult Intellectual Assessment.* Boston: Allyn and Bacon, 1987.

183. Kaufman, A.S., and Kaufman, N.L. *Kaufman Adolescent & Adult Intelligence Test*. Circle Pines, MN: American Guidance Service, 1993.

184. Guilmette, T.J., and Kastner, M.P. "The Prediction of Vocational Functioning from Neuropsychological Data." In *Ecological Validity of Neuropsychological Testing,* eds. R.J. Sbordone and C.J. Long. DelRay Beach, FL: GR Press/St. Lucie Press, 1996, pp. 387–411.

185. Heinrichs, R.W. "Current and Emergent Applications of Neuropsychological Assessment: Problems of Validity and Utility." *Professional Psychology* 21, no. 3 (1990): 171–76.

186. Wilson, B. "Ecological Validity of Neuropsychological Assessment After Severe Brain Injury." In *Ecological Validity of Neuropsychological Testing,* eds. Sbordone and Long, pp. 414–28.

187. Hannay, H.J., et al. "Outcome Measures for Patients With Head Injuries: Report of the Outcome Measures Subcommittee." *Journal of Head Trauma Rehabilitation* 11 (1996): 41–50.

188. Stanczak, D.E., Gouvier, W.D., and Long, C.J. "Rival Hypotheses Concerning the 'Nonorganic' Sequelae of Cerebral Trauma." *Clinical Neuropsychology* 5, no. 4 (1983): 16–18.

189. Ewing, R., et al. "Persisting Effects of Minor Head Injury Observable During Hypoxic Stress." *Journal of Clinical Neuropsychology* 2 (1980): 147–55.

190. Fordyce, D.J., Roueche, J.R., and Prigatano, G.P. "Enhanced Emotional Reactions in Chronic Head Trauma Patients." *Journal of Neurology Neurosurgery, and Psychiatry* 46 (1983): 620–24.

191. Thomsen, I.V. "Late Outcome of Very Severe Blunt Head Trauma: A 10–15 Year Second Follow-Up." *Journal of Neurology, Neurosurgery, and Psychiatry* 47 (1984): 260–68.

192. Long, C.L., Gouvier, W.D., and Cole, J.C. "A Model of Recovery for the Total Rehabilitation of Individuals with Head Trauma." *Journal of Rehabilitation* 50, no. 1 (1984): 39–45, 70.

193. Gouvier, W.D. "Quiet Victims of the Silent Epidemic: A Comment on Dlugokinski." *American Psychologist* 41 (1986): 483–84.

194. Prigatano, G.P., et al. "Neuropsychological Rehabilitation after Closed Head Injury in Young Adults." *Journal of Neurology, Neurosurgery, and Psychiatry* 47 (1984): 505–13.

Outcome Questionnaire for Traumatic Brain Injury

This questionnaire establishes pre-TBI baseline function, against which current status is evaluated to assess overall neurological health.

I. *Baseline:* Native or foreign origin; location and extent of education; family conditions and other aspects of development, including marital status; preexisting personality, medical, and substance abuse conditions; family and social status; employment level and persistence; relevant personality qualities.

II. *Description of the accident and traumatic brain injury:* Head injury; other injuries; alterations of consciousness; recovery conditions and length; any residual somatic injury, loss of limb use, dysfunction.

III. *Interval since injury:*

IV. *Trauma-related disorders:* Indicate whether patient is in treatment, not in treatment, whether treatment is possible, whether disorder is accident-related, preexisting, or exacerbated.
  A. General medical and endocrinological:
  B. Somatic trauma:
  C. Neurological:
  D. Stress:
  E. Dental and pharyngeal:
  F. Disorders of consciousness:
  G. Conditions needing examination:

V. *Neuropsychological summary:* May be organized by findings in the Neurobehavioral Taxonomy.
  A. Impairing symptoms—*positive* (compares well with baseline):
  B. Impairing symptoms—*negative* (less effective than baseline):

VI. *Current employment status:*
  Performance is graded in terms of current level, expressed as deviation from baseline. *Disabled* should mean total incapacity to work. If partially disabled, then there should be a criterion (relative to former employment, or with specified restrictions). For example, if the patient is partially employed at the former job, indicate that patient is capable of less skilled work, or detail the number of hours patient can perform at work. Indicate any employment accommodations needed: special physical, mental, or other work conditions.
  A. Adults employed, or actively seeking work
    Currently Employed: Yes ❏ No ❏
      1. No objective or subjective signs of impairment or distress
      2. Functions at pre-injury baseline with complaints
      3. Partially disabled, some reduced competence with impairment documented
      4. Significantly reduced competence with documented impairment.
  B. Adult rated totally disabled with documented impairment:
      5. Can only function in a sheltered workshop
      6. Treatable medical condition, potentially employable (specify)
      7. Incapable of performing any productive activity for the foreseeable future (specify).
  C. Adult unemployed, impairment not firmly documented:
      8. Reduced motivation
      9. Firmly documented evidence for malingering or secondary gain
      10. under study: claim of inability to work not yet documented.
  D. Current academic status of students at time of injury:
      1. Returned to school at baseline
      2. Returned to school below baseline (specify)
      3. Did not return to school (specify).

VII. *Quality of Life:* Mood, personality, and daily activities.
  A. *Economic status:* Reduced funds diminish treatment, domicile, and usual activities.
  B. *Embarrassing symptoms:* Scarring; dysarthria; anomia; social deficits due to neuropsychological impairment.

C. *Restricted by injury:* Loss of limb or range of motion; loss of audition or vision.

VIII. *Independence and residence:*
1. Competent to take care of self and family
2. Needs some assistance at work or home
3. Needs great assistance at work or home, not ambulatory at home or in the community, loss of eye-hand skills due to sensory or brain trauma problems
4. Requires home supervision for safety
5. Requires institutional care.

IX. *Prognosis:* In terms of age, known late developing conditions, and documented dysfunctions or diseases.

X. *Recommendations:* A. Need for vocational and domestic retraining; B. Safety and support at home; C. Medical care and further examination; D. Psychotherapy, counseling, further study, psychotropic medication; family counseling. E. Outside assistance: disability, legal advice.

25

Long-Term Outcome Follow-Up of Postacute Traumatic Brain Injury Rehabilitation: An Assessment of Functional and Behavioral Measures of Daily Living

Mark J. Ashley, Craig S. Persel, and David K. Krych

ASSESSING THE PROBLEM

One of the most important questions facing the field of traumatic brain injury (TBI) rehabilitation today has to do with the long-term outcomes of persons with TBI. Over 500,000 people suffer severe head injuries annually, resulting in significant disability for a large percentage of those individuals.[1] Long-term outcome studies aid in determination of the effectiveness of rehabilitation technologies that have evolved over time.[2] In an era of medical cost containment, the costs of rehabilitation are met increasingly with more conservative funding and increased demands for accountability.[3–5]

Outcome studies suggest that postacute TBI rehabilitation can be effective in reducing overall disability, improving independence, and achieving functional gains.[6–12] For many studies, the average length of follow-up is 12 months, which is a relatively short period of time, given that the average age range of persons sustaining TBI is 15–30 years.[13] Harrick et al. reported stability at three years' follow-up in functional status as measured by participation in productive activity, financial support, place of residence, and level of supervision required ($N = 21$). Loneliness and depression were noted to increase over time and were the two most frequently reported problems at the three-year follow-up.

The purpose of this study was to look at the effects of postacute TBI rehabilitation on the functional and behavioral activities of daily living over a period of time extending up to 15 years. This longer follow-up interval might indicate the effectiveness of the rehabilitation therapies and provide a basis for the utilization of large databases to predict the outcomes of similar groups in the TBI population. Ongoing examination of

large databases can provide the necessary information for the most efficacious rehabilitation in life-care planning.[14] Such planning will suggest the most cost-effective and satisfactory rehabilitation therapy for the individual client.

METHOD

Subjects

The initial pool of subjects for this study included all persons treated between August 1980 and April 1994 ($N = 689$). Only persons with a length of stay greater than 30 days (considered more than an evaluation period) and an elapsed time of six months postdischarge were included in the study. In all, 332 persons representing the 332 clients were contacted and cooperated in completing the survey.

Treatment Setting

Treatment was conducted for all clients at two postacute rehabilitation clinics with inpatient residential and outpatient service capabilities. Clients participated in therapy for up to six hours per day, five days per week, on a one-to-one (therapist-to-client) basis. Therapeutic programming was continued with residential therapy during the evenings and weekends. Residential programming was initially conducted on a one-to-one basis until the client developed sufficient skills to allow a reduced level of supervision.

Study Design

A 127-item questionnaire was developed for use in a telephone survey of subjects of this study. An independent firm was utilized to conduct the survey to control for study bias and provide increased validity of collected data. The tele-

J Rehabil Outcomes Meas, 1997, 1(4), 40–47
© 1997 Aspen Publishers, Inc.

phone survey was utilized due to its comparatively low cost contrasted to face-to-face interviews.[15] Telephone surveys tend to have higher response rates compared to mail surveys and lower interviewer bias than face-to-face surveys.[16,17] The firm was authorized to use extraordinary measures to locate persons for whom available address and telephone records were insufficient. Respondents to the survey consisted of a close and involved family member or caretaker or the person having sustained the TBI.

Three rating scales were utilized to evaluate long-term stability of skills following discharge from postacute TBI rehabilitation programming. The three rating scales were the Disability Rating Scale,[18] the Living Status Scale, and the Occupational Status Scale. The Disability Rating Scale (DRS) measures a person's general level of disability on a 30-point scale ranging from "none" to "extreme vegetative state." The DRS measures a person's status in areas of awareness, self-care, dependence on others, and employability. It has been shown to be a reliable and valid assessment of a person's general level of functioning.[19] The Living Status Scale (LSS) measures the amount of required living supervision on a 10-point scale (see box entitled "Living Status Scale"). The Occupational Status Scale (OSS) documents a person's educational or vocational involvement on a 16-point scale (see box entitled "Occupational Status Scale").

The LSS and the OSS are scales that have been utilized for over 15 years in the study facilities as evaluative tools of the therapeutic process. These three scales were determined to most closely match the outcome variables of level of disability, level of living supervision, and vocational status, which were of greatest interest to the people served, their families, and financially responsible parties.

Survey Instrument

Thirteen main categories were covered by the survey questionnaire and consisted of the following:

Living Status Scale (LSS)

0 Unknown
1 Private living quarters, independent
2 Private living quarters, supervision
3 Private living quarters, active family help
4 Private living quarters, active professional help
5 Senior citizen center
6 Board and care/group home
7 Long-term care facility
8 Acute or rehabilitation hospital
9 Locked facility
10 Deceased

Occupational Status Scale (OSS)

0 Unknown
1 Full-time, former or equal job
2 Formal education at level of former job
3 Part-time, former or equal job
4 Full-time, lesser position
5 Formal education at a level below former job
6 Part-time, lesser position
7 On-the-job training, paid
8 On-the-job training, unpaid
9 Sheltered employment, paid
10 Volunteer position
11 Multiple jobs for brief period of time
12 Not working, vocational counselor involved
13 Not working, active legal case or payments contingent on unemployment
14 Not working, placement precludes work
15 Hospitalization for physical illness
16 Not working, cognitive and/or physical disabilities preclude employment

---

Activities of daily living
Behavior and emotional issues
Community activities
Economic status
Educational status
Marital status
Medication
Recreational activities
Safety
Sleep
Therapeutic activities
Transportation
Vocational status

Statistical Analysis

Statistical analysis was completed using analysis of variance (ANOVA) for repeated measures for parametric data (DRS scores) and the Wilcoxon Matched Pairs Signed Rank test for nonparametric data.

RESULTS

Demographic

A total of 332 persons were contacted and cooperated with completing the survey. Age ranged from 10 to 75 years with a mean of 34.94 years. Of the persons contacted, 81.3 percent were male, 18.7 percent female. Educationally, 24.7 percent did not finish high school, 61.0 percent finished high school, and 14.3 percent had college courses or a college education. Of the injuries, 77.4 percent were closed-head injury, 9.3 percent open head injury, 3.5 percent anoxia, 8.4 percent stroke, and 1.3 percent other.

Treatment

Treatment latency ranged, for the group, from 11 to 8,898 days (24.4 years) with a mean of 524.74 days (1.4 years). The mean time elapsed from discharge to follow-up was 1,947.88 days (5.3 years) with a range of 0.57 to 14.2 years. The mean time elapsed from injury to follow-up was 2,615.64 days (7.1 years) with a range of 1.3 to 39.1 years.

Mean length of stay in rehabilitation programming was 220.2 days with a mean program cost of $132,085 (all amounts converted to 1996 rates). Of the persons contacted, 84.5 percent received inpatient programming, while 15.5 percent received outpatient services; 49.4 percent had workers' compensation coverage, 35.2 percent accident and health coverage, 5.1 percent private pay, 0.3 percent were in a health maintenance organization (HMO), and 10 percent had other insurance.

Follow-up

As can be seen in Table 1, there were no significant differences between follow-up and discharge score for the DRS and LSS scores. The OSS scores, however, were significantly higher at follow-up from the time of discharge, indicating a decrease in vocational status.

Analysis of the OSS scores was conducted, breaking out those persons who received vocational rehabilitation services from those who did not. Those persons receiving vocational rehabilitation services had a median score of 15 at admission, 10 at discharge, and 14 at follow-up, while those not receiving vocational rehabilitation services had a median score of 15 at admission, discharge, and follow-up (Table 2).

It can be seen that those persons receiving vocational rehabilitation services fared better at discharge than those not receiving such services. Those persons receiving vocational rehabilitation services experienced a statistically significant

Table 1. Admission, discharge, and follow-up scores on the three rating scales

	DRS (Mean) n = 258	LSS (Median) n = 279	OSS (Median) n = 232
Admission	7.11	8	15
Discharge	4.03	1	12
Follow-up	4.30	1	15*

*Significant difference, Wilcoxon Matched Ranks $z = 3.59$, $p < .05$.

Table 2. Median scores on OSS by grouping for having vocational rehabilitation (VOC-REHAB) and those that did not (NO VOC-REHAB)

	VOC-REHAB n = 143	NO VOC-REHAB n = 166
Admission	15	15
Discharge	10	15
Follow-up	14*	15

*Significant difference, K-Related Samples, $p < .05$

decline at follow-up, while those not receiving vocational rehabilitation services did not change at follow-up.

Financial Status

Economic status was reviewed with the finding that 83.9 percent were financially "getting by" or better at follow-up; 0.06 percent were in a critical financial state, 2.9 percent were "not getting by," and 12.5 percent were "barely getting by" (Table 3). Table 4 shows that 82.6 percent reported no increase in indebtedness at the time of follow-up contrasted to pre-injury status; 16.1 percent experienced increased indebtedness; 92.6 percent required no public assistance for medical costs, while 7.4 percent required public assistance; 96.5 percent required no public assistance for living expenses, while 3.5 percent required public assistance; 92.7 percent required no public assistance for child care services, while 1.2 percent did.

A review of family employment indicated that, in 90.7 percent of the cases, there was no job separation required for care by a family member. The estimated monthly loss for personal earnings averaged $1,058 while the mean household earnings loss averaged $402.

Financial management was reviewed with reference to ability to handle expenses, money, checkbooks, and bill payment. While 49.4 percent were independent with these activities, 11.2 percent were slightly dependent, 8.2 percent were moderately dependent, and 31.3 percent required maximum assistance.

Medications

Fifty percent of those surveyed were prescribed medications by a physician at the time of follow-up. Of those taking

Table 3. Financial status of group at follow-up (Part I)

Financially getting by or better	83.9%
Barely getting by	12.5
Not getting by	2.9
Critical financial state	0.06

Table 4. Financial status of group at follow-up (Part II)

No increase in indebtedness since injury	82.6%
Increased indebtedness	16.1
No public assistance for medical costs	92.6
Required public assistance for medical costs	7.4
No public assistance for living expenses	96.5
Required public assistance for living expenses	3.5
No public assistance for child care	92.7
Required public assistance for child care	1.2

medications, 91.1 percent were always or virtually always compliant with prescription, whereas 2.4 percent had occasional lapses, and 6.5 percent were usually not or were never compliant with prescription (Table 5). Of those requiring medications, 60.3 percent were independent with medications, 13.5 percent had a slight dependence, 5.1 percent had a moderate dependence, and 20.5 percent required maximum assistance for medications (Table 6).

Household Activities

The vast majority of individuals contacted were independent for activities (range 62 percent–70 percent). By contrast, 12.0 percent–14.7 percent of individuals required maximum assistance in one or more of these household activities (Table 7).

Family Status

A review of marital status indicated that 26.1 percent of respondents were never married, 41.1 percent were married, 2.2 percent were separated, 25.8 percent were divorced, 1.9 percent were widowed, and 2.9 percent were cohabitating. Nearly 74 percent of those surveyed had no change in their marital status since the time of discharge.

Emotional Status

The survey included a review of emotional status: 54 percent of respondents indicated that there were symptoms of emotional distress, sadness, or a lack of emotional control observed in the last 30 days. Only 34.6 percent reported that there was never any interference with ongoing tasks by emotional distress, whereas 42.0 percent reported occasional interference, 15.2 percent frequent interference, 8.2 percent

Table 5. Medication compliance of group at follow-up

Compliant	91.1%
Occasional lapses of compliance	2.4
Usually not or never compliant	6.5

Table 6. Independence with medications of group at follow-up

Independent	60.3%
Slight dependence	13.5
Moderate dependence	5.1
Maximum assistance	20.5

very frequent interference, and 2.9 percent extremely frequent interference. Looking at potential for harm, 91.3 percent of respondents had never threatened to harm themselves, while 8.7 percent had threatened to harm themselves. Of those who had made threats, 87 percent had no plan or means for carrying out the threat, while 13 percent had a plan or means. This equated to 1.1 percent of the total population studied. Regarding harming others, 86.6 percent of respondents had never threatened to harm others; 8.7 percent had occasionally (1–8 times per month) threatened to harm others, 2.2 percent very frequently (30–57 times per month) threatened to harm others, and 2.2 percent extremely frequently (58 or more times per month) threatened to harm others.

Vocational Status

Of those surveyed, 72.1 percent worked 30–40 hours per week, 20.6 percent worked 20–29 hours per week, 2.9 percent worked 10–19 hours per week, and 4.4 percent worked 1–9 hours per week (Table 8).

Of those surveyed, 23.4 percent received compensation for work performed. Of those employed, 28.0 percent were in managerial, supervisory, professional, or self-employed positions. In skilled labor or higher level clerical positions were 24.4 percent, and 47.6 percent were in semi-skilled, unskilled labor, or low-level clerical positions. For those individuals working, employment compensation comparisons were made. Table 9 shows the distribution of such comparisons.

A similar comparison was made for employment responsibility and Table 10 shows those results. In general, it appeared as though respondents perceived that they had reduced responsibility as a group and slightly less pay compared to pre-injury status.

Employment setting showed that 73.9 percent of the respondents employed were in competitive employment, 7.2 percent were in supported employment, 8.7 percent in sheltered work or special arrangement settings, 5.8 percent in on-the-job-training setting, 1.4 percent in a nonpaid work trial setting, and 1.4 percent in formal vocational training. A review of postdischarge employment duration demonstrated that mean job duration for the first employment setting was 33.73 weeks. Mean job duration for the second employment setting was 68.42 weeks.

Table 7. Levels of independence for four household activities: laundry, shopping, meal preparation, and cleaning

	Independent	Slight dependence	Moderate dependence	Maximum dependence
Laundry	70%	11.4%	6.5%	12.0%
Shopping	62	15.0	8.5	14.7
Meal preparation	63	13.4	9.1	14.0
Cleaning	70	12.0	5.2	13.3

Educational Status

A review of preinjury achievement showed that 2.1 percent of respondents had elementary or junior high education, 13.8 percent had some high school, 47.0 percent completed high school, 22.3 percent had some college programming or an associate's degree, 9.6 percent had a bachelor's degree, 3.9 percent had a master's degree, and 0.8 percent had a doctoral degree. For those involved in educational activities at the time of follow-up, two persons were participating in a master's level college preparation course. Eleven were in a four-year degree program, 12 were in a two-year degree program, 2 were in a home-based study program, and 10 were in special education programming. Those respondents participating in educational activities at the time of follow-up reported their current performance: 16.7 percent reported their academic performance to be about the same as preinjury, 25.0 percent reported their performance to be slightly better, 12.5 percent slightly worse, 8.3 percent moderately lower, 35.4 percent far lower or worse. Comparisons of academic effort to preinjury status were such that 6.5 percent indicated that academic pursuits required about the same effort, 4.3 percent indicated their required effort was moderately less, 4.3 percent slightly less, 39.1 percent moderately more, and 43.5 percent far more. A comparison of academic participation showed that 14.6 percent of the respondents had been in school at the time of injury and, at follow-up, 11.2 percent were in school.

Recreational Activity

Respondents were asked to rate the number of hours the person spent doing quiet versus active recreational activities in an average week. Those results are listed in Table 11.

Table 8. Number of hours worked by the group at follow-up

30–40 hrs./week	72.1%
20–29 hrs./week	20.6
10–19 hrs./week	2.9
1–9 hrs./week	4.4

Of all respondents, 58.2 percent did not participate in religious services, 38.2 percent spent 1–3 hours weekly doing so, 3.0 percent spent 4–9 hours, and 0.7 percent spent 10–19 hours. Participation in clubs, organizations, or church/community meetings was not undertaken at all by 72.1 percent of the respondents; 15.5 percent of the respondents did so 1–3 hours per week, 4.6 percent did so 4–9 hours per week, and 1.3 percent did so 10–29 hours per week.

Finally, respondents indicated that 67.5 percent of the persons spent 4–8 hours either sleeping or in a prone position, resting; 27.6 percent spent greater than 8 hours; 1.9 percent spent 2–4 hours; and 2.6 percent indicated less than 2 hours per day.

DISCUSSION

The results of this study were consistent with past research investigating the long-term outcome of persons with TBI who have received specialized postacute rehabilitation services.[8–12,20–25] In the present study, many of the functional and behavioral gains achieved by the time of discharge remained stable through the postdischarge time frame until the time of follow-up contact. This period of time averaged 5.3 years for the current study.

Vocational status was found to be an unstable variable at follow-up. Further investigation into these findings revealed that, while persons who received vocational rehabilitation services fared better at the time of discharge than those who did not, over time, those persons as a group worsened, approaching the level of vocational involvement of those individuals who did not receive vocational rehabilitation

Table 9. Distribution of change in compensation for work

Greatly reduced	30.8%
Somewhat reduced	10.3
Slightly reduced	15.4
About the same	17.9
Slightly increased	10.3
Moderately increased	14.1

Table 10. Employment responsibility at follow-up

Greatly reduced	33.8%
Somewhat reduced	8.8
Slightly reduced	10.0
About the same	22.5
Slightly increased	7.5
Moderately increased	17.5

services. The group that did not receive vocational rehabilitative services was not significantly worse at the time of follow-up; though this may represent a "ceiling" effect of the rating scale wherein higher scale scores (lower vocational status) were not available because of the scale's upper limit.[7] On the other hand, there exists the possibility that further efforts or innovative techniques may need to be developed to provide a better outcome from vocational rehabilitation in patients with TBI.

These findings of vocational instability are consistent with the findings of other authors. Ponsford, Olver, and Curran demonstrated that DRS score was the greatest contributor to prediction of employment status two years postinjury.[24] It will be interesting to conduct further analysis of this data to determine the degree to which DRS scores, or other scales, predicted the vocational outcome of the study population.[26]

The results of this study were somewhat encouraging. The majority of individuals (83.9 percent) were financially "getting by" or better. Of those employed, nearly 74 percent were in a competitive employment setting. Again, the majority of individuals showed good functional skills at the time of follow-up: 66 percent of the individuals were independent in carrying out household activities. Marital status was fairly stable at nearly 74 percent unchanged at the time of follow-up.

Of concern was the fact that nearly 54 percent of the individuals responding suffered from some emotional distress, and that 8.7 percent had threatened to harm themselves. This indicates the need for continuing counseling in some form in the years following discharge. The data support the idea that "peer" and/or social activities may be sparse for persons with TBI.

• • •

It can be concluded that rehabilitation outcomes achieved via postacute rehabilitation can be expected to have good long-term stability for functional and behavioral measures. Levels of supervision required at discharge can be expected to remain the same for a number of years postdischarge. Conversely, this study demonstrates that persons sustaining TBI and undergoing postacute rehabilitation programming have, nonetheless, substantial difficulties in returning to work and, more specifically, in maintaining a work position. Additionally, these individuals appear to be experiencing what may be an untoward amount of emotional distress as a group, perhaps arising from social isolation.

Of the 689 original subjects in the sample, 357 (51.8 percent) were lost at follow-up. This is higher than other studies with rates of around 40 percent,[27] although most of these studies were one-year follow-ups compared to the 15-year range of this study. Still, the systematic bias created by subjects lost at follow-up must be considered. Corrigan et al. concluded that subjects with a history of substance abuse were more likely to be lost at follow-up than those without.[27] The effects of substance abuse and other "drop out" factors on overestimating the positive results of longitudinal studies need to be taken into account.

This study group is also subject to a degree of selection bias on the basis of the fact that the majority of individuals referred to the treating facilities would be classified in a higher severity of disability category and would also have funding to pay for rehabilitation programming. It is possible that positive economic support and social/emotional difficulties have an adverse impact on vocational status, though lack of regular vocational involvement implicates reduced socialization.

This study supports assertions of earlier studies referencing stability of outcome as late as three years and extends the length of stability to an average of five years postdischarge. This positive trend in long-term stability of rehabilitation outcomes helps to demonstrate the overall cost effectiveness of postacute rehabilitation services. The results also indicate that continued monitoring of psychosocial and vocational issues may be required postdischarge and that further efforts are needed in the postacute rehabilitation milieu to address these issues. It appears that it may be advisable to develop schemes for addressing psychological and emotional issues as well as vocational issues postdischarge in an effort to maintain stability in those arenas.

Table 11. Percentage engaging in quiet versus active recreational activities per week at follow-up

	Not at all	*1–3 hrs.*	*4–9 hrs.*	*10–19 hrs.*	*20–29 hrs.*	*30–39 hrs.*	*40+ hrs.*
Quiet pursuits	4.1	8.5	14.6	21.4	23.7	12.9	14.9
Active pursuits	9.7	15.3	24.7	21.3	15.7	9.0	4.3

REFERENCES

1. Swiercinsky, D., Price, T., and Leaf, L. *Traumatic Head Injury: Cause, Consequence, and Challenge.* Shawnee, KS: Head Injury Association of Kansas, 1987.

2. Malec, J., et al. "Outcome Evaluation and Prediction in a Comprehensive Integrated Outpatient Brain Injury Rehabilitation Programme." *Brain Injury* 7, no. 1 (1993): 15–29.

3. Melia, R. "Research, Consumer Involvement, and Models of Care." *Neurorehabilitation* 7, no. 3 (1996): 203–10.

4. Malkmus, D., and Johnson, P. "Dedicated Management of Outcome, Quality, and Value: Internal Case Management." *Journal of Head Trauma Rehabilitation* 7, no. 4 (1992): 57–67.

5. Papastrat, L. "Outcome and Value Following Brain Injury: A Financial Provider's Perspective." *Journal of Head Trauma Rehabilitation* 7, no. 4 (1992): 11–23.

6. Harrison-Felix, C., et al. "Descriptive Findings from the Traumatic Brain Injury Model Systems National Data Base." *Journal of Head Trauma Rehabilitation* 11, no. 5 (1996): 1–14.

7. Hall, K., et al. "Functional Measures after Traumatic Brain Injury: Ceiling Effects of FIM, FIM + FAM, DRS, and CIQ." *Journal of Head Trauma Rehabilitation* 11, no. 5 (1996): 27–39.

8. Ashley, M.J., Persel, C.S., and Krych, D.K. "Changes in Reimbursement Climate: Relationship Among Outcome, Cost and Payor Type in the Postacute Rehabilitation Environment." *Journal of Head Trauma Rehabilitation* 8, no. 4 (1993): 30–47.

9. Evans, R., and Ruff, R. "Outcome and Value: A Perspective on Rehabilitation Outcomes Achieved in Acquired Brain Injury." *Journal of Head Trauma Rehabilitation* 7, no. 4 (1992): 24–36.

10. Cope, D.N., et al. "Brain Injury: Analysis of Outcome in a Post-Acute Rehabilitation System. Part 1: General Analysis." *Brain Injury* 5, no. 2 (1991): 111–25.

11. Johnson, M., and Lewis, F. "Outcomes of Community Re-entry Programmes for Brain Injury Survivors. Part 1: Independent Living and Productive Activities." *Brain Injury* 5, no. 2 (1991): 141–54.

12. Fryer, L.J., and Haffey, W.J. "Cognitive Rehabilitation and Community Re-adaptation: Outcomes from Two Program Models." *Journal of Head Trauma Rehabilitation* 2, no. 3 (1987): 51–63.

13. Rimel, R., Jane, J., and Bond, M. "Characteristics of the Head Injured Patient." In *Rehabilitation of the Adult and Child with Traumatic Brain Injury*, eds. M. Rosenthal, E. Griffith, M. Bond, and J. Miller. 2nd ed. Philadelphia: F.A. Davis Co., 1990.

14. Evans, R. "Commentary and an Illustration on the Use of Outcome in the Life Care Planning for Persons with Acquired Neurological Injuries." *Neurorehabilitation* 7, no. 2 (1996): 157–62.

15. Korner-Bitensky, N., et al. "Health-related Information Postdischarge: Telephone Versus Face-to-Face Interviewing." *Archives of Physical Medicine and Rehabilitation* 75 (1994): 1,287–96.

16. Narins, P. "Choosing the Right Administration Method for Your Research." *Keywords* 56 (1995): 6–7.

17. de Leeuw, E., and van der Zouwen, J. "Data Quality in Telephone and Face-to-Face Surveys: A Comparative Meta-Analysis." In *Telephone Survey Methodology*, eds. R. Groves, et al. New York: Wiley, 1988.

18. Rappaport, M., et al. "Disability Rating Scale for Severe Head Trauma: Coma to Community." *Archives of Physical Medicine and Rehabilitation* 63 (1982): 118–23.

19. Gouvier, W.D., et al. "Reliability and Validity of the Disability Rating Scale and the Levels of Cognitive Functioning Scale in Monitoring Recovery from Severe Head Injury." *Archives of Physical Medicine and Rehabilitation* 68, no. 2 (1987): 94–97.

20. Masson, F., et al. "Prevalence of Impairments 5 Years after a Head Injury, and Their Relationship with Disabilities and Outcome." *Brain Injury* 10, no. 7 (1996): 487–98.

21. Harrick, L., et al. "Stability of Functional Outcome Following Transitional Living Programme Participation: 3-year Follow-up." *Brain Injury* 8, no. 5 (1996): 439–48.

22. Hall, K.M., and Cope, N. "The Benefit of Rehabilitation in Traumatic Brain Injury: A Literature Review." *Journal of Head Trauma Rehabilitation* 10, no. 1 (1995): 1–13.

23. Sbordone, R., Liter, J., and Pettler-Jennings, P. "Recovery of Function Following Severe Traumatic Brain Injury: A Retrospective 10-year Follow-up." *Brain Injury* 9, no. 3 (1995): 285–300.

24. Ponsford, J., Olver, J., and Curran, C. "A Profile of Outcome: 2 Years After Traumatic Brain Injury." *Brain Injury* 9, no. 1 (1995): 1–10.

25. Schalen, W., et al. "Psychosocial Outcome 5–8 Years After Severe Traumatic Brain Lesions and the Impact of Rehabilitation Services." *Brain* Injury 8, no. 1 (1994): 49–64.

26. Sander, A., et al. "A Multicenter Longitudinal Investigation of Return to Work and Community Integration Following Traumatic Brain Injury." *Journal of Head Trauma Rehabilitation* 11, no. 5 (1996): 70–84.

27. Corrigan, J., et al. "Systematic Bias in Outcome Studies of Persons with Traumatic Brain Injury." *Archives of Physical Medicine and Rehabilitation* 78, no. 2 (1997): 132–37.

26

Justification of Postacute Traumatic Brain Injury Rehabilitation Using Net Present Value Techniques: A Case Study

Mark J. Ashley, John D. Schultz, Velda L. Bryan, David K. Krych, and Dennis R. Hays

THE PRESSURE TO SHORTEN TREATMENT

Developments in managed care and the resulting need for providers to be more accountable have had a substantial impact on rehabilitation services. Recent pressure to reduce time spent in rehabilitation may result in a patient's rehabilitation potential not being fully met. The apparent aim of these developments has been to reduce both length of stay (LOS) and per diem cost of care. The perspective has been that these two methods will result in cost savings to the financially responsible parties.

A number of studies have been published that address the efficacy of traumatic brain injury (TBI) rehabilitation.[1-3] In general, TBI rehabilitation is thought to be advantageous in reducing disability and in enhancing functional outcome. Few studies, however, have reviewed the relationship between rehabilitation and short- and long-term cost benefit ratios, perhaps because of the relative inexperience the health care community has with cost/benefit analysis.

A comprehensive review of TBI outcome studies can be found in Hall and Cope.[4] Some studies suggest that the approach of reducing length of stay and per diem costs may not be maximally effective in management of the catastrophically injured patient. Blackerby[5] reviewed the effects of brain injury rehabilitation intensity on length of stay, showing that when rehabilitation intensity was increased from five to eight hours per day, length of stay was reduced by 31 percent. Ashley and colleagues reviewed the outcomes of 218 consecutive cases of traumatic brain injury following postacute rehabilitation programming.[6] The authors reported significant reductions in overall disability, reductions in re-

quired levels of supervision, and improved occupational status. The authors also pointed to Total Lifetime Savings (TLS) ranging from one to seven million dollars realized for the majority of cases when long-term cost of care was considered following rehabilitation programming. Ashley and colleagues pointed to a relationship between length of stay and program intensity as measured by program cost and outcome wherein longer lengths of stay and greater program intensity resulted not only in higher program costs but better outcomes.[7] The authors concluded that there appeared to be a relationship between achievable outcomes and the amount of time spent in therapy and type of therapy provided. Spivack and colleagues examined rehabilitation effort and its relationship to outcome in acute rehabilitation.[8] Rehabilitation intensity was classified into high and low intensity groups based on a median split of treatment hours in the first month of treatment. These authors noted that outcomes for patients who received higher intensity of rehabilitation treatment surpassed those of persons who received low intensity treatment. Length of stay was shown to be an important factor in achievement in physical performance, higher level cognitive skills, cognitively mediated physical skills, and improvement as measured by the Rancho Los Amigos Scale.

Taken together, the above studies raise serious question about whether trends toward shorter lengths of stay and reduced per diem costs will result in true lifetime cost savings. In fact, since rehabilitation seeks to reduce both short- and long-term impairment associated with TBI, it may be appropriate to consider cost savings in a more sophisticated fashion.

The case study presented herein seeks to do so. The purpose of this case study review is to evaluate the rehabilitative and cost effectiveness of postacute rehabilitation for persons suffering from traumatic brain injury via TLS and Net Present Value (NPV) analyses.

J Rehabil Outcomes Meas, 1997, 1(5), 33–41

MEDICAL HISTORY

On January 1, 1990, Mr. M., then a 33-year-old roofer, fell from a structure and sustained multiple severe injuries including a traumatic brain injury and spinal cord injury (SCI). Upon admission to the emergency room, he was unresponsive with no movement in the lower extremities. Painful stimulus elicited flexor posturing in the upper extremities. Glasgow Coma Scale score was 6.

The initial emergency room and subsequent acute medical diagnoses included a right parietal subdural hematoma and frontal contusion; left temporal hemorrhagic contusions; a large right temporo-occipital skull fracture; severe comminuted fracture at T8; vertebral body fracture at T12, and transverse processes fractures at T8, T9, T10; multiple rib fractures; fracture of left scapula; and complete spinal cord compromise at T8.

Over the initial days of acute care, medical management was required for severe cerebral edema, intracranial pressure elevation, blood pressure instability, and pansinusitis. Internal fixation for thoracic spine stabilization was not elected. The alternative SCI management was via rotorest bed. He gradually improved and began to awaken.

On January 29, 1990, Mr. M. was transferred to an acute rehabilitation hospital and was eventually weaned from the ventilator on February 14, 1990. A fenestrated trach allowed initial verbalizations and an estimated 50 percent response accuracy was recorded. By April 3, 1990, the tracheostomy was removed. Swallowing difficulties subsequently led to replacement of the nasogastric tube with a gastrostomy tube. In a thoracolumbar spine orthotic brace, sitting tolerance increased and he began to self-propel a wheelchair.

As mobilization increased, agitated behavior increased, which hindered advancement in bowel and bladder training and therapies. Psychoactive medications were introduced to attempt behavior management. The first grand mal seizure occurred in May, 1990, and Dilantin was introduced. At that time, medications included Mellaril, Haldol, Valium, Baclofen, and Didronel.

An oral feeding program was initiated with assisted self-feeding. By mid-June, 1990, the gastrostomy tube was removed. By early July, 1990, Mr. M. was discharged from the first acute rehabilitation hospital and admitted to a second acute rehabilitation hospital. Agitated behaviors were described as "extreme" and had not responded to earlier behavior modification and medications.

In October of 1990, Mr. M. was discharged from the second acute rehabilitation hospital and admitted to the first postacute rehabilitation program. Cognitive and speech deficits and dependency in activities of daily living were to be addressed in more structured therapeutic sessions. Breakthrough seizures continued secondary to subtherapeutic combined doses of Dilantin and Tegretol. By late October of 1990, he was discharged from the postacute rehabilitation program and admitted to a third acute rehabilitation hospital.

In early 1991, Mr. M. was transferred to a second postacute rehabilitation program. Behaviors had escalated to frequent, severe verbal and physical outbursts. Psychoactive medications and a behavior modification program continued in an attempt to manage the patient. However, effective progress in rehabilitation was significantly compromised. Emergency room admissions occurred secondary to repeated traumatic self-removal of a suprapubic catheter, leaving the inflated portion in the bladder.

In May, 1991, evaluation by a third postacute rehabilitation facility was requested by the case manager as an option to placement in an extended care facility for long-term care. At that time, Mr. M. remained semidependent for self-care activities and lacked adequate mobility skills secondary to cognitive, perceptual, and motor planning deficits and interruptive behavioral episodes. Behavioral episodes occurred virtually continually and consisted of verbal outbursts, threats, swearing, spitting, hitting, throwing objects, and self-abuse. Disability Rating Scale (DRS)[9] score was 13, indicating a severe level of disability (Appendix). Several medical issues were also in need of evaluation and treatment. These factors combined hindered progress toward realistic rehabilitation goals and greater independence.

Mr. M. was admitted on June 4, 1991, for postacute rehabilitation with inpatient residential services. Mr. M. participated in therapy for up to six hours per day, five days per week, on a one-to-one (therapist-to-client) basis. Therapeutic programming was continued with residential therapy addressing ADLs and behavioral issues during the evenings and weekends. Residential programming was initially conducted on a one-to-one basis until the client developed sufficient skills to allow a reduced level of supervision.

Admission occurred 540 days postinjury. After 14 months, Mr. M. was successfully discharged, with the aid of his parents and other family members, to a home environment. DRS score at discharge was 5, indicating a moderate level of disability. Follow-up at 32 months postdischarge indicates that Mr. M. resides in an apartment with his sister. He currently attends computer classes and participates in a home exercise program and other activities of daily living with limited paid attendant care. Behavioral dyscontrol has continued to improve beyond discharge. DRS score at follow-up was 4. No paid attendants are used, though the sister takes some responsibility for Mr. M.'s care.

METHOD

Prior to Mr. M.'s admission and at the request of the case manager, an evaluation was performed documenting Mr. M.'s status, the proposed rehabilitation approach, and the projected functional outcome. Based on the evaluation, the postacute rehabilitation program cost was predicted. Two potential outcome scenarios were developed representing a best and worst case as possible outcomes following the postacute rehabilitation program. The best possible outcome prediction consisted of placement with Mr. M.'s family with five to seven hours, per day, of paid attendant care (Supervised Home Placement). The worst possible outcome prediction consisted of placement in a behavioral group home (Behavioral Group Home Placement). The annual cost for each scenario was calculated and annual lifetime costs after rehabilitation for each outcome scenario were projected.

Cost of care projections were completed following a specified format that considered costs for 15 areas (see box). This format was used for all cost projections, allowing subsequent comparisons of costs to be prepared in an equally comprehensive and consistent manner. Four separate cost projections were completed.

The first projection assumed no further rehabilitative intervention and placement in a previously identified extended care facility, the only placement available willing to admit the patient while simultaneously being acceptable to the patient's family (Annual Life Care Cost Without Rehabilitation). A second cost projection provided review of anticipated costs of additional rehabilitation in a third postacute rehabilitation facility (Projected Postacute Rehabilitation Program Cost). This review considered not only per diem costs of the postacute rehabilitation program, but all other costs as well. A third cost projection was completed for a projected discharge placement (best case) following the postacute rehabilitation program, consisting of placement with Mr. M.'s family and provision of five to seven hours per day of paid attendant care (Annual Life Care Cost With Supervised Home Placement). The fourth cost projection was completed for a projected discharge placement (worst case) in a behavioral group home (Annual Life Care Cost With Behavioral Group Home Placement) (Table 1).

Two financial measures were used in this study: Total Lifetime Savings and the Net Present Value of the TLS resulting from postacute TBI rehabilitation. TLS represents the total dollars saved as a result of the decrease in living costs following rehabilitation when compared to living costs before rehabilitation. The annual savings is multiplied by the injured individual's number of projected remaining years of life to yield TLS. In prior studies, this was typically the ex-

---

Cost Consideration Format

A. Nursing and Attendant Needs
B. Medical/Allied Health Services
C. Emergency Services
D. Medical Procedures
E. Medications
F. Anticipated Hospitalization Needs
G. Bed and Accessories
H. Wheelchair and Accessories
I. Bathing/Hygiene Equipment
J. Incontinence Management Supplies
K. Transportation Needs
L. Housing Needs
M. Feeding Supplies
N. Per Diem Charges
O. Miscellaneous

---

tent of the financial analysis used to justify the expense of rehabilitation.

NPV is a more sophisticated analysis that takes the time value of money into account.[10] Financial decisions should be considered using an NPV approach to compare the cost to be expended today and the anticipated savings (or profits to be realized) that will result from a given program (Figure 1). In a scenario where the anticipated savings are projected to be $20,000 per year for 20 years, today's value of $20,000 to be received in future years is less due to the time value of money. This is similar to a loan when one borrows $20,000 and pays back $20,000 plus interest over the term of the loan. The sum of the payments represent the total amount spent over the time period of the loan and the $20,000 represents the present value of the future payments. NPV calculation mathematically adjusts the total dollars to be saved over a specified period of time back to today's value. If the cost of a program is greater than the value of the anticipated savings (or profits), a negative NPV is reached (Figure 2). If the value of the anticipated savings (or profits) is greater than the cost of the program, a positive NPV is reached (Figure 3). Two programs that both produce either a negative or positive NPV can be compared by the amount of the NPVs. If the NPV is greater than $1.00, the cost effectiveness of the rehabilitation investment is confirmed, although the larger the

---

Table 1. Costs of care and treatment options

Annual Life Care Cost Without Rehabilitation	Projected Postacute Rehabilitation Program Cost	Annual Life Care Cost with Supervised Home Placement	Annual Life Care Cost with Behavioral Group Home Placement
$222,600	$450,000	$49,688	$84,082

Net Present Value

"... Allows evaluation of initial costs with
long-term savings in today's dollars ..."

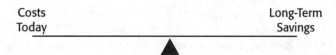

Figure 1. Costs applied today break even with long-term savings;
rehabilitation now does not save long-term cost.

Negative Net Present Value

Costs Outweigh Savings

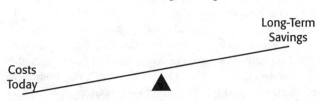

Figure 2. Costs applied today outweigh the cost of long-term care
without rehabilitation.

NPV, the stronger the financial incentive for the financially
responsible party to make the rehabilitation investment.

With this analysis, all rehabilitation costs *and* future savings resulting from the rehabilitation program are presented
in current dollar values. Future savings are discounted back
to today's dollar value using an appropriate cost of capital
(discount rate). The cost of rehabilitation should be deducted
from the future savings, expressed in current dollars, to yield
the NPV of the savings resulting from the rehabilitation investment.

Prior to admission, the attained figures above were analyzed as part of the decision-making process of determining
whether further postacute rehabilitation programming would
be pursued. The comparative analysis was conducted by
NPV calculations contrasting the Annual Life Care Cost
Without Rehabilitation to both the Annual Life Care Cost
with Supervised Home Placement and the Annual Life Care
Cost with Behavioral Group Home Placement.

Following discharge, the analysis above was repeated using the actual cost of the postacute rehabilitation program
and the actual annual cost of care with the achieved discharge placement.

COST EXPENDITURES PRIOR TO POSTACUTE ADMISSION

Mr. M. had been cared for at one acute hospital, three
acute rehabilitation hospitals, and two postacute rehabilitation facilities prior to his admission to the final postacute rehabilitation facility. The costs of his care were reviewed
from payer records (see box).

PREDICTED ANNUAL LIFE-CARE COST AND OUTCOME EXPECTED FOLLOWING THE THIRD POSTACUTE REHABILITATION ADMISSION

The Annual Life Care Cost without Rehabilitation, which
excluded further postacute rehabilitation, was calculated for
Mr. M. estimating the annual costs of his ongoing care after
taking into account the status of his disability and significant

behavioral problems. Using an Extended Care Facility model,
the proposed long-term care site, it was determined that the total costs for Mr. M.'s care would average $222,663 per year. It
should be understood that the extended care facility willing to
admit Mr. M. required 24-hour nursing care attendants as a
condition of his admission due to the complexity of his care and
behavioral dyscontrol. This requirement added substantially to
the annual cost of care. With a projected life expectancy of 42
years (Statistical Forecast of the United States, 1993),[11] the
Total Lifetime Cost of Mr. M.'s care would approximate
$9,351,846 without considering the impact of inflation and rising medical costs. It may be more reasonable, given the nature
of Mr. M.'s injuries, to reduce life expectancy by 15 percent to
35 years.[12] The Total Lifetime Cost of Mr. M.'s care without
further rehabilitation would approach $7,791,000.

The TLS and NPV analysis was prepared using a 35-year
estimate for life expectancy. This analysis predicted a Total
Lifetime Savings of between $4.85 million and $6.0 million
(Tables 2 and 3). The NPV was determined to be between
$2.2 million and $2.88 million in today's dollars, assuming
the third postacute rehabilitation program was effective and
depending upon which discharge scenario was achieved.

ACTUAL COST AND OUTCOME OF THIRD POSTACUTE REHABILITATION ADMISSION

The actual costs for Mr. M.'s 14-month postacute rehabilitation program were as follows: facility fees, $390,800; phy-

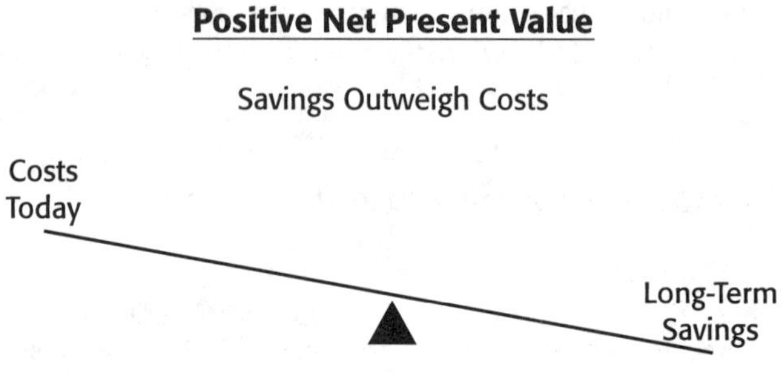

Positive Net Present Value

Savings Outweigh Costs

Figure 3. Costs applied to rehabilitation today result in significant
long-term savings.

<table>
<tr><td colspan="2">Costs of Care</td></tr>
</table>

Costs of Care	
1 Acute Hospital	$ 95,100
3 Acute Rehabilitation Hospitals (Total)	372,000
2 Postacute Rehabilitation Facilities (Total)	51,000
Air Ambulance	18,000
Miscellaneous Physician Charges	3,500
TOTAL:	$540,000

(All amounts are rounded)

sician fees, $2,300; other ancillary expenses, $22,600; for a total of $415,700. Predicted program costs were $450,525 prior to admission; however, the actual costs were $34,300 less.

The actual Annual Life Care Cost With Supervised Home Placement was determined to be $42,255, resulting in a TLS of $6.3 million over 35 years (Table 4). NPV for this figure was determined to be $3.0 million. The revised projection was calculated with actual annual cost figures provided by review of payer records.

Follow-up data collected for this individual at 5.2 years postinjury (2.7 years postdischarge) indicated that the level of disability remained stable with a DRS score of 5 at discharge and 4 at follow-up. Level of supervision required also remained stable with supervision by family in private living quarters at discharge and follow-up. These data suggest long-term stability in the rehabilitation outcome achieved. The broader review conducted by Ashley and colleagues[13] points to the long-term stability of postacute rehabilitation outcomes in general.

• • •

It should be noted that this program was not typical of most on the basis of cost. The average program cost for patients discharged from this postacute facility in 1991 was $93,587 and, in 1992, was $91,568. In fact, mean admission DRS was 5.44 and chronicity was 499 days for patients discharged in 1991 and 1992.

The chronicity of this case reduces the likelihood that observed improvements were due to spontaneous recovery. Additionally, the achieved outcomes strongly suggest that further rehabilitative efforts may be warranted even in cases where substantial rehabilitation effort has already been expended together with substantial financial expenditure.

A sum of $540,000 had been expended for Mr. M.'s treatment prior to the last postacute rehabilitation admission. Expenditure of another $415,700 resulted in substantial functional improvement and financial savings.

The chronicity of injury, the number of rehabilitation programs, and the financial expenditures prior to the third postacute admission would have been sufficient in many cases to dissuade pursuit of yet another rehabilitation program. It is interesting to note the substantial benefit realized, however, pursuant to the last rehabilitation effort. Additionally, it could be argued that a portion of the initial $540,000 expended prior to this admission could have been saved by earlier referral to a facility more experienced in addressing the types of medical and severe neurobehavioral problems Mr. M. experienced. It is, likewise, conceivable that the $415,700 expended for this admission might have been reduced by earlier referral.

As can be seen from the above review, application of appropriate postacute TBI rehabilitation can be extremely cost effective for catastrophically injured persons facing lifetime medical care. It can be useful for the case manager to investigate comprehensive projections of rehabilitation costs for purposes of conducting a cost-benefit analysis of a proposed rehabilitation plan, especially when treatment proposals require stringent cost justification. Cost projections must be conducted for likely discharge outcomes as a part of the cost-benefit analysis. The rehabilitation program that will be accountable for achieving likely discharge outcomes within projected costs should be involved in preparation of the cost-benefit analysis. Experienced providers should be capable of projecting total costs and length of stay for their recommended program of therapy as well as the realistic outcome goals.

Applying NPV techniques allows the parties to evaluate rehabilitation proposals from a quantitative perspective, giv-

Table 2. Behavior group home placement, projected net present value 35 years, 4 percent discount

		Cost before rehab	*Cost of rehab*	*Cost after rehab*
Total cost of care		$222,663	$450,525	$84,082
Annual savings				$138,581
Number of years				35
Discount rate				4%
"Net" cost of rehabilitation	$190,751			
		Annual savings year 2–35		$138,581
		Total lifetime dollars saved		$4,850,335
		Net Present Value		$2,247,686

Table 3. Supervised home placement, projected net present value 35 years, 4 percent discount

		Cost before rehab	Cost of rehab	Cost after rehab
Total cost of care		$222,663	$450,525	$49,688
Annual savings				$172,975
Number of years				35
Discount rate				4%
"Net" cost of rehabilitation	$190,751			
		Annual savings year 2–35		$172,975
		Total lifetime dollars saved		$6,051,920
		Net Present Value		$2,883,363

ing appropriate weight to initial rehabilitation costs and long-term cost savings, thus avoiding the effects of initial rehabilitation "sticker shock" and allowing the carrier to focus on the overall "investment" in rehabilitation and the eventual economic "return."

The total dollars to be expended on a proposed treatment plan should be considered in tandem with dollars that would be expended without the proposed treatment plan for the same time period. In this way, the "net" program cost can be calculated. For example, Mr. M.'s Annual Life Care Cost Without Rehabilitation was projected to be $222,663. The Actual Postacute Rehabilitation Program Cost was $415,700 for 14 months. The cost of the rehabilitation program was annualized to allow a direct comparison to the Annual Cost of Care Without Rehabilitation. Therefore, the "net" program cost was actually only $155,926 (Table 4). Another way to view this is to consider the incremental dollars to be placed "at risk" in association with pursuit of a proposed treatment plan.

The advantages associated with the prerehabilitation cost justification approach include the following:

1. Clear, comprehensive delineation of treatment and outcome expectations and projected costs for the treaters, case manager, financially responsible party, family, and patient.

2. An objective review of the financial ramifications associated with pursuit or lack of pursuit of a proposed treatment plan and alternatives.
3. An objective review of the financial ramifications of projected outcomes comparing both costs and projected future savings in today's dollars.
4. An objective comparison of predicted and actual treatment and outcome costs.
5. A method for objective validation of the success of a proposed treatment plan.

A decided disadvantage to this approach is the risk that treatment plans will be viewed only from the perspective of cost savings versus quality of life issues. There are clearly many examples where one would not be well advised to have medical care decisions based solely upon financial criteria without due consideration of quality and quantity of life issues. At the same time, it could be argued that one measure of increased quality could be found in the overall decrease in costs of care over the long term achieved by the stable rehabilitative outcome.

While the specific case reviewed herein was covered by a workers' compensations policy, the financial realities of the case can be generalized to many cases, regardless of whether those cases were publicly or privately funded. Should managed care result in provision of lesser rehabilitative intensity

Table 4. Supervised home placement, achieved at discharge, net present value 35 years, 4 percent discount

		Cost before rehab	Cost of rehab	Cost after rehab
Total cost of care		$222,663	$415,700	$42,255
Annual savings				$180,408
Number of years				35
Discount rate				4%
"Net" cost of rehabilitation	$155,926			
		Annual savings year 2–35		$180,408
		Total lifetime dollars saved		$6,314,280
		Net Present Value		$3,014,935

Table 5. Matched group (MG) compared to K.M. for age, cost, length of stay, and DRS

	Age	Cost	LOS	DRS (admission)	DRS (discharge)
MG (*n* = 9)	34	190,753	226	13	6.7
KM	34	414,593	387	13	5

MG: Matched on DRS (admission), male, age, TBI, completed program, inpatient.

in the short term, this and other published data[6-8] strongly suggest greater levels of disability and higher levels of required supervision as a result, both of which translate to higher long-term costs in both public and private sectors.

When Mr. M's case is compared to a group of others matched on DRS at admission, age, sex, diagnosis (TBI), and inpatient status, it is seen that Mr. M. had a longer LOS, a higher program cost (all converted to 1991 rates) and a better outcome as measured by DRS at discharge (Table 5). This finding is consistent with earlier research, which pointed to a relationship between outcome, dollars expended, and length of stay.[7]

REFERENCES

1. Cope, D.N., et al. "Brain Injury: Analysis of Outcome in a Post-Acute Rehabilitation System. Part 1: General Analysis." *Brain Injury* 5, no. 2 (1991): 111–25.

2. Jones, M., and Evans, R.W. "Rating Outcomes in Post-Acute Rehabilitation of Acquired Brain Injury." *The Case Manager* (January 1991): 44–47.

3. Johnston, M., and Lewis, F. "Outcomes of Community Re-Entry Programmes for Brain Injury Survivors. Part 1: Independent Living and Productive Activities." *Brain Injury* 5 (1991): 141–54.

4. Hall, K.M., and Cope, D.N. "The Benefit of Rehabilitation in Traumatic Brain Injury: A Literature Review." *Journal of Head Trauma Rehabilitation* 10, no. 1 (1995): 1–13.

5. Blackerby, W.F. "Intensity of Rehabilitation and Length of Stay." *Brain Injury* 4, no. 2 (1990): 167–73.

6. Ashley, M.J., Krych, D.K., and Lehr, R.P. Jr. "Cost/Benefit Analysis for Post-Acute Rehabilitation of the Traumatically Brain-Injured Patient." *Journal of Insurance Medicine* 22, no. 2 (1990): 156–61.

7. Ashley, M.J., Persel, C.S., and Krych, D.K. "Changes in Reimbursement Climate: Relationship Among Outcome, Cost, and Payor Type in the Postacute Rehabilitation Environment." *Journal of Head Trauma Rehabilitation* 8, no. 4 (1993): 30–47.

8. Spivack, G., et al. "Effects of Intensity of Treatment and Length of Stay on Rehabilitation Outcomes." *Brain Injury* 6, no. 5 (1992): 419–34.

9. Rappaport, M., et al. "Disability Rating Scale for Severe Head Trauma: Coma to Community." *Archives of Physical Medicine and Rehabilitation* 63 (1982): 118–23.

10. Horngren, C.T. *Cost Accounting: A Managerial Emphasis.* Englewood, NJ: Prentice-Hall, Inc., 1982.

11. *Statistical Abstract of the United States.* 113th ed. Washington, DC: Government Printing Office, 1993.

12. Samsa, G.P., Patrick, C.H., and Feussner, J.R. "Long-Term Survival of Veterans with Traumatic Spinal Cord Injury." *Archives of Neurology* 50 (1993): 909–14.

13. Ashley, M.J., Persel, C.S., and Krych, D.K. "Long-Term Outcome Follow-Up of Post-Acute TBI Rehabilitation: An Assessment of Functional and Behavioral Measures of Daily Living." *Journal of Rehabilitation Outcomes Measurement* 1, no. 4 (1997): 40–47.

Disability Rating (DR) Scale[*]

Name _____ Sex _____ Birthdate _____ Brain Injury Date _____

Cause of Injury: _____ MVA/MCA* _____ Head Trauma** _____ Infection _____ Stroke _____ Anoxia

_____ Developmental (Congenital) _____ Degenerative _____ Metabolic _____ Drowning

_____ Other (Specify) _____

*MVA = Motor Vehicle Accident; MCA = Motorcycle Accident. *Circle one.*
**Gun shot, blunt instrument, blow to head, fall, etc.

DATE OF RATING

CATEGORY	ITEM▲								
Arousability	Eye Opening[1]								
Awareness and	Communication Ability[2†]								
Responsivity**	Motor Response[3]								
Cognitive Ability for	Feeding[4]								
Self Care	Toileting[4]								
Activities	Grooming[4]								
Dependence on Others***	Level of Functioning[5]								
Psychosocial Adaptability	"Employability"[6]								
COMMENTS:	**Total**								

[1]Eye Opening
0   Spontaneous
1   To Speech
2   To Pain
3   None

[2]Communication Ability†
Either Verbal; Writing or Letter Board;
or Sign (viz. eye blink, head nod, etc.)
0   Oriented
1   Confused
2   Inappropriate
3   Incomprehensible
4   None

[3]Best Motor Resp.
0   Obeying
1   Localizing
2   Withdrawing
3   Flexing
4   Extending
5   None

[4]Cognitive Ability for Feeding, Toileting, Grooming
(Does patient know how and when? Ignore motor disability.)
0   Complete
1   Partial
2   Minimal
3   None

†In presence of tracheostomy (plate T next to score); for voice or speech dysfunction (place D next to score if there is dysarthria, dysphonia, voice paralysis, aphasia, apraxia, etc.)

[5]Level of Functioning
(Consider both physical & cognitive disability)
0   Completely independent
1   Independent in special environment
2   Mildly dependent   – (a)
3   Moderately dependent   – (b)
4   Markedly dependent   – (c)
5   Totally dependent   – (d)

[6]"Employability"
(As a full time worker, homemaker or student)
0   Not restricted
1   Selected jobs, competitive
2   Sheltered workshop, non-competitive
3   Not employable

Disability Categories

Total DR Score	Level of Disability
0	None
1	Mild
2–3	Partial
4–6	Moderate
7–11	Moderately severe
12–16	Severe
17–21	Extremely severe
22–24	Vegetative state
25–29	Extreme vegetative state
30	Death

a	**needs limited assistance (non-resident helper)**
b	**needs moderate assistance (person in home)**
c	**needs assistance with all major activities at all times**
d	**24-hour nursing care required**

[*]Rappaport et al. Disability Rating Scale for Severe Head Trauma Patients: Coma To Community. Arch Phys Med Rehab. 63:118–123, 1982
**Modified from Teasdale, Jennett, Lancet 2:81–83, 1974
***Modified from Scranton et al. Arch Phys Med Rehab. 51:1–21, 1970

▲Item definitions available from M. Rappaport, Brain Function Laboratory, San Jose, California

Source: Reprinted with permission from M. Rappaport et al., Disability Rating Scale for Severe Head Trauma Patients: Coma To Community, *Archives of Physical Medicine and Rehabilitation,* Vol. 63, pp. 118–123, © 1982, W.B. Saunders Company.

27

Longitudinal Assessment of Stroke Survivors' Handicap

Mary E. Segal and Marian Gillard

How are individuals with disabilities doing as a result of rehabilitation interventions?" is the most general form of the question that rehabilitation outcome measurement seeks to answer. Until recently, emphasis focused on disability or the effects of one or more impairments on an individual's normal level of skill or ability. Currently, interest is increasing in measuring handicap. *Handicap* has been defined by the World Health Organization (1980) as the net effects of disabilities, in interaction with the physical and social environment, on an individual's performance of normal social roles, such as moving freely about the home and community, working, and interacting socially with others.

This article extends earlier work at the Moss Rehabilitation Research Institute on the appropriateness of the Craig Handicap Assessment and Reporting Technique (CHART; Whiteneck, Charlifue, Gerhart, Overholser, & Richardson, 1992) for stroke survivors. Validation for stroke patients is necessary because the CHART was originally developed for and validated with spinal cord injury (SCI) patients, who tend to be young and male and can be expected to have social roles that differ from older populations.

In an earlier study, a sample of former inpatient rehabilitation stroke patients was assessed in-person at 6 months postonset with the CHART (Segal & Schall, 1995). Primary caregivers were asked to respond as proxies for survivors in concurrent assessments conducted separately. In the present study, stroke survivors' and caregiver proxies' CHART scores were again obtained for a subset of the original sample contacted by telephone 1 year later.

This study had four purposes. First, stroke survivors' and caregiver proxies' CHART scores were again assessed for agreement, and results on agreement were compared with

those obtained by in-person administration 1 year earlier. Second, CHART scores of stroke survivors at 18 months postonset were compared with their earlier scores to determine if the sample had significantly improved, deteriorated, or remained stable. Third, the variability of change in the CHART dimensions and predictive value of 6-month CHART dimensions' scores for the 18-month scores were examined. Finally, the internal consistency of the construct of handicap as measured by the CHART was determined for both the telephone and in-person administrations.

Of particular interest was the issue of proxy agreement because, as other reports from this laboratory have suggested, it is important to be able to collect accurate proxy data for populations who often suffer cognitive deficits, such as stroke patients (Segal & Schall, 1994). While good proxy agreement was found for in-person administration of the CHART (Segal & Schall, 1995), a Medline literature search found no reports comparing the proxy agreement of in-person and telephone interviews for any outcome measure used in rehabilitation. Nevertheless, it is also important to be able to collect outcomes information in a reliable manner over the telephone, given the inefficiency of conducting in-person interviews for determining follow-up status of rehabilitation patients.

The accuracy of telephone reporting has been an important issue in health outcomes assessment. Epidemiological studies have compared rates of specific kinds of responses and found that in-person and telephone assessments produce

No commercial party having a direct or indirect interest in the subject matter of this article has or will confer a benefit upon the authors or upon any organization with which the authors are associated.

This research was supported by a grant from the Moss Rehabilitation Research Institute and was approved by the MossRehab Hospital Institutional Review Board.

Top Stroke Rehabil, 1997, 4(1), 41–52

similar data with some exceptions. A few studies have compared telephone and in-person assessments of rehabilitation outcomes using the same group of subjects. Studies of the Functional Independence Measure (FIM; Hamilton, Granger, Sherwin, Zielezny, & Tashman, 1987), for example, have shown that telephone administration is an acceptable and efficient substitute for in-person interview, with the exception of a few FIM items, around the time of discharge from geriatric in-patient rehabilitation (Jaworski, Kult, & Boynton, 1994) and at 3 to 10 months postdischarge from inpatient stroke rehabilitation (Smith, 1995). For longer term follow-up (1–5 years), Korner-Bitensky, Wood-Dauphinee, Siemiatycki, Shapiro, and Becker (1994) obtained good intermodal (telephone compared to in-person) agreement for a protocol including the Reintegration to Normal Living Index (Wood-Dauphinee, Opzoomer, Williams, Marchand, & Spitzer, 1988), a measure of global function, and the Barthel Index (Mohoney & Barthel, 1965), a measure of physical disability.

The purposes of the study in addition to the telephone proxy agreement are relevant because, given the current emphasis on cost-effective delivery of health care services, it can be expected that long-term outcomes will become increasingly important in documenting the effectiveness of rehabilitation. However, longitudinal follow-up analyses, especially for periods exceeding a year postdischarge, are relatively rare in the stroke rehabilitation literature, whether at the level of impairment, disability, or handicap.

METHODS

Subjects

Twenty-five community-living stroke survivors were recruited by telephone from a sample of 38 stroke survivors who had participated, with their primary caregivers, in separate but concurrent in-person assessments and interviews 1 year earlier. In this study, as in the earlier one, survivors with moderate to severe cognitive deficits were excluded because the proxy agreement aspect required a high level of cognitive function. Thirteen (34%) of the 38 original subjects were not available for this subsequent study. Reasons were patient or caregiver refusal, 7 (18%); inability to contact because of disconnected telephone, 2 (5%); severe ill health or hospitalization, 2 (5%); and death of former patient, 2 (5%).

Demographically, the 25 survivor/proxy pairs in this study were very similar to the subjects in the earlier study. Median age of the subjects in the first study was 65 years. One year later, the median age was 64 years. Table 1 presents demographic data for both studies. No differences were statistically significant when assessed by Mann-Whitney (M-W) U tests or by chi-square analysis.

Subjects in this study also were representative of the earlier study in terms of their 6-month CHART scores. The original 38 subjects and the 25 subjects recruited for this study were compared using M-W tests on the four CHART dimensions used in this study and also on a summary score. There were no statistically significant differences for either

Table 1. Numbers (percentages) of stroke survivors and caregivers in demographic categories for 6 months postonset (*N* = 38) and 18 months postonset (*N* = 25) studies of handicap

Characteristics	Earlier study (N = 38)		Later study (N = 25)	
	n	*(%)*	*n*	*(%)*
Survivors				
Male	17	(45)	11	(44)
African American	23	(61)	15	(60)
Married	25	(66)	16	(64)
Divorced/widowed	11	(29)	7	(28)
Less than 12 years education	25	(66)	15	(60)
Employed full time prestroke	8	(21)	5	(25)
Index stroke location				
Right	20	(53)	12	(48)
Left	16	(42)	11	(44)
Index stroke was first	22	(58)	14	(64)
Caregivers				
Male	7	(18)	5	(20)
Married	27	(71)	18	(72)
Less than 12 years education	12	(32)	8	(32)
Employed full time prestroke	20	(53)	12	(48)

stroke survivor or caregiver ratings. *P*-values ranged from .65 to .99, with a median of .80. In addition, the following variables associated with statistically significantly greater handicap in the original sample were also statistically significant for this subsample: lower educational status; occurrence of stroke prior to the index stroke; and right hemisphere lesion in survivors whose index stroke had been their first. Thus, the subsample appeared to represent the original sample well.

The Measure: CHART

The CHART assesses five dimensions of social disadvantage or handicap, as suggested by the World Health Organization: (1) physical independence (PhysInd), (2) mobility (Mob), (3) occupation (Occ), (4) social integration (SocInt), and (5) economic self-sufficiency (Econ). Because of difficulty in obtaining Econ scores for this sample over the telephone, and also its lack of demonstrated relationship with other handicap dimensions (Segal & Schall, 1995; Whiteneck et al., 1992), it was not used in this study. A total of the other four dimensions was computed as a summary score.

Each CHART dimension is scaled from 0 to 100, with 0 corresponding to total handicap and 100 to absence of handicap. Complete descriptions of the dimensions and their items are available elsewhere (Whiteneck et al., 1992).

Procedure

During the summer of 1994, the second author contacted the subjects to arrange the telephone interviews. The first and second authors alternated in interviewing either the stroke survivor or caregiver. Two other measures, the FIM and the Frenchay Activities Index (Wade, Leigh-Smith, & Hewer, 1985), were also part of the protocol. Results for these measures are not included in this report. All procedures were reviewed and approved by the Institutional Review Board at the first author's facility.

At recruitment and again before the data collection, the purpose of a proxy agreement study was explained to the subjects, and each was requested to assure that the other member of the survivor/caregiver pair was not present during the telephone interview. The first author, who had experience with the CHART in other studies and is collaborating with the team that developed the instrument, trained the second author in its use. Interrater reliability was not assessed for the two raters for the telephone administration. However, for the earlier in-person administration, interrater reliability as assessed by methods described elsewhere (Segal & Schall, 1995) was excellent: the intraclass correlation (ICC) for the total CHART scores was .97.

Data Analysis

Data were analyzed using SYSTAT (1992). CHART agreement between stroke survivors and proxy caregivers was analyzed with ICCs, according to the method described by Winer (1971) to measure the reliability of a single rater or informant. (Note that this method unavoidably confounded interrater reliability with proxy agreement. However, as described above, we assumed good interrater reliability and that any important differences were due to differences between stroke survivor and proxy caregiver responses.) Because the CHART distributions were skewed, medians and interquartile ranges were calculated to describe score distributions. M-W *U* tests were used to test differences in CHART subscale and total score distributions according to demographic variables. Wilcoxon sign-ranked tests were used to test for differences between earlier scores obtained at 6 months postonset and scores at 18 months postonset. Associations between CHART dimensions were assessed with Spearman rho correlations.

RESULTS

Proxy Agreement

Table 2 shows ICCs for agreement between stroke survivors and proxy caregivers on CHART dimensions for the following:

- the total sample of 38 survivor/proxy pairs obtained during the 6-month post-onset in-person assessment, which have been reported earlier (Segal & Schall, 1995)
- this study's subsample of 25 pairs obtained during the 6-month postonset in-person assessment
- the subsample of 25 pairs obtained during the 18-month postonset telephone assessment

Longitudinal Assessment of Handicap

Median scores according to the 25 survivors and their caregivers on each of the four dimensions of handicap are shown in the stacked bars of Fig 1, for both 6 months and 18 months postonset.

Wilcoxon signed-rank tests showed that caregiver proxy scores for SocInt were significantly higher at the later assessment ($z = 2.52$, $p < .02$). Median SocInt score by caregiver report was 65 for the 6-month assessment and 90 for the 18-month assessment. Survivors' scores were 79 and 85 respectively, a nonsignificant difference. Caregivers' summary scores were also significantly higher at the later assessment ($z = 2.52$, $p < .02$). Median summary score according to caregivers' reports was 252 for the 6-month assessment and 288 for the 18-month assessment. Survivors' scores were 259 and 272 respectively, a nonsignificant difference.

Table 2. Intraclass correlations (confidence intervals) for CHART dimensions' proxy agreement

| | 6 mos. postonset in-person assessment | | 18 mos. postonset telephone assessment |
	Total sample n = 38	Subsample n = 25	Subsample n = 25
CHART dimension			
PhysInd	0.35 (0.05–0.60)	0.65 (0.35–0.83)	0.51 (0.16–0.75)
Mob	0.65 (0.43–0.80)	0.58 (0.25–0.79)	0.74 (0.49–0.88)
Occ	0.68 (0.47–0.82)	0.67 (0.39–0.84)	0.61 (0.29–0.80)
SocInt	0.27 (–0.05–0.54)	0.28 (–0.11–0.60)	0.26 (–0.14–0.59)
Summary score	0.68 (0.47–0.82)	0.73 (0.47–0.87)	0.66 (0.37–0.83)

Otherwise, there were no significant differences from the 6-month to the 18-month assessment according to either survivor or caregiver reports. However, the relative stability of medians shown in Fig 1 masks some variability in individual survivors' change scores. Fig 2 plots the medians, interquartile ranges (middle 50%), and interdecile ranges (middle 90%) of these change scores for each of the four dimensions.

Effects of Demographic Variables on CHART Dimension Scores at 18 Months

As described earlier, statistically significant differences on the CHART had been found at the 6-month postonset assessment for educational status of survivor, occurrence of stroke prior to the index stroke, and location of lesion. These differences were preserved at the 18-month assessment in the following manner:

1. *Lower educational status of survivor:* Summary scores, PhysInd, and Occ showed significantly greater handicap for both survivors' and caregivers' reports and SocInt for caregivers' reports (survivors' reports were consistent with this direction).
2. *Stroke prior to the index stroke:* Summary scores showed significantly greater handicap for caregivers' reports (survivors' reports were consistent with this direction) and SocInt for both survivors' and caregivers' reports.
3. *Right hemisphere lesion for those who had sustained first strokes:* Summary scores showed significantly

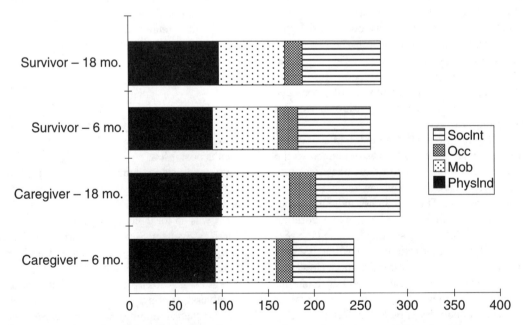

Figure 1. Median CHART dimension and summary scores for stroke survivors and caregivers at 18 months postonset.

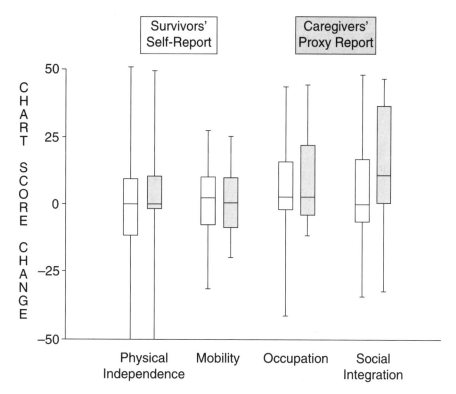

Figure 2. Median, interquartile range, and interdecile range for change in stroke survivors' CHART dimension scores from 6 months to 18 months postonset.

greater handicap for caregivers' reports (survivors' reports were consistent with this direction).

Two demographic variables were associated with differences in SocInt scores, but not summary scores, only at the 18-month assessment. These were (1) caregiver gender and (2) relation of caregiver to survivor:

1. *Caregiver gender:* According to caregivers' reports, SocInt scores of survivors with male caregivers were higher than for those with female caregivers (M-W $U = 78$, $p < .05$). Median SocInt score for the five survivors with male caregivers was 100; for those with female caregivers, 83. Differences according to survivors' reports were consistent with this direction although not statistically significant.
2. *Relation of caregiver to survivor:* According to survivors' reports, SocInt scores of survivors cared for by spouses were higher than for those cared for by children (M-W $U = 62$, $p < .05$). Median SocInt score for the survivors cared for by spouses was 90; by children, 58. Differences according to caregivers' reports were consistent with this direction although not statistically significant.

Effects of Demographic Variables on Change Scores from 6 Months to 18 Months

Only one demographic variable was associated with differences in CHART dimension change scores, as reported consistently by survivors and caregivers. Gender of caregiver was associated with differences in Mob changes for both survivors' and caregivers' reports (M-W $U = 20$, $p < .05$). According to caregivers' reports, median Mob scores for survivors cared for by men decreased from 87 at 6 months to 74 at 18 months. Median Mob scores for survivors cared for by women increased from 67 at 6 months to 78 at 18 months. Survivors' reports showed similar changes.

Associations between CHART Dimensions and Prediction of 18-month Scores from 6-month Scores

Table 3 shows the intercorrelations between the four CHART dimensions and the summary scores, all at the 18-month assessment. When the intercorrelations were computed for the 6-month assessment for these 25 subjects (not shown here), 17 of the 20 correlations were higher (although not necessarily significantly higher) at the 18-month assessment. The three that did not follow this pattern were from caregivers' data and included correlations between PhysInd and Mob, PhysInd

Table 3. Intercorrelations of survivors' scores on CHART dimensions at 18 months poststroke as assessed by survivors (caregivers in parentheses)

	PhysInd	Mob	Occ	SocInt
PhysInd	—			
Mob	0.79*	—		
	(0.53)*			
Occ	0.79*	0.80*	—	
	(0.59)*	(0.61)*		
SocInt	0.50	0.48	0.44	—
	(0.34)	(0.50)	(0.48)	
Summary score	0.92*	0.88*	0.88*	0.62*
	(0.72)*	(0.80)*	(0.90)*	(0.64)*

*$p < 0.05$, one-tailed, with Bonferroni's correction applied for multiple significance tests.

and SocInt, and Mob and the summary score. The general pattern of higher intercorrelations, suggesting greater internal consistency of the handicap assessment, for the later data set is reflected in the Cronbach alphas calculated for each assessment. For the CHART summary scores at the 6-month assessment, the alpha for survivors' data was .61 (.73 for caregivers). At 18 months, the alpha was .80 (.79).

The correlation between the 6-month and the 18-month summary scores was 0.70 for survivors' report (0.82 for caregivers'). For Phys, the correlation was 0.51 (0.56); Mob, 0.55 (0.82); Occ, 0.81 (0.70); and SocInt, 0.38 (0.38). Except for the two SocInt coefficients, all were statistically significant, $p < .05$, one-tailed, with Bonferroni's correction applied for multiple significance testing.

DISCUSSION

Proxy Agreement

The subsample of stroke survivors and their caregivers was representative of the original sample used in the 6-month postonset study. Not surprisingly, ICCs for the 6-month proxy agreement study for this subsample were similar to those for the larger sample. Only the subsample ICC for PhysInd was not similar to the point estimate for the larger sample. Otherwise, the subsample ICCs were well within the confidence intervals for the larger sample. The PhysInd ICC for the subsample was considerably higher than for the original sample. However, this probably chance occurrence did not result in any major difference between the total sample and subsample on the CHART summary score ICC at 6 months postonset.

The ICCs for proxy agreement for the telephone study at 18 months postonset were similar to those reported for the subsample's in-person agreement at 6 months postonset, al-

though in general somewhat lower. This is not surprising, as telephone assessment precludes many of the body language clues that convey important information in-person about respondents' confidence in their answers, suggesting to the data collector the need to probe. Another, less compelling explanation is that caregivers' ability to provide proxy information may decrease as time postonset increases. However, it is difficult to suggest a mechanism to explain such an effect.

In general, the ICCs obtained in the telephone assessment were adequate, particularly because caregiver/proxy agreement was confounded with rater agreement, as in the earlier 6-month assessment. The ICC for summary proxy score agreement was .66, which suggests an adequate scale and compares favorably with other assessments of patient/proxy agreement; for example, Wood-Dauphinee et al. (1988) obtained an ICC of .62 for the Reintegration to Normal Living Index for in-person proxy agreement. The telephone assessment replicated the poor agreement for SocInt obtained in the earlier in-person assessment. Examination of the individual items on this dimension revealed particularly poor agreement for the heavily weighted item for number of friends contacted, rather than relatives, associates, or strangers. However, trade-offs between items (e.g., associates and friends) were not evident. Rather, it appeared that there was a generalized effect within a pair for over- or underreporting across all items of the SocInt dimension.

Longitudinal Assessment of Handicap

Handicap summary scores changed little from the 6-month to the 18-month assessment. Survivors reported a median gain of 19 (caregivers 24) on a 400-point scale for the summary score. For caregivers, this was statistically significant, resulting from the significant gain of 10 points they reported for survivors on the 100-point SocInt dimension. Inspection of the SocInt items showed that caregivers and patients both reported increases in number of friends they were in contact with once a month, rather than relatives or organizational associates with whom they were in contact or strangers to whom they talked. The other three dimensions, however, showed very small changes in median scores.

This overall trend toward stability masks some variability in individual change scores. As shown in Fig 2, the average interquartile range for the four dimensions' changes was 20 points. Thus, 50% of the distribution at 18 months scored, on average, within 20 points of their scores at 6 months on the dimensions, and 50% at 18 months scored more than 20 points from their scores at 6 months.

The lability in handicap may be attributable to environmental changes, as handicap is defined as disability interacting with the environment to affect social role functioning. The largest interquartile range for change scores was for SocInt, the only dimension not shown in the earlier study to be correlated with physical disability as measured by the FIM (Segal & Schall, 1995).

Of course, the apparent stability is not representative of the general stroke population but those in our sample who survived and were doing fairly well at 18 months. Of the original 38 subjects in the 6-month postonset study, at least 4 (11%) had suffered adverse events (death, severe illness) and were not part of the sample. As noted above, the inclusion criteria for the original subjects required relatively high functioning. Nevertheless, these data suggest that for stroke survivors in the community at 18 months postonset, large decrements in handicap are not apparent when compared with their functioning 1 year earlier.

Effects of Demographic Variables on CHART Dimension Scores at 18 Months and on Change Scores from 6 Months to 18 Months

Predictors of differences in handicap at 6 months were all still present at 18 months, including the association of lower educational status, prior strokes, and brain lesions on the right side with greater handicap. These effects, particularly for educational status, were strong ones not ameliorated by time for this sample. It is tempting to speculate that the higher SocInt scores at 18 months for the 5 female survivors with male (husband) caregivers and also the 13 survivors cared for by spouses may be an artifact of the SocInt dimension, which allots 30 of the 100 points for being married. However, there was no direct effect on the SocInt dimension for being married when 3 additional married survivors cared for by others than their spouses were added to the 13 cared for by spouses and compared with unmarried survivors. The small numbers in this sample suggest the necessity for further research on the association between having a male caregiver and social integration after disability.

The discrepancy in Mob score changes between the five married women cared for by male caregivers (husbands) and other survivors cared for by female caregivers is interesting. The mobility of survivors cared for by men decreased, while mobility of survivors cared for by women increased. The Mob item that contributed the greatest decrease and increase was the number of days per week the subjects went outside the home. Number of hours out of bed, nights away from home, and access within the home and to transportation were all relatively unchanged. However, the small sample of survivors cared for by men again suggests that further research is necessary.

Associations between CHART Dimensions and Prediction of 18-month Scores from 6-month Scores

The intercorrelations of survivors' scores on CHART dimensions at 18 months replicated the finding for this sample at 6 months. The PhysInd, Mob, and Occ dimensions were all significantly and substantially intercorrelated for this sample, suggesting they represent facets of a single dimension, probably physical disability. There was no statistically significant relationship between SocInt and the other CHART dimensions. The relationship of SocInt to handicap appears more complex. It may be influenced relatively more by social circumstances than physical disability to a greater extent than is true for the other dimensions.

The higher Cronbach alphas for the 18-month assessment, compared to the 6-month assessment, suggest that, as the course of disability proceeds for community-living stroke patients, the dimensions of handicap are more intercorrelated than earlier in the course of disability. It is interesting to speculate on some causes of this phenomenon. Possibly, during early phases of adjustment to disability, attempts are made to preserve premorbid patterns. Then, as adjustment to disability proceeds, trade-offs may bring the way time is spent in activity patterns, social exchanges, and ability to be mobile into closer correspondence.

In general, there were modest associations between handicap at 6 months postonset and 1 year later. The average Spearman rank coefficient was .56. However, there were clear differences among the dimensions, with Mob and Occ showing more predictive value than PhysInd and SocInt. Because of the ordinal nature of the data, it was not possible to test for differences between these Spearman rank correlation coefficients.

● ● ●

Rehabilitation outcome measurement for stroke patients needs to progress beyond the level of disability. The CHART, especially its scales for physical independence, mobility, and occupation, is an instrument that appears to have good construct validity for documenting follow-up status of stroke rehabilitation patients at the level of handicap.

REFERENCES

Hamilton, B.B., Granger, C.V., Sherwin, F.S., Zielezny, M., & Tashman, J.S. (1987). A uniform data system for medical rehabilitation. In M.J. Fuhrer (Ed.), *Rehabilitation outcomes* (pp. 137–147). Baltimore: Paul H. Brookes Publishing.

Jaworski, D.M., Kult, T., & Boynton, P.R. (1994). The functional independence measure: a pilot study comparison of observed and reported ratings. *Rehabilitation Nursing Research,* 141–147.

Korner-Bitensky, N., Wood-Dauphinee, S., Siemiatycki, J., Shapiro, S., & Becker, R. (1994). Health-related information post-discharge: telephone versus face-to-face interviewing. *Archives of Physical Medicine and Rehabilitation, 75,* 1,287–1,296.

Mohoney, F.I., & Barthel, D.W. (1965). Functional evaluation: the Barthel index. *Maryland Medical Journal, 14,* 61–65.

Segal, M.E., & Schall, R.R. (1994). Determining functional/health status and its relation to disability in stroke survivors. *Stroke, 25,* 2,391–2,397.

Segal, M.E., & Schall, R.R. (1995). Assessing handicap of stroke survivors: a validation study of the Craig handicap assessment and reporting technique. *American Journal of Physical Medicine and Rehabilitation, 74,* 276–286.

Smith, P. (1995, July). Intermodal agreement of follow-up telephone functional assessment using the functional independence measure (FIM) in patients with stroke. Paper presented at the Conference on Functional Assessment, Buffalo, NY.

SYSTAT for Windows. (1992). Version 5. Evanston, IL.

Wade, D.T., Leigh-Smith, J., & Hewer, R.L. (1985). Social activities after stroke: Measurement and natural history using the Frenchay activities index. *International Rehabilitation Medicine, 7,* 176–181.

Whiteneck, G.G., Charlifue, S.W., Gerhart, K.A., Overholser, J.D., & Richardson, G.N. (1992). Quantifying handicap: A new measure of long-term rehabilitation outcomes. *Archives of Physical Medicine and Rehabilitation, 73,* 519–526.

Winer, B.J. (1971). *Statistical principles in experimental design* (2nd ed.). New York: McGraw-Hill.

Wood-Dauphinee, S.L., Opzoomer, A., Williams, J.I., Marchand, B., & Spitzer, W.O. (1988). Assessment of global function: The reintegration to normal living index. *Archives of Physical Medicine and Rehabilitation, 69,* 583–590.

World Health Organization. (1980). *Classification of impairments, disabilities and handicaps: A manual of classification relating to the consequences of disease.* Geneva, Switzerland: Author.

28

Stroke Transition after Inpatient Rehabilitation

Gary Goldberg, Mary E. Segal, Stephen N. Berk, Richard R. Schall, and Arthur M. Gershkoff

The need to identify cost-effective means for delivering health care to the survivors of a stroke is an issue of concern to health care planners and providers throughout the industrialized Western world (Russell, Hamilton, & Tweedie, 1993; Wolfe, Beech, Ratcliffe, & Rudd, 1995; AHCPR, 1995). Several deficiencies with current models of stroke rehabilitation delivery of services can be identified. Stroke rehabilitation programs tend to provide patient-centered care with a focus on medical stabilization and the optimization of physical functioning in the protected environment of an inpatient setting. Stroke care is typically hospital- rather than community-based, thus limiting care for home-bound patients and patients without access to adequate transportation. The current system of care tends to be crisis driven rather than prevention oriented. While community support programs are available, they are generally not centrally coordinated or well publicized, and tend to provide little more than disjointed, limited services, often without access to opportunities for therapeutic recreation and other avocational pursuits that draw the patient and caregiver back into the community. Stroke survivors and their caregivers frequently have difficulty obtaining timely access to stroke-related information and educational activities. There is also a general lack of knowledge available regarding the long-term psychosocial adjustment issues and, consequently, a lack of understanding of the support service needs of patients and their caregivers following discharge to the community. There is, however, a significant accumulation of data suggesting that the availability of a stable social support system can have a significant beneficial effect on functional outcome following stroke (Anderson, 1992; Glass & Maddox, 1992; Glass, Matchar, Belyea, & Feussner, 1993).

Top Stroke Rehabil, 1997, 4(1), 64–79

RATIONALE FOR THE STUDY

In his comprehensive longitudinal study of 173 stroke patients and their caregivers in Greenwich, England, Anderson (1992) noted that caregivers were disappointed in the lack of continuity of care, particularly in the area of social support services, after the patient was discharged home from the hospital. An active, case-managed approach directed toward early intervention and preventive services has generally not been available to stroke survivors and their caregivers following discharge from the hospital. The authors reasoned that coordinated community-based delivery of services to stroke survivors could ease the transition from hospital back to community. It had been our informal observation that, in spite of carefully devised discharge plans, the stress of leaving the protected inpatient environment and transitioning back into the community, particularly for the primary caregiver, frequently led to recurrent hospitalizations and health problems, respectively, for the patients and their caregivers. The provision of coordinated services to ease this transition was felt to be important, particularly in view of ongoing changes in the ways in which hospital-based stroke care is being funded.

More of inpatient rehabilitation program and available time is necessarily devoted to the medical stabilization of the patient, as prospective payment for acute care services leads

The authors thank the following individuals for their contributions: Stephen Braverman; John Whyte, MD, PhD; Susan Riddle, MSW, project coordinator for the study and case manager for the experimental group; Katherine Elokdah, who provided therapeutic recreation interventions for the experimental group and assisted in program review; and Lenore Spiegel, PhD, data collector. The study was supported by grants from the William Penn Foundation and from the Moss Rehabilitation Research Institute.

to rapid transfer of patients from the acute care hospital to the inpatient rehabilitation setting. Restrictions in reimbursement have forced reductions in the length of stay for inpatient rehabilitation and have limited the provision of hospital-based psychosocial services to older stroke patients funded through Medicare. For these reasons, the current model of care for stroke survivors, with its focus on the inpatient phase of care, is noticeably deficient in terms of the organization, monitoring, effectiveness, and focus on the psychosocial factors that impact significantly on recovery and maintenance of general health in both the patient and their primary caregiver(s). The authors therefore sought to develop a systematic follow-up program for stroke survivors and their caregivers during the first year after discharge from inpatient rehabilitation, and to test a new model of delivery of health services to this population.

DESCRIPTION OF THE PROGRAM

In this research, the authors innovated and tested a new model of care that proposed to improve post-discharge services to stroke survivors and their families by monitoring the general health status of stroke survivors and their caregivers in the first year following discharge to the community, and by mobilizing existing hospital and community-based resources to support family-based care for the patient in the home. The STAIR program (Stroke Transition after Inpatient Rehabilitation) sought to improve postdischarge care for the stroke survivor by

- providing case-managed care that was home-based;
- documenting and attending to psychosocial stressors affecting both the patient and the caregiver;
- providing ready access to information and support as needed;
- identifying problems at an early stage in their development and directing appropriate intervention; and
- advocating for the patient and mobilizing existing community resources on behalf of the patient and primary caregiver.

An important emphasis of the STAIR program was the recognition of the importance of the well-being of the caregiver as well as the stroke survivor.

Subjects were randomized to either the experimental group or the control group. Each patient in the experimental group received weekly phone contact and monthly home visits from the research program case manager; home-based treatment as needed from therapeutic recreation, social work, and psychology consultants; and special access to educational resources, including a stroke educational manual with associated printed materials and a stroke "hot-line" telephone number. Hour-long bimonthly reviews were conducted on the experimental group patients by the case manager together with the research treatment team. The treatment team included the project physiatrist, psychologist, and recreational therapist, in addition to the case manager who was also a social worker. Problems and progress were briefly reviewed and discussed for each patient in the experimental group along with specific action plans. Concerns and questions of a medical nature were referred to the project physiatrist who worked closely with the case manager and the patient's primary care physician to resolve identified issues.

It was hypothesized that the STAIR system of care could serve to verify and guarantee adherence to the elements of the discharge plan, stabilize the community placement and reintegration of the stroke survivor, attend specifically to psychosocial stressors and prevent significant psychosocial problems from accelerating, assure adequate support and improve the quality of life for both patient and caregiver, and, in the end, obtain a better functional recovery for the stroke survivor while helping to prevent health problems in the caregiver(s).

DESCRIPTION OF THE TRIAL METHODOLOGY

All patients entered into the trial were 65 years of age or older at the time of their stroke. All patients had sustained a recent well-documented stroke (2 weeks to 3 months prior to enrollment) and had been transferred to the inpatient rehabilitation unit of the MossRehab Stroke Center for poststroke rehabilitation. All patients had a home to which to return and a readily identified primary caregiver and were discharged back to the community from the rehabilitation center. All patients were able to give informed consent to participate in the study and agreed to remain involved in the follow-up program for 1 year after their discharge from the rehabilitation center. Patients were excluded if they had severe premorbid or co-morbid conditions sufficient to impact significantly on their capacity to recover from the qualifying stroke. Patients were also excluded if residual cognitive or communicative impairment prevented adequate participation in the follow-up interviews. Caregiver proxy for information about the status of the patient was not utilized. The study protocol and consent form received full approval of the Institutional Review Board of MossRehab Hospital.

All qualifying patients admitted to the MossRehab Stroke Center were approached along with their caregivers regarding their willingness to participate in the study. Informed consent was sought from those patients or caregivers who expressed a desire to participate in the research. Once this was obtained, subjects were randomized using a random number table to either the experimental group, which received the STAIR program, or to a control group, which did not. Both groups received standard outpatient follow-up services, which included routine medical follow-up visits and, when indicated, outpatient rehabilitation services. Both the experimental and the control group were assessed in their homes at 1 week (baseline evaluation [BE]), 6 months (6M), and 1 year (1Y) postdischarge with a variety of instruments designed to measure disability, physical health, available socioeconomic resources, and activity level, as well as social and emotional functioning. The specific measures utilized in the follow-up assessments are listed and described briefly in the two boxed items. (Abbreviations for each of the instruments used are provided.)

The case manager set up appointments for data collection in the subjects' homes. The data collector was a licensed PhD-level psychologist. She visited the subjects' homes and administered the 2 to 3 hour assessment. Blinding of the data collector was attempted, although this was difficult to consistently accomplish and maintain, since the subjects clearly could not be blinded to their own treatment. Both the data collector and the case manager visited the subjects' homes for the assessments. Attempts were made in the process of the assessment to collect the data in separate interviews with the patient and the caregiver without allowing them to overhear each other's responses.

The case manager maintained detailed qualitative assessments and narrative notes documenting the interactions between her and each patient-caregiver dyad in the experimental group, all significant events, and all major issues not otherwise captured by formal data collection. The case manager also recorded nonprogram health care utilization and, particularly, rehospitalization or institutionalization events for both the experimental and the control groups.

Subjects and their caregivers in the experimental group participated in exit interviews to assess the extent to which they felt the case manager's involvement and the STAIR intervention as a whole were helpful. The exit interviews were conducted by the study psychologist and by the case manager. Complete exit interviews were obtained on 15 participants in the experimental group.

HYPOTHESES TO BE TESTED

Specific hypotheses to be tested included the following: when compared to the control group, the experimental group would have (1) increased level of functioning; (2) reduced incidence of rehospitalization or institutionalization; (3) reduced health care costs through reduction of unnecessary and preventable utilization of the health care system; (4) improved quality of life for both the patient and caregiver; (5) improved levels of psychosocial functioning for patients and caregivers; and (6) improved activity levels of patients and their caregivers. Data were also analyzed for (1) changes in functional status and quality of life measures over time; (2) differences in these measures associated with demographic variables such as gender and race, and medical variables such as rate of rehospitalization; and (3) associations between the various functional and quality of life measures that were obtained.

DATA ANALYSIS MEASURES

Descriptive statistics were employed for initial data characterization. Nonparametric tests were generally used since most continuous variables were not normally distributed across the study sample. Wilcoxon tests and the Mann-

---

Assessment Instruments for Patient Functioning

Functional Independence Measure (FIM)
Eighteen-item scale in 6 subscales (self-care, sphincter control, mobility, locomotion, communication, social cognition) with scoring range from complete dependence (1) to complete independence (7). Scales assess physical functioning (eg, self-care, sphincter control, mobility, locomotion) and cognitive functioning (eg, communication, social cognition).

Frenchay Activities Index (FAI)
Fifteen different instrumental activities of daily living (ADL) (eg, gardening, washing dishes, social outings, etc) rated on a 4-point frequency scale with higher scores indicating greater frequency.

The Active Lifestyle: Efficacy Expectancies Scale (EFF)
Measures the perception of one's own ability to perform a standard set of tasks. Twenty-four questions about various activities (eg, getting out of the home, feeling comfortable socializing with friends, etc) with respondents rating their certainty of their ability to perform the activity on a scale from 1 to 10.

The Center for Epidemiologic Studies—Depression Scale (CES-D)
Respondents use a 4-point scale to rate the frequency with which they have experienced 20 different mood states in the previous week (eg, "I felt lonely," "I enjoyed life," etc). Sixteen items describe negative affect states while 4 items describe positive affect states and are reverse-scored. Higher scores indicate greater depressed affect.

The Older American Resources and Services Scales—Physical Health (OARS-PH)
Questions about medical conditions and physical functioning in last month. Summarized on a 6-point scale ranging from excellent physical health (1) to total impairment (6).

The Older American Resources and Services Scales—Activities of Daily Living (OARS-ADL)
Fifteen questions about activities such as using the telephone, traveling, shopping, cooking, feeding, dressing, bathing, etc. Summarized on a 5-point scale ranging from excellent functioning (1) to total impairment (5).

Additional Assessment Instruments

Caregiver functioning

The Questionnaire on Resources and Stress (QRS)

Eleven scales of 6 true-false questions examining a variety of constructs believed to contribute to caregiver stress including family disharmony, financial stress, dependency and management, lack of personal reward, perceived personal burden, etc.

The Center for Epidemiologic Studies—Depression Scale (CES-D)

See previous box for description.

Social resource assessment

The Older American Resources and Services Scales—Social Resources (OARS-SR)

Measures extent and perceived adequacy of social contacts with friends and family, presence of a confidant, availability of help from friends in times of need, etc. Information

from 9 questions is summarized on a 6-point scale ranging from excellent social resources (1) to total lack of social resources (6).

Social system functioning

The Social Functioning Examination (SFE)

Twenty-eight items that assess social functioning including social activities, living environment, family relationships, etc. Each item rated on a 3-point scale: satisfactory functioning (0), moderate problems (1), or severe difficulties (3).

Economic resources

The Older American Resources and Services Scales—Economic Resources (OARS-ER)

Assesses work status, sources and amount of family income, health insurance status, adequacy of financial resources to meet basic needs, etc.

Whitney U (M-W-U) test were used for pairwise comparisons of variables, and Friedman's test was used to assess changes over time in the repeated measures sampled at 1 week, 6M, and 1Y after discharge. Chi-square statistics were used for analysis of categorical variable relationships. Multiple regression models were used to look at the prediction of FIM and FAI scores at 6M and 1Y assessments.

All data sheets were checked by the case manager for general accuracy and referred back to the data collector for any identified problems or inconsistencies. Data entry and analysis were performed on personal computers. Data were entered into spreadsheets in Microsoft Excel 4.0 where information was checked for missing data and incorrect coding. Data were then imported into SYSTAT for Windows, Version 5.0, for analysis.

RESULTS

Fifty-five subjects were recruited during the period from July 1992 through February 1994. There were 27 subjects

randomized to the experimental group, while 28 subjects were randomized to the control group. Of all patient/caregiver dyads who were eligible, 45% agreed to participate. Complete follow-up data were obtained for 75% of the patients entered into the study. Reasons for patient attrition included (1) medical deterioration of the patients; (2) subject/caregiver loss of interest in continued participation in the project (encountered especially in the control group); and (3) difficulties with scheduling appointments for data collection in the home.

There were no significant differences between the experimental and control groups at baseline with regard to demographic variables, educational level, and reported per capita household income. Summarized in Table 1, this would indicate that the randomization procedure was effective. Baseline FIM and CES-D scores also showed no significant differences between the experimental and control groups.

The complete final subject sample included 21 men and 20 women with an average age of 72 years (range 65–84). Twenty-five (61%) were Caucasian and 16 (39%) were Afri-

---

Table 1. Descriptive statistics for experimental and control groups

	Experimental group (N = 21)	Control group (N = 20)
Gender (frequency)*	10 (48%) male	11 (55%) male
Age (median)†	72 (65–84)	72 (65–81)
Race (frequency)*	12 (57%) Caucasian	13 (65%) Caucasian
Caretaker relationship to patient	13 (62%) spouses	16 (80%) spouses
Educational status (frequency)*	11 (52%) high school grads	9 (45%) high school grads
Per capita income (median)†	$11,000 ($3500–35000)	$8,500 ($2500–29000)

* = percent; † = range

can-American. For 29 (71%) of the subjects, the primary caregiver was the patient's spouse. The only significant effects among the demographic variables were for income according to educational status and age according to race. Those who had not completed high school had incomes lower than those who had completed high school or gone beyond (M-W-U = 112, $p < 0.03$). African-American subjects were significantly younger than Caucasian subjects (M-W-U = 291, $p < 0.04$). The median age of the African-American subjects was 70.0 while that of the Caucasian subjects was 72.5.

Looking at the entire sample, significant improvement was noted in the FIM (Friedman's test = 34.355, $p < 0.001$) and the FAI (Friedman's test = 43.829, $p < 0.001$). Applying the Wilcoxon test, significant differences were seen in assessments between the BE and 6M and between the BE and 1Y, but not between the 6M and 1Y assessments. This finding is consistent with reports that show most of the improvement in stroke patients occurs within approximately the first 6 months (eg, Jorgensen et al., 1995). The OARS-ADL and physical health (OARS-PH) measures did not show significant change and were not helpful to the study since they reflected changes that were more sensitively captured by the FIM; this is consistent with the fact that these scales were designed to assess the well elderly who are fully ambulatory in the community.

A total of 11 patients, 8 in the experimental group and 3 in the control group, sustained strokes subsequent to the index stroke. Of the 49 patients for whom BE data were available, 22% had a subsequent stroke. Of these, 73% were in the experimental group and 27% were in the control group. The differ-

ence was not statistically significant using the chi-square test. Sixteen patients (33%) were rehospitalized while being followed at 1 year after discharge. Of these, 9 were in the experimental group and 7 were in the control group. These included all of the 11 patients with recurrent strokes. The difference between the control and experimental groups for rehospitalization was not significant. Four patients (8%) were placed in nursing homes. They included three patients who sustained a recurrent stroke subsequent to the index stroke. Two were in the experimental group and two were in the control group. Of these, two dropped out of the study, one from the experimental group and one from the control group.

Looking at the association between outcome measures and various independent variables for the entire sample revealed some interesting findings. The median score for caregiver stress on the QRS was lower, indicating less caregiver stress for Caucasians than for African-Americans at 6M (M-W-U = 102.5, $p < 0.02$) and at 1Y (M-W-U = 94.0, $p < 0.01$). Caregiver stress at one week was not significantly lower for Caucasians as compared to African-Americans ($p > 0.1$). Depression scores for caregivers showed significant differences according to race at 6M (M-W-U = 105, $p < 0.03$) and at 1Y (M-W-U = 18, $p < 0.05$) with scores lower (indicating less depression) for Caucasian as compared with African-American caregivers. Caregiver stress scores as measured by the QRS were lower for spouses than for nonspouse caregivers at 6M (M-W-U = 93.5, $p < 0.04$). By the 1Y assessment, the caregiving stress of caregivers who were not spouses had decreased and was not significantly different from caregiving stress for spouses (see Figure 1). At 1Y, the depression scores were substantially higher for female subjects than

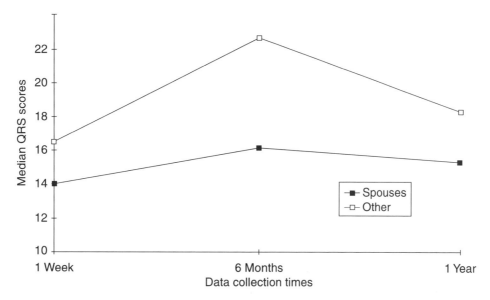

Figure 1. Median QRS scores for spouses and other caregivers for STAIR patients.

for males (M-W-U = 116.5, $p < 0.02$). The mean CES-D for female subjects was 9.5 (range 0–34) and that for males was 2 (range 0–9).

Patients who suffered second strokes while in the study did not differ on any demographic variable from patients who did not suffer subsequent strokes. Stress associated with caregiving, however, was significantly greater at the 6M assessment (M-W-U = 200, $p < 0.05$). At the 6M assessment, mean QRS score was 23 (range 12–36) for caregiver stress associated with patients who suffered subsequent strokes, and 16 (range 6–29) for patients who did not. At the 1Y assessment, QRS scores were also significantly different for caregivers for these two groups (M-W-U = 219.5, $p < 0.01$). As would be expected, the FIM and FAI scores also differed significantly for these two groups at the 1Y assessments. For the FIM, median score was 82 (range 48–123) for patients who suffered subsequent strokes, and 117 (range 33–126 for patients who did not. This was a significant difference (M-W-U = 78.5, $p < 0.04$). For the FAI, median score was 23 (range 15–37) for patients who suffered subsequent strokes and 33 (range 15–57) for those who did not, which was also a significant difference (M-W-U = 61.5, $p < 0.02$).

Multiple regression models were used to identify variables at the BE assessment that best predicted differences at 6M and 1Y for the FIM and the FAI, the two measures that changed significantly between BE and 6M, as well as BE and 1Y. For FIM scores at both 6M and 1Y, the best predictors were the BE FIM scores. After the BE FIM score was entered in the model, the BE FAI score added significant additional predictive value (see Table 2). The predictive value of the models was high.

After BE FAI scores were included for multiple regression models predicting 6M and 1Y FAI scores, there was a significant effect for EFF scores at BE. After the EFF scores were entered, a significant effect was found for the study group (experimental versus control) of the subjects for the prediction of FAI at 6M ($p < 0.05$). At 1Y, the significance of the variation of FAI with the study group was somewhat less ($p = 0.063$). Again, the predictive value of the models was high. The proportion of variance of the FAI scores (adjusted for sample size), which was accounted for at 6M, was 0.63, and at 1Y it was 0.40. There was thus evidence to suggest that the STAIR intervention enabled the experimental group to achieve higher levels of activity and more frequent performance of instrumental ADL at the 6M assessment as assessed by the FAI, given equivalent baseline activity levels and perceptions of self-efficacy (see Table 2, item A). A strong trend toward a significant effect of the STAIR intervention on FAI score was also seen at the 1Y assessment (see Table 2, item B).

At the 6M and 1Y assessment points, strong interrelationships existed between the FIM, the QRS measure of caregiver stress, and the FAI (see Tables 3–5 and Figure 2). Disability, activity level, and caregiver stress were all strongly and consistently related to each other. The strongest correlation was between FIM and FAI at the 1Y assessment. The personal efficacy (EFF) scores were strongly and positively related to the FAI at 6M and 1Y but not at BE. In turn, the EFF was inversely related to the OARS-SR at 1Y, suggesting that the greater the available social resources (and thus the lower the OARS-SR score), the greater the sense of effectiveness (EFF) eventually correlates at the 1Y assessment. As would be expected, caregiver stress (QRS) was directly correlated to the caregiver depression score at 6M and 1Y as well as inversely related to the actual patient functional level as measured by the FIM (see Figure 2, Tables 3 and 4).

Analysis of the exit interview results showed that 80% of the respondents felt that the case manager's involvement was valuable and neither too frequent nor too infrequent. Thirty-five percent felt that the phone contact was more helpful than the in-home visits and another 60% felt the phone contacts

---

Table 2. Multiple regression models

Variable	St Coeff*	Multiple R†	Multiple R²	R² Change	Probability (from t-test)
A. *FAI scores at 6M predicted from 1-week baseline data*					
1-week FAI	0.640	0.669	0.448	—	< 0.001
1-week EFF	0.423	0.784	0.615	0.167	< 0.001
Study group‡	0.215	0.811	0.658	0.043	0.039
B. *FAI scores at 1Y predicted from 1-week baseline data*					
1-week FAI	0.550	0.560	0.313	—	< 0.001
1-week EFF	0.299	0.621	0.386	0.073	0.025
Study group	0.246	0.665	0.443	0.057	0.063

* = standardized coefficient; † = multiple regression correlation coefficient; ‡ = the factor of group (experimental or control) to which the patient was assigned—i.e., whether or not the patient received the STAIR program intervention.

Table 3. Spearman correlation coefficients for STAIR measures at baseline assessment

	Patient CES-D	Caregiver CES-D	FIM	FAI	EFF	SF	OARS-SR	QRS
Patient								
CES-D	1.00							
Caregiver								
CES-D	0.06	1.00						
FIM	−0.22	−0.21	1.00					
FAI	−0.16	−0.14	0.45	1.00				
EFF	−0.45	−0.08	0.30	0.29	1.00			
SF	0.30	0.23	−0.38	−0.49	−0.48	1.00		
OARS-SR	0.28	0.03	−0.08	−0.12	−0.15	0.16	1.00	
QRS	0.46	0.44	*−0.52**	−0.41	−0.29	0.40	0.23	1.00

*Intercorrelations in italics are statistically significant at the $p < 0.001$ level.

were at least as helpful as the in-home visits. Aspects of the STAIR intervention that were mentioned most frequently as beneficial included education about stroke and available resources (35%), the positive value of regular, scheduled contacts (25%), and the emotional and moral support provided by the case manager (20%). Additional positive aspects of the program noted by patients and caregivers during the exit interview included the recreational therapy input, emphasis on improved socialization, the role of the case manager as patient advocate, the growth of the ability to see things from a different perspective, and participation in supervised community outings. Services other than case manager activities that were felt to be helpful included working with the recreational therapist (73%) and the rehabilitation psychologist (47%). Only 20% of the patient/caregiver dyads did not find the STAIR program to be helpful in some way. Interestingly, 95% believed that the telephone calls were either as helpful or more helpful than the in-home visits, suggesting that future interventions might be just as effective and certainly more efficient and less expensive if focus is on the use of telephone calls for patient monitoring rather than in-home visits.

DISCUSSION

While this study did not conclusively demonstrate an improvement in general health or reduction in subsequent risk of stroke in the patients who received the STAIR intervention, a number of important findings can be identified. This was not a severely disabled sample due to the study inclusion criteria. Patients had to be able to cognitively understand the questions in the interview protocol since a decision was made to not allow proxy responses from caregivers (see

Table 4. Spearman correlation coefficients for STAIR at 6M assessment

	Patient CES-D	Caregiver CES-D	FIM	FAI	EFF	SF	OARS-SR	QRS
Patient								
CES-D	1.00							
Caregiver								
CES-D	0.27	1.00						
FIM	−0.26	−0.34	1.00					
FAI	−0.17	−0.23	*0.66**	1.00				
EFF	−0.43	−0.24	0.46	0.62	1.00			
SF	0.37	0.29	−0.36	−0.23	−0.44	1.00		
OARS-SR	0.46	0.16	−0.26	−0.26	−0.35	*0.56*	1.00	
QRS	0.32	*0.63*	*−0.72*	−0.56	−0.42	0.41	0.22	1.00

*Intercorrelations in italics are statistically significant at the $p < 0.001$ level.

Table 5. Spearman correlation coefficients for STAIR measures at 1Y assessment

	Patient CES-D	Caregiver CES-D	FIM	FAI	EFF	SF	OARS-SR	QRS
Patient CES-D	1.00							
Caregiver CES-D	0.02	1.00						
FIM	−0.12	−0.24	1.00					
FAI	−0.16	−0.41	*0.80**	1.00				
EFF	−0.32	−0.09	*0.62*	*0.66*	1.00			
SF	0.22	0.00	−0.29	−0.17	−0.24	1.00		
OARS-SR	0.46	0.11	−0.40	−0.46	*−0.56*	0.35	1.00	
QRS	0.15	*0.58*	*−0.53*	*−0.63*	−0.46	0.07	0.18	1.00

*Intercorrelations in italics are statistically significant at the $p < 0.001$ level.

Segal & Schall, 1995). The FAI was low initially, however, in spite of relatively high FIM scores. This finding is consistent with previous reports (Segal & Schall, 1994). The question of whether the STAIR intervention would be more efficacious for more impaired patients cannot be directly answered by this work but may merit further research. It is also more likely that a significant effect of the intervention could be detected in a more initially-impaired population.

Based on multiple regression models predicting FIM and FAI scores, it appears that the STAIR intervention does lead to higher eventual activity levels (measured by the FAI) as compared to the control group when baseline FAI and EFF are kept constant. However, psychosocial functioning and quality of life were not significantly improved by the STAIR

program as compared to controls in this sample. There was no evidence indicating a reduced rate of recurrent stroke, rehospitalization, or institutionalization in the STAIR-treated patients, as had been initially hypothesized. This could be due to the relatively small sample size. Alternatively, it is possible that the type of interventions used in this study do not significantly alter the risk of subsequent stroke or other conditions necessitating rehospitalization.

Burden of care (as measured by the FIM) and caregiver stress and depression (as measured by the QRS and the Caregiver CES-D) were higher for African-Americans in the sample than for Caucasians. These differences were not apparent at the BE evaluation. This suggests that the process for adaptation and for the development of caregiver stress

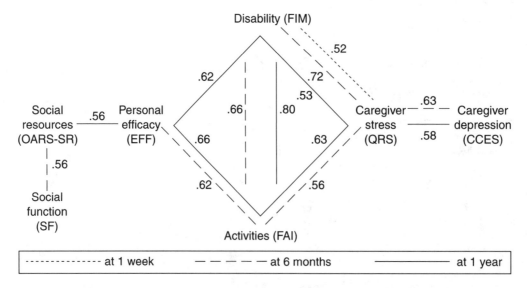

Figure 2. Significant intercorrelations ($p < 0.001$) among STAIR measures at the same point in time, for the three data collection points.

appears to be different between the two groups. These differences cannot be readily explained by differences in educational level or socioeconomic status since these factors were not significantly associated with race in this population.

Caregiver stress and the associated increase in caregiver depression scores appear to be reactions that develop over time, rather than being present from the start of the adaptation process. These appear to be in reaction to the very real FIM differences in the patient, not due to some inherent psychosocial make-up or support system differences.

Another interesting finding was the difference in apparent coping between caregivers who are children or siblings of the patient as opposed to caregivers who are married to the patient. There was a small amount of stress associated with spousal caregiving, as compared with nonspousal caregiving. This may be related to societal expectations, financial arrangements, or the additional responsibilities that a child of an elderly disabled patient may carry. Interestingly, nonspousal caregiver stress had decreased by 1 year and was not significantly different from caregiving stress in spouses at this point, suggesting that nonspousal caregivers had found some means to adapt (see Figure 1).

Strong correlations existed between FIM, QRS, FAI and EFF at 6M and 1Y assessments that were not apparent at the BE assessment. The association between the FIM and the FAI at 1 year was the strongest in the entire study, supporting the finding that disability is strongly and consistently related to activity level and handicap (Schuling, de Haan, Limburg, & Groenier, 1993). Perception of efficacy scores is also related strongly to activity level and disability at 1 year but not before that point. This would suggest that the patients' sense of their own ability to be effective may gradually come into line with the objective measure of disability as the course of their recovery proceeds.

There are several limitations that can be identified for this pilot study. This was a relatively small, albeit intensively studied, sample of stroke survivors. Given the wide range and variety of sequelae following stroke, it is not surprising that the STAIR intervention produced few statistically significant differences in such a small sample. This highlights some of the difficulties in doing controlled clinical trials of this nature in stroke patients. There is a large variety of levels and forms of involvement. If one attempts to restrict the sample by using limiting inclusion criteria to make the sample more uniform and ensure participation in this type of protocol, then the sample size is decreased significantly if the available pool of patients remains the same; the generalizability of the results also is diminished. Because of restrictive inclusion criteria, this sample was not excessively disabled, even though their scores on the activity level measure (FAI) tended to be low. The incidence of depression in the sample appeared low for both patients and caregivers, possibly because of selection criteria. Had there been greater disability, depression, or

poorer social functioning in the sample at baseline, the STAIR interventions may have proven more clearly efficacious. However, such a sample may not have been able to participate adequately in the study protocol.

The protocol did not attempt to measure any adaptive personality traits of the patient or caregiver. These variables might be important mediating factors in the recovery process. They could also influence outcome, although the randomization procedure used in this controlled clinical trial should have distributed such factors equally between control and experimental group. In addition, with a small sample size, there is low statistical power, and the probability of detecting a statistically significant effect of an intervention is relatively limited as a result unless the effect size is large. While the attrition of subjects from the trial was disappointing, it was not especially surprising. In many longitudinal studies of chronic disability that require repeated observations over an extended period of time, an attrition rate of 15% to 25% is generally expected.

An attempt was made to blind those individuals making critical data measurements regarding the assignment of patients to the experimental or control groups. Data collection was generally done by an individual who had no explicit knowledge regarding the group to which the patients had been assigned. It was difficult to maintain blinding, however, since the patients themselves could not be blinded to their treatment assignment and could be expected to reveal evidence to the data collectors regarding their program-related activities.

Finally, while this study was structured as a controlled clinical trial, the control group did receive significant rehabilitation services through the Stroke Center. These included outpatient therapy services and home care, when indicated, as well as medical follow-up. Had the control group not had access to these services, it is likely that differences between the two groups would have been more pronounced. Withholding standard medical care from the control group would have been clearly unethical and unacceptable.

RECOMMENDATIONS FOR FUTURE STUDY

Examination of the study results and exit interviews has implications for designing and testing future similar interventions. One factor with a strong effect in this study was race: African-American participants experienced greater disability, more caregiver stress, and more caregiver depression than Caucasians. These differences did not appear attributable to differences in educational or socioeconomic factors. A future study might focus on this issue with involvement of an African-American case manager and service providers to help avoid potential recruitment bias.

Information from the exit interviews suggested that phone contact was perceived to be as effective as in-home visits by the case manager. The case management system of a future study could consist of weekly or twice-monthly telephone contacts supplemented by a home visit every 4 to 6 months. This would greatly reduce the cost of the intervention and the monitoring, without a significant loss of effectiveness. Outcome measures could be adapted for application through telephone interviews rather than home visits.

Finally, because of the large number of potential subjects who had to be excluded because of residual cognitive or communicative deficits, outcome measures might be restricted to more "objective" measures, which could be reliably answered by caregiver proxy. Such measures might include the physical abilities scale of the Short-Form-36 of the Medical Outcomes Study (Segal & Schall, 1994), as well as some scales from the Craig Handicap Assessment and Reporting Technique (Segal & Schall, 1995). In this way, it would be possible to open up the STAIR intervention to a larger pool of subjects who would be more impaired and could potentially benefit more from it. Similarly, it would be of interest to examine a younger group of stroke survivors. For the sake of consistency, this study was restricted to patients aged 65 and older. Younger stroke patients have very different psychosocial needs and issues than older patients. Given these differences, it would be important to explore whether interventions similar to the STAIR program could ameliorate the medical and psychosocial sequelae of stroke for younger patients.

CONCLUSIONS

Several items present themselves as logical conclusions from this study.

1. The strongest benefit of the STAIR program was an increase in the level of general social activity and in the frequency of performance of instrumental ADL as measured by the FAI (Wade, Leigh-Smith, & Hewer, 1985). This effect was found to be strongest and most significant at 6M postdischarge and less pronounced at 1Y postdischarge.
2. The STAIR program did not have significant beneficial effects in preventing rehospitalization or institutionalization of patients who had been placed in the community, and no benefit could be demonstrated for improvement in functional status or quality of life for the patient or caregiver.
3. Caregiver stress was generally lower for spousal caregivers as compared with nonspousal caregivers at 6M postdischarge but not at 1Y postdischarge.
4. Tendency toward depression was greater in female patients as compared to male patients at 1Y postdischarge.

5. Caregiver stress was generally greater among caregivers looking after patients who suffered a stroke subsequent to the index stroke, as compared to caregivers looking after patients who had no further strokes during the year following discharge from inpatient rehabilitation.
6. Strong intercorrelations were found between caregiver stress, residual disability of the patient (as assessed by the FIM), and the social activity level of the patient (as assessed by the FAI). Caregiver stress was also found to correlate with the caregiver depression score.
7. Multiple regression models showed that the patient activity level (FAI) at 6M was significantly greater for patients who received the STAIR program compared to those who did not, when baseline FAI and perception of personal efficacy (EFF) were taken into account.
8. African-Americans in the sample experienced a lesser degree of poststroke recovery and a greater degree of caregiver stress as compared to the Caucasians in the sample. This finding should be investigated further in future studies.
9. Participants in the experimental group felt that telephone contact was as efficacious as in-home visits, suggesting that the STAIR intervention could be as effective with significantly fewer visits to the home and more reliance on telephone contact. This could substantially reduce the cost of the intervention.
10. The current sample had an inadequate size to fully address all of the study hypotheses. Future research in this area may require broadening sample selection and inclusion criteria to allow a greater range of cognitive and physical impairment. The use of patient measures obtained by caregiver proxy may be required. Multicenter cooperation may be necessary to mount a trial that has a truly adequate sample size.

REFERENCES

Agency for Health Care Policy Research. (1995). *Post-stroke rehabilitation. Clinical practice guidelines* (No. 16, AHCPR Publication No. 95-0662). Rockville, MD: U.S. Government Printing Office.

Anderson, R. (1992). *The aftermath of stroke. The experience of patients and their families.* Cambridge: Cambridge University Press.

Glass, T.A., & Maddox, G.L. (1992). The quality and quantity of social support: stroke recovery as a psycho-social transition. *Social Science & Medicine, 34,* 1249–1261.

Glass, T.A., Matchar, D.B., Belyea, M., & Feussner, J.R. (1993). Impact of social support on outcome in first stroke. *Stroke, 24,* 64–70.

Jorgensen, H.S., Nakayama, H., Raaschou, H.O., Vive-Larsen, J., Stoier, M., & Olsen, T.S. (1995). Outcome and time course of recovery in stroke. Part II: Time course of recovery. The Copenhagen Stroke Study. *Archives of Physical Medicine and Rehabilitation, 76,* 406–412.

Russell, I.T., Hamilton, S., & Tweedie, V. (1993). Models of health care for stroke. *Scottish Medical Journal, 38*(3 Suppl), S15–17.

Schuling, J., de Haan, R., Limburg, M., & Groenier, K.H. (1993). The Frenchay Activities Index: assessment of functional status in stroke patients. *Stroke, 24,* 1173–1177.

Segal, M.S., & Schall, R.R. (1994). Determining functional/health status and its relation to disability in stroke survivors. *Stroke, 25,* 2391–2397.

Segal, M.S., & Schall, R.R. (1995). Assessing handicap of stroke survivors.

A validation study of the Craig Handicap Assessment and Reporting Technique. *American Journal of Physical Medicine and Rehabilitation, 74,* 276–286.

Wade, D.T., Leigh-Smith, J., & Hewer, R.L. (1985). Social activities after stroke. Measurement and natural history using the Frenchay Activities Index. *International Rehabilitation Medicine, 7,* 176–181.

Wolfe, C., Beech, R., Ratcliffe, M., & Rudd, A.G. (1995). Stroke care in Europe. Can we learn lessons from the different ways in which stroke is managed in different countries? *Journal of the Royal Society of Health, 115,* 143–147.

29

Outcomes Management through a Spinal Treatment Evaluation Process

Trudy Millard Krause, Jeffrey Kozak, and Nancy Claiborne

THE NEED FOR SPINAL TREATMENT OUTCOMES MANAGEMENT

The prevalence and incidence of spinal injuries, along with the medical and indemnity costs associated with such injuries, reinforce the need for spinal treatment outcomes management. Successful outcomes management works in a collaborative manner in the provision of comprehensive treatment from multidisciplinary providers that will optimize the outcome and facilitate the delivery of cost-effective, outcomes-driven quality care for the spinal-injured patient.

Successful spinal treatment outcomes are evaluated not merely by surgical or technical results such as the radiographic evidence of a solid fusion. Successful outcomes are also measured by patient-reported improvement in quality of life, return to work and/or functionality, and cost-effectiveness. The psychological and emotional state of a patient greatly impacts treatment and rehabilitation.

IMPACT OF SPINE INJURIES: PREVALENCE AND COST

To best understand the benefits of spinal outcomes management, it is important to recognize the impact of spine injuries on the health care system. Low back pain is recognized as the number one cause of disability for workers under the age of 45.[1] At any given time, 1 out of 100 Americans is chronically disabled, and another 1 out of 100 is temporarily off work due to a back injury.[2] Additionally, low back pain accounts for 40 percent of all lost workdays a year.[3] In 1994, the Agency for Health Care Policy and Research noted that the total annual cost of back pain in the United States ranged from $20 billion to $50 billion. The annual national cost associated with back pain was identified as $8.3 billion related to medical costs, $7.1 billion in disability and indemnity payments, and $7.8 billion in indirect costs.[3] Other estimates ran from $20–$100 billion annually for medical, indemnity, and social costs associated with back pain.[4,5]

The average cost per low back pain claim in Texas in 1995 was $14,564, with $6,631 for indemnity and $7,933 in medical costs, as reported by the Research and Oversight Council on Workers' Compensation Claim Costs in Texas. This average counts all claims, including those that had no medical costs associated with them, as well as surgical cases. The average cost of surgery is estimated between $32,000 and $50,000 per case, with $6 billion spent annually on U.S. back surgeries. Approximately 90 percent of claims are acute and are resolved within three months at low cost. However, the 10 percent that become chronic account for 90 percent of the total costs associated with back injuries. Over 250,000 lumbar spinal operations are performed in the United States annually.[6] The lifetime prevalence for spine surgery is three to four percent, with the most frequent procedure being a surgical excision of lumbar disc.[6]

IMPACT OF SPINE INJURIES: WHO GETS HURT?

It is important to realize that 80 percent of the population will experience low back pain at some time in their lives.[6] Chronic or episodic low back pain is experienced by 10 percent–20 percent of the population. Studies show that 80 per-

This research was conducted through the Spinal Treatment Evaluation Process of Texas Orthopedic Hospital in Houston, Texas, with the assistance of the Fondren Orthopedic Group physician practice.

J Rehabil Outcomes Meas, 1997, 1(4), 15–22

cent of these incidences improve within one month and 90 percent improve within 3 months.[7]

The normal spinal degenerative process begins at age 20 and most often results in nonsymptomatic disorders. A recent study in California of 98 asymptomatic individuals found that magnetic resonance imaging (MRI) studies revealed that only 36 percent had normal discs. Of these asymptomatic individuals, 79 percent had pathology: 52 percent with bulging discs and 27 percent with discs protruding beyond the vertebrae.[8] It is this normal, asymptomatic degenerative process that makes it difficult to predict or prevent on-the-job back injuries. An existing degenerative disorder may be aggravated by an action or event that occurs at work, which causes it to become a work-related injury.

The Bureau of Labor[9] has identified the following causes of on-the-job back injuries by percentage of total work injuries:

Overexertion—lifting	16.9
Fall	15.7
Overexertion—not lifting	11.3
Repetitive motion	4.2
Slip or trip	3.7
Contact with an object or equipment	27.3
Harmful substance exposure	5.0
Other	15.9

Other studies ascribe lifting as the cause for 18 percent–39 percent of on-the-job back injuries.[10,11] Improper lifting and lifting bereft of appropriate use of ergonomics or other actions aggravate or cause back injuries. One reason is overloading. The excessive torque and poor body mechanics place strain on the spine and spinal muscles. Extended work in a flex position applies added stress. Sudden movement related to stops, starts, or jolts can create trauma to the spine. Sudden shifting or loss of control of a load also produces mechanical stress or shock. Additionally, poor body mechanics associated with lifting and twisting or asymmetric movement creates ergonomic insult with potential for injury.

COMPENSATION EFFECT

As noted, the inappropriate management or use of proper ergonomics related to job tasks can aggravate the normal degenerative process as well as create injury. The onset of spinal pain on the job causes the patient to assume the injury and pain are tied to the identified "cause," such as lifting at work. This is referred to as the "compensation effect," which goes beyond identifying a "cause" to creating a sense of "fault." The compensation effect creates a belief that external forces caused the

injury, therefore "they" should "fix" it, thus eliminating any internal or personal responsibility.[12]

The compensation effect results not only in the loss of personal responsibility, but also in a sense of distrust and blame. Furthermore, it can create an incentive for illness behavior because of increased expectations of return to 100 percent of previous pre-injury state. The potential for secondary gain issues is also increased. All these factors contribute to the perpetuation of the medical cycle and to the potential for chronicity.

Several studies have shown that on-the-job injuries last longer than similar not-on-the-job injuries. Greenough conducted a study of 150 compensable and 150 noncompensable spine injuries and found that the median time off work was 12 months for noncompensable injuries and 21 months for compensable injuries.[7] A study of railroad workers found that those with on-the-job injuries were off work for 14.9 months, while those with matched not-on-the-job injuries returned in 3.6 months.[13] A study of surgical disc patients showed that on-the-job injuries were off 9.3 months and not-on-the-job injuries were off 4.4 months.[14]

THE STEP PROGRAM

The Spinal Treatment Evaluation Process (STEP) is a program initiated at Texas Orthopedic Hospital in Houston to assess outcomes and to identify the barriers to recovery and rehabilitation. The STEP program was initially conceived by three spinal surgeons who had identified that positive outcomes in patients with spinal disorders were not solely reliant on surgical expertise. The STEP program was developed to provide a multidisciplinary evaluation and assessment of spine patients through comprehensive physical, therapeutic, psychological, psychosocial, and vocational assessments, as well as a review of general health and medical status. The multidisciplinary team of the STEP program consists of the physician or chiropractor, a doctoral level specialist in occupational health, a psychologist, a social worker, an orthopedic nurse educator, an exercise physiologist, a physical therapist, an occupational therapist, and a vocational counselor. The program provides education, evaluation, and case management on an outpatient basis over four days. The components of the program include: back education, treatment options, psychological testing and diagnosis, assessment for chemical dependency, assessment for sleep disorders, pain profile, comprehensive physical therapy evaluation, exercise, lumbar stabilization, body mechanics, health and nutrition, activities of daily living, sexuality, pain management, coping skills, relaxation, family coping skills, and prevention techniques. These components have been shown to be important in the assessment and treatment of patients with spinal disorders.[15]

Central to the philosophy of the STEP program is the concept of locus of control. Locus of control is a learning theory that attributes one's tendency to take action based on his or her belief that he or she is able to impact the outcomes.[1] It has been demonstrated in health research in the areas of epilepsy, diabetes, hypertension, hemodialysis, weight loss, and other health conditions that those with a more internal sense of control have a more positive outcome.[16,17]

The sense of control is mediated by knowledge and understanding of both external environmental forces, and internal adaptation and situation management skills. In the STEP program the patient is shown the results of the evaluations and assessments of his or her medical condition to facilitate an understanding of the diagnosis. He or she is presented with education regarding the anatomy, pathology, and treatment options related to his condition. Additionally, he or she is provided with training in coping skills, pain management skills, and personal insight on adaptation strengths. With the philosophy that a fully informed patient will gain a sense of internal control and work toward his or her recovery, the patient then becomes a partner in his or her treatment decisions and plan.

The four days of the program are presented in a logical sequence that follows the patient's ability to accept and process information. Day One of the program focuses on physical evaluations related to the spinal condition and the limitations incurred due to the impairment or pain. Elements in Day One include: comprehensive physical therapy evaluation, functional capacity evaluation, assessment of physical and aerobic capacity, psychological testing, pain profile, vocational assessment, and back education. Day Two introduces the concept of pain as a physical and psychological "experience" and focuses on the psychosocial components to a greater degree. Relaxation training, spinal stabilization, back education, body mechanics, and other instruction focus on prevention of further injury and minimization of pain from activity. Day Three pulls together the physical and psychological components of spinal injury and provides a focus on coping, locus of control, quality of life, and management of pain. Frank discussion of the risks and benefits of treatment options are discussed, with encouragement for the patient to make informed choices.

The program is concluded with a case conference among the treating team and the physician or chiropractor, to report on findings and recommendations and the patient decision. From this meeting, a comprehensive treatment plan is developed that identifies expected steps in the health care continuum and projected outcomes. The recommended treatment plan is developed with consideration of the factors that promote positive outcomes as well as the barriers to recovery.

The STEP program is recommended for the complex spine patient who has reached the chronic stage without relief of symptoms (usually three months or more). In the one-year period reviewed, the STEP program provided services to a total of 340 patients. The mean age of this group was 41. The majority of the patients (61 percent) were male. The racial distribution was 57 percent white, 23 percent African American, and 20 percent Hispanic. Eighty-nine percent were injured on the job (workers' compensation), and the median time since the date of injury was 372 days. Patients are referred to the program by orthopaedic surgeons, spinal surgeons, neurosurgeons, chiropractors, primary care physicians, occupational medicine physicians, or otherwise directed by the employer or insurance case manager.

Not all STEP patients are surgical candidates, as only 41 percent come into the program as potential surgical patients. Of the others, 30 percent are considered nonsurgical and 29 percent are undetermined. As a result of the comprehensive evaluation and education in STEP, 27 percent of the patients initially evaluated are referred to surgery. Of the remaining, 45 percent are nonsurgical and their case is resolved through case closure. Another 28 percent are referred to alternative conservative treatment or preliminary interventions such as psychiatric treatment, other medical referrals (such as urology, gynecology, rheumatology, or internal medicine), focused physical therapy, epidural steroids, or work hardening programs.

Analysis of patient evaluations of the program show that 94 percent of the patients stated that they were very satisfied with the program and 95 percent stated that they benefited from participation. The STEP program has enjoyed success and satisfaction not only from the patient perspective but also from the physicians and referral sources, who have stated that their patients subsequently participate more in treatment, have more realistic expectations, and report greater satisfaction with their medical care. The primary reason STEP is successful in outcomes management is because it addresses the patient as a whole. It is known that spinal treatment options are many and vary in approaches, and as such the medical cycle can be perpetuated.[3–5,7,15,18] The multidisciplinary collaboration in STEP can break this time-consuming cycle, which utilizes resources and increases costs. Secondly, back injury and chronic pain are multifactorial. The potential for chronicity and disability is high due to the complexity of the patient and the many factors related to the injury and its impact.

The high satisfaction and sense of resolution from the STEP program come from meeting both the patient's needs and the medical team's needs. The patient develops a sense of control in the situation through increased knowledge and understanding. This informed choice and participation in decision making leads to more realistic expectations and acceptance of personal responsibility in rehabilitation. The physicians and providers maximize outcomes through the development of a treatment plan that considers the multifactorial issues of the patient and confronts the barriers to positive outcomes.

IMPACT OF SPINE INJURIES: QUALITY OF LIFE

Once a back injury occurs and has become chronic without relief of symptoms, the patient has already experienced personal impacts in addition to pain. Common experience related by STEP patients include debilitation due to pain but also due to loss of function, general health, and well-being, the essential factors of quality of life. Increased pain leads to decreased quality of life, which leads to increased pain. This is known as the chronic pain cycle, where psychosocioeconomic factors magnify stress and pain.[19,20]

Elements of the chronic pain cycle include pain behaviors for conscious or unconscious secondary gain, deconditioning (loss of muscle tone, increased weight), isolation, loss of social and leisure activities, family stress, decreased income, financial stress (possible loss of home, car, job), depression, anxiety, irritability, stress, and insomnia. All elements of the chronic pain cycle aggravate the pain and increase its effects, thus perpetuating the cycle.

QUALITY OF LIFE IN STEP PATIENTS

The MOS SF-36 (Medical Outcomes Trust, Boston, Massachusetts) is an instrument that measures patient perception of quality of life indicators related to general health, function, and well-being. It is a widely utilized and extensively validated instrument in medicine to measure outcomes, based on patient perspectives and impact of rehabilitation on quality of life.[21,22] It is an instrument used by the American Academy of Orthopedic Surgeons, as well as other physician specialty groups and database services such as Focus on Therapeutic Outcomes, Inc.

The STEP program uses this tool as a measure of the impact of chronic spinal injury on quality of life, as well as an outcome measurement at designated time intervals following participation in the STEP program. The SF-36 reports the patient perception of quality of life in eight domains: general health, physical functioning, role limitations due to physical state and role limitations due to emotional state, social func-

tioning, mental health, energy and fatigue, and relief from bodily pain. Scores are reported in a range of 0–100, with 100 as ideal. The mean scores at admission in the study group are shown in Table 1, along with the scores of certain other population groups. As noted, the scores in all eight domains for the STEP patients are considerably lower than the general population, and are frequently lower than serious chronic medical conditions with complications and psychiatric disorders.

It is evident from the scores illustrated below that the chronic spinal patient suffers from a perception of a poor quality of life, as measured nearly one year after date of injury. If the assumption could be made that the injured person was comparable to those in the general population prior to the injury, the decrease in quality of life is dramatic. This chart is presented as an illustration of this very assumption: that a chronic back injury impacts many aspects of an individual's life.

Chronic back injury and/or pain is multifactoral in its causes, its costs, its complications, and its effects on the injured person.[19,20,23–26] Proper treatment must focus on the whole person, not just the spine. It is for this reason that outcomes management is so important. Outcomes management of spine injuries, then, orchestrates the delivery of quality outcomes-driven care based on the needs and limitations of the whole person.

OUTCOME MEASURES FOR SPINE INJURIES

Orthopaedic outcomes are measured not only by the surgical or technical results, but also by the patient perception of change, return to work, and cost-effectiveness. The surgeon attempts to evaluate the patient globally but often has the tendency to assess outcome by evidence of healing. The patient assesses his perceived quality of life. The employer aims for return to work, and the insurance carrier or payer wishes to minimize cost.

The technical outcomes are measured primarily by radiographic indications. The surgeon reviews radiographs or MRI

Table 1. Comparison of SF-36 Scores

SF-36 domain	STEP	General population	Serious medical patients	Psychiatric patients
General health	47	80	49	58
Physical functioning	30	93	57	81
Social functioning	37	92	80	65
Role limitations—emotional	33	91	76	41
Role limitations—physical	8	90	44	56
Mental health	56	78	78	53
Energy	33	69	48	45
Relief from body pain	22	83	65	63

reports to determine (for example) if the fusion is solid or the herniation is improved. The physician may also measure results by patient-reported clinical pain relief. However, technical repair may not equate to pain relief, due to complications from other patient factors. Technical outcomes are also influenced by patient factors, both physical and psychosocial. Smoking, obesity, age, and comorbidities can complicate the patient's recovery.[4,5,15,27] The complexity and extent of pathology may obviate the probability for positive outcomes from specific procedures. Even the choice of procedure can affect technical outcome. For example, it has been demonstrated that laminectomies are largely ineffective as a sole treatment method for back pain only.[5]

The importance of psychological factors in determining the outcome in spinal treatment has been demonstrated by many studies.[24,27–32] Psychological factors that may impact patient compliance in rehabilitation are overreliance on narcotic pain medication, secondary gain, unrealistic expectations, and certain personality features. Studies have shown that poor indicators for spine surgery include history of physical or sexual abuse, severe depression, paranoia, thought disorders, and elevated scales on histrionic and narcissism.

These known complicating factors indicate a need for appropriate patient selection for spinal surgery. Identifying the right patient for the right surgery is important to the promotion of positive outcomes. The surgeon has the obligation to "select" carefully those patients with high probability of success, limited risk for complications, and reasonable cost. All too often the usual indication for surgery is pain, radiographic pathology, and patient desire. But few surgeries are essential other than those required for cauda equina syndrome and progressive neurological deficit.[3]

Nationally, 15 percent of patients who had surgery for disc herniation become "failed back" cases.[3] Inappropriate selection of the patient or an inappropriate selection of a treatment approach account for 98 percent of these failures. Therefore, the surgeon can benefit from the early identification of important contraindications for surgery, as revealed in the STEP program. Examples of such contraindications include:

1. Certain psychological conditions or personality features
2. Secondary gain issues, conscious or unconscious and personal or emotional
3. Compensation effect
4. Wrong or inconclusive diagnosis
5. Conflicts in patient complaints and clinical presentation, patient behaviors, and diagnostic studies
6. Inconsistent presentation among disciplines or over time
7. Abnormal illness behaviors
8. General health conditions, potential complications from comorbidities
9. Complications with past history of anesthesia or surgery
10. Patient anxiety level, history of panic attacks
11. Discrepancy in patient and physician expectations
12. Patient failure to accept responsibility in rehabilitation

PATIENT PERCEPTION OF OUTCOME

When STEP patients are asked what they desire as an outcome, the usual and initial response is "I want my life back." The second response is "pain relief." No patient has ever stated, "I want a solid fusion at L4/L5 on my radiograph." Clearly, the patient's measure of a positive outcome is different from the physician's.

"I want my life back" refers to the elements of the quality of life. The eight domains of the SF-36 that measure the three areas of quality of life (general health, function, and well-being) cannot be "healed" by the physician through surgery or other clinical procedures. Certainly, if a technical improvement in the source of pain is realized, then quality of life elements may improve. However, the improvement in these areas is directly related to the patient's actions, beliefs, and approach to rehabilitation.

Quality of life factors are influenced by an individual's position on the continuums of action, beliefs, and psychological state. Actions are affected by one's perception of disability. Does an individual define himself by his abilities or his disabilities? Does he acknowledge his limitations and take action based on the knowledge of the difference between hurt and harm?

Beliefs affect actions, and beliefs are impacted by the locus of control. Locus of control refers to one's perceived ability or inability to impact results. If one believes he can impact results by his actions, he is more likely to take action than if he feels hopeless and helpless. A person with a strong internal locus of control is more likely to take action to improve his quality of life instead of waiting for something else or someone else to "rescue" him.

Finally, the patient's perception of improvement will be influenced by his emotional and psychological state. Some chronic pain sufferers find benefit in emotional or social rewards received from the sick role. Illness behaviors and victimization perpetuate the compensation effect. For example, it is not uncommon for those who have been longtime caregivers to welcome receiving care once injured themselves.

Clinical personality patterns that guide an individual's approach in life are unlikely to be easily changed. Severe clinical syndromes such as disturbed thoughts, schizophrenia, paranoia, mania, dysthymia, and depression will alter one's perception, action, and behaviors to a potentially inappropriate or threatening level.

RETURN TO WORK

Successful outcomes from a spine injury can be measured in terms of clinical improvement, enhancement of quality of life, and productivity and return to work. The optimal vocational outcome is to return to the same line of work with the same employer. In many cases this may not be possible, so outcome is measured by return to productivity and optimal functioning. Some of the factors that measure the potential and likelihood for return to work include functional capacity (the ability to perform the work), ease of changing occupation or job (which is related to skill or education level), number of days off work, and compensation effect: work-related injury or non–work-related injury, and secondary gain issues related to perceived benefits of work avoidance.

Studies have shown that the longer one is off of work, the less likely he or she is to return to work. For those who are early in their injury and have been off work for less than six months, the probability of return to work is 50 percent. The odds drop to 25 percent after six months, and diminish to less than 10 percent after one year.[33] The factors that provide the best prognosis for return to work include:

1. Early intervention and rehabilitation
2. Positive medical response
3. Positive work history
4. No major psychopathology
5. No narcotic dependency
6. No secondary gain, including litigation.

Research has shown that barriers to return to work are not physical or pain-related. Rather, the identified barriers include: age, time off work, ease of change of occupation, activities of daily living, psychological profile, and locus of control. The most significant factors are time off work, ease of changing occupation, and elevated psychological measures in hysteria, hyperchondriasis, and thought disorder.[33]

Despite the influence of compensation effect, it is important to recognize that frank malingering is rare and is evident in less than 10 percent of injured patients.[33] However, compensation neurosis, the unconscious maintenance or exaggeration of physical or emotional symptoms, can become a barrier to rehabilitation. An unconscious fear (fear of failure, re-injury, increased pain, or the unknown) or unconscious need (need for comfort, attention, or control) is maladaptive and can sabotage positive outcomes.

COST AND TIME OUTCOMES

Finally, in this age of health care, recognition of costs and allocation of resources is an important outcome measurement for the provider as well as the insurer. In the case of spine-injured patients, particularly workers' compensation patients, time becomes cost due to the perpetuation of the medical cycle. As noted earlier, costs are measured not only by actual dollars spent on medical care but also on indemnity expense and indirect costs.

Use of the STEP program as an outcomes management tool can effectively intervene in the costs associated with spine injury. In a study of the patients of a major insurance company, it was determined that outcomes management through the STEP program saved an average of $42,000 on their cases. This was deduced by a review of reserves and projected expenses per case before participation in STEP and projected expenses following the development of the treatment plan from STEP. Cost savings came from early intervention, case closure, patient choice of treatment, appropriate selection of treatment option, and patient involvement and commitment to treatment recommendations.

Furthermore, the development of a treatment plan that is agreed upon by the patient, the physician, and the multidisciplinary treatment team provides for consensus on actions and time lines, which facilitate outcomes management. Establishing patient expectations promotes compliance and thereby decreases time and increases results.

Finally, for surgical patients, participation in the STEP program clarifies expectations pre- and postsurgery along the clinical path. A recent internal review of surgical and inpatient charts of STEP patients and matched non–STEP cases revealed significant differences. The STEP patients had a hospital stay that was 14 percent less than non–STEP patients. STEP patients ambulated 10 hours earlier than non–STEP patients (ambulation is a critical indicator of recovery). STEP patients had a lower pain rating and spent 25 percent less time in PACU recovery. These observed differences ultimately account for cost savings as well as improved outcome rates.

•   •   •

The need for outcomes management of spine injuries is evident through the review of the costs and complications involved. The STEP program has demonstrated an enhanced outcomes effect. The outcomes management process utilizes the evaluations of a multidisciplinary team to maximize treatment outcomes, as viewed by all constituencies.

The STEP program does this through the evaluation and education of the patient, during which the team identifies any barriers to recovery. These barriers are diminished through the provision of psychological assessment, instruction on coping skills, breaking the chronic pain cycle, facilitating return to work, and appropriate identification of expectations, as well as through physical therapy and other treatments.

Outcomes management through the STEP program orchestrates all the influential factors of the whole person into the development of an informed treatment plan that will lead to case resolution. Selection of the right treatment option for the right patient leads to a win–win situation for all. Above all, the patient benefits from the education and empowerment he or she receives while becoming a partner in his or her recovery.

REFERENCES

1. Roberts, N., et al. "Health Beliefs and Rehabilitation After Lumbar Disc Surgery." *Journal of Psychosomatic Response* 28 (1984): 139–44.

2. Bigos, S.J., and Battie, M.C. "The Impact of Spinal Disorders in Industry." In *The Adult Spine: Principles and Practice,* ed. J.W. Frymoyer. New York: Raven Press, 1991.

3. Hanley, E.N. Jr. "The Cost of Surgical Intervention For Lumbar Disc Herniation." In *Clinical Efficacy and Outcome in the Diagnosis and Treatment of Low Back Pain*, ed. J.N. Weinstein. New York: Raven Press, 1992.

4. Weinstein, J.N., ed. *Clinical Efficacy and Outcome in the Diagnosis and Treatment of Low Back Pain.* New York: Raven Press, 1992.

5. Hadler, N. "'Conservative Care' for Low Back Pain." In *Clinical Efficacy and Outcome in the Diagnosis and Treatment of Low Back Pain*, ed. J.N. Weinstein. New York: Raven Press, 1992.

6. Grazier, K.L., et al. *The Frequency of Occurrence, Impact and Cost of Musculoskeletal Conditions in the United States.* Chicago: American Academy of Orthopaedic Surgeons, 1984.

7. Keller, R.B. "Tracking Physician Practice: Small Area Analysis Techniques." In *Clinical Efficacy and Outcome in the Diagnosis and Treatment of Low Back Pain*, ed. J.N. Weinstein. New York: Raven Press, 1992.

8. Jensen, M.C., et al. "Magnetic Resonance Imaging of the Lumbar Spine in People without Back Pain." *New England Journal of Medicine* 331, no. 2 (1994): 69–73.

9. U.S. Department of Labor, Bureau of Labor Statistics. *Occupational Injuries and Illnesses: Counts, Rates, and Characteristics, 1993.* Washington, DC: Government Printing Office, 1996.

10. Snook, S.H., Campanelli, A., and Hart, J.W. "A Study of Three Preventive Approaches to Low-Back Injury." *Journal of Occupational Medicine* 20 (1978): 478–81.

11. Stobbe, T.J., and Plummer, R.W. "Sudden Movement/Unexpected Loading as a Factor in Back Injuries." In *Trends in Ergonomics/Human Factors*, ed. V. Amsterdam. Elsevier Science Publishers, 1988.

12. Hadler, N.M. "Occupational Illness: The Issue of Causality." *Journal of Occupational Medicine* 26 (1984): 586–93.

13. Sander, R.A., and Meyers, J.E. "The Relationship of Disability To Compensation Status In Railroad Workers." *Spine* 11 (1984): 141–43.

14. Walsh, N., and Dumitru, D. "The Influence of Compensation on Recovery From Low Back Pain." In *Occupational Back Pain*, ed. Richard Deyo. Hanley & Belfus, Inc., Philadelphia, 1996.

15. Martin, R.D. "Secondary Gain, Everybody's Rationalization." *Journal of Occupational Medicine* 16 (1974): 800–01.

16. Frymoyer, J.W., and Cats-Baril, W.L. "An Overview of the Incidences and Costs of Low Back Pain." *Orthopaedics Clinics of North America* 22 (1991): 262–71.

17. Wallston, K.A., and Wallston, B.S. "Health Locus of Control Scales." In *Research with the Locus of Control Construct,* vol. 1, *Assessment Methods,* ed. H.M. Lefcourt. New York: Academic Press, 1981, pp. 189–243.

18. Report of the Quebec Task Force on Spinal Disorders. "Scientific Approach to the Assessment and Management of Activity-Related Spinal Disorders. A Monograph for Clinicians." *Spine* 12 (1987): S1–S59.

19. Waddell, G., et al. "Chronic Low Back Pain, Psychological Distress and Illness Behavior." *Spine* 9 (1984): 209–13.

20. White, A.H., and Schofferman, J.A. *Spine Care,* vol. 1, *Diagnosis and Conservative Treatment.* St. Louis, MO: Mosby, 1995.

21. Ware, J.E. Jr., et al. *SF-36 Health Survey Manual and Interpretation Guide.* Boston: The Health Institute, New England Medical Center, 1993.

22. McHorney, C., Ware, J., and Raczek, A. "The MOS 36 Item Short Form Health Survey (SF-36): II. Psychometric and Clinical Tests of Validity in Measuring Physical and Mental Health Constructs." *Medical Care* 31, no. 3 (1993): 247–63.

23. Mayer, T., et al. "Contemporary Concepts in Spine Care, Spine Rehabilitation, Secondary and Tertiary Nonoperative Care." *Spine* 20, no. 18 (1995): 2,060–64.

24. Polatin, P., et al. "A Psychosociomedical Prediction Model of Response to Treatment by Chronically Disabled Workers with Low Back Pain." *Spine* 14, no. 9 (1988): 956–61.

25. Taylor, W., Stern, W., and Kubiszyn, T. "Predicting Patient's Perceptions of Response to Treatment for Low Back Pain." *Spine* 9, no. 3 (1984): 313–16.

26. Tollison, C.D., and Satterthwaite, J. "Multiple Spine Surgical Failures: The Value of Adjunctive Psychological Assessment." *Orthopaedic Review* 29, no. 12 (1990): 1,073–77.

27. Flynn, S. "Performance of the MMPI in Predicting Rehabilitation Outcome: A Discriminant Analysis, Double Cross-Validation Assessment." *Rehabilitation Literature* 38 (1977): 12–15.

28. Deyo, R., and Diehl, A. "Psychosocial Predictors of Disability in Patients with Low Back Pain." *The Journal of Rheumatology* 15, no. 10 (1988): 1,557–64.

29. Doxey, N.C., et al. "Predictors of Outcome in Back Surgery Candidates." *Journal of Clinical Psychology* 44, no. 4 (1988): 611–22.

30. McNeill, T., Sinkora, G., and Leavitt, F. "Psychological Classification of Low Back Pain Patients: A Prognostic Tool." *Spine* 11, no. 9 (1986): 955–59.

31. Oostdam, E.M.M., and Duivenvoorden, H.J. "Predictability of the Result of Surgical Intervention in Patients with Low Back Pain." *Journal of Psychosomatic Research* 27, no. 4 (1983): 273–81.

32. Riley, J.L., III, Robinson, M.E., and Geisser, M.E. "Relationship Between MMPI-2 Cluster Profiles and Surgical Outcome in Low Back Pain Patients." *Journal of Spinal Disorders* 8, no. 3 (1995): 213–19.

33. Gallagher, R., et al. "Determinants of Return to Work Among Low Back Pain Patients." *Pain* 39 (1989): 55–67.

PART V

Speech-Language Outcomes

30

The Development of a Functional Outcomes System: A First Look at Speech-Language Pathology Outcome Data

Cecelia M. Lux, Lea Chiaromonte, and Shawn Johns

THE PRESSING NEED FOR OUTCOMES DATA

For years, speech-language pathologists, like their rehabilitation team counterparts, physical, occupational, and respiratory therapists, have been a part of the helping professions in health care. They have explained their craft, theoretical implications of disease and injury, and taken their place with others as they lobbied for health care dollars and for their patients. Efficacy studies were rejected in most research situations because of the ethical dilemma of withholding treatment in a control group. As a result we asked the world to take us at face value that our services were necessary and worth the dollar expenditure. With the changing directions of health care and the shrinking of the availability of the health care dollar, consumers and third-party payers are not as willing as they once were to accept our statements of value. What is more, rehabilitation professionals have struggled and failed to adequately describe our services, predict the results of those services, and justify the continued need of those services. We see it happening everywhere. Most states face yearly challenges to the ongoing funding of basic care, including speech-language pathology services. Physicians are being asked to monitor Medicare dollars or face losing control over funding practices.

In long-term care (LTC), an added challenge is the physicians' and caregivers' belief that we just need to warehouse "these people." Managed care in many cases does not consider speech-language pathology (SLP) to be a basic service, but an outlier to be denied or limited severely. In part, the responsibility for this is within our own field. We have failed at the marketing game to substantiate what we do in terms that appeal to the managed care organizations. Other payers are responding, such as Medicare, and we are seeing a sizable increase in Medicare denials of SLP services in the LTC setting. Professionals in this field are beginning to see the need for development of standard methods of collecting and analyzing data regarding rehabilitation services, including SLP services. The American Speech-Language-Hearing Association (ASHA) has had a task force on the development of outcomes for the last few years. ASHA has been searching for methods to standardize measurements and collection of data from various provider settings. This is an enormous task that will take time and resources to accomplish. At the time of this writing, the American Occupational Therapy Association is attempting similar activities on behalf of its membership. In the private sector, which may have limited access to funded university-based research support, several entities have attempted to develop systems to answer the challenges of health care. The purpose of this article is to detail one such effort and share a preliminary look at some of the data being collected.

HISTORY

Significant changes in the health care industry, such as the expansion of managed care and Medicare reimbursement models (including the development of diagnosis-related groupings for acute hospital reimbursement), demanded greater accountability from health care providers to deliver cost-effective services with functional outcomes. Both payers and health care providers were challenged to develop systems to measure clinical outcomes and the costs associated with service delivery.

One attempt to categorize the outcome of rehabilitation interventions was the Functional Independence Measure (FIM[SM]),[1] which was developed to capture *discipline-free* outcomes information. The FIM has been widely used in the

J Rehabil Outcomes Meas, 1997, 1(1), 45–55

acute hospital setting by multiple health care providers ranging from nursing to rehabilitation clinicians as an indicator of a patient's *overall* functional performance. While the FIM is useful to rehabilitation providers to demonstrate patient performance from an interdisciplinary perspective, there was an additional need for a *discipline-specific* outcomes measurement tool, which would provide pertinent, real-time data for various rehabilitation settings.

In response to the growing need to develop such an outcome measurement tool, particularly for settings other than acute care, South Coast Rehabilitation Services (SCRS), a subsidiary of Regency Health Services, Inc., based in Laguna Hills, California, developed the Rehabilitation Outcome Measurement-I (ROM-I)[2] in 1994. SCRS provides physical therapy (PT), occupational therapy (OT), speech-language pathology (SLP), audiology, and respiratory therapy (RT) services to more than 180 subacute and LTC settings in 14 states. Below is a description of SCRS and its ROM scales.

SCRS: A CLOSER LOOK

SCRS provides PT, OT, SLP, audiology, and RT services primarily to subacute LTC facilities. Operational since 1987, SCRS currently has more than 1,000 full- and part-time therapists within the company, as well as two other divisions, Pulse Point Technologies (software development and support) and Therapy International (recruitment). Pulse Point Technologies (PPT) is the information systems division with which our corporate clinical team works closely to develop and revise our measurement tool, as well as collect, maintain, and distribute our national outcomes database information. Therapy International (TI) is the recruiting division that has 20 recruiters. Therapists are given the option of full-time, part-time, interim, independent contractor, or travel assignments.

SCRS and PPT have developed the OMS Network,[3] a multiuser information system, which has both clinical and managerial applications. It is a user-friendly, point-of-service system that provides real-time (i.e., billing, documentation, etc.) decision resource information for both users and managers.

In a recent company acquisition, SCRS obtained a documentation software package that computerizes the Health Care Financing Administration Series (HCFA's recommended evaluation and plan of treatment form). This component of the system is proving to be an asset not only for SCRS clinicians, but also for PPT's clients. Time savings during the documentation process approximate 35–40 minutes, based on time studies conducted. The ROM is another integral part of the OMS network. It, too, is licensed by PPT clients as well as utilized by SCRS clinicians.

RESEARCH AND DEVELOPMENT OF THE ROM-I

The ROM was developed as a discipline-specific deficit measurement tool, designed by clinicians for use by clinicians. It allows PTs, OTs, and SLPs to rate subacute and long-term care patients regarding their level of function for specific discipline-related deficit areas on a seven-point rating scale (see Table 1).

The ROM was developed by a core team of clinicians (representing speech, occupational, and physical therapy) from SCRS. Because no instrument of its kind existed, development of the ROM was based on clinical experience and research of existing industry standards for the measurement and description of patient performance. Each core team member assembled a task force comprising clinicians actively involved in patient care in the subacute and long-term care settings. Uniform terminology was established to provide a means by which a patient's functional performance could be measured and described.

CLINICAL UPGRADES TO THE ROM-I

Following a year and a half of ROM-I usage and collection of clinical feedback regarding the scales' content, revisions were made; hence, the ROM-II. The ROM-II expanded the number of scales in each discipline to capture deficit areas such as skin integrity, physical restraints, and home management. After six months of revisions, and following feedback and participation of approximately 100 clinicians in the SCRS ranks, ROM-II was ready for use.

ROM-II CERTIFICATION TRAINING

Important to the development of any measurement tool are the foundations to ensure the development of reliable, clinically repeatable measures. The ROM Certification Training program is a comprehensive program designed to systematically train clinicians to use the ROM for the purpose of accurate data collection and clinical outcomes reporting. Certification training is available to SLPs, registered occupational therapists (OTRs), certified occupational therapy assistants (COTAs), PTs, and physical therapist assistants (PTAs).

Training consists of discipline-specific, as well as discipline-free, information. Discipline-specific training (i.e., deficit area rating) was done by trainers from within the same discipline as the trainees. Discipline-free sections (i.e., historical perspective) were taught in an interdisciplinary setting. Only clinicians certified by a certified ROM trainer may use the system.

Table 1. Rehabilitation Outcome Measure: Deficit Area Overview

Speech therapy		Occupational therapy		Physical therapy	
Functional levels	*Deficit areas*	*Funtional levels*	*Deficit areas*	*Functional levels*	*Deficit areas*
Profound	Auditory	Total assistance	Bathing	Dependent	Bed mobility
Severe	comprehension	Maximum	Bed mobility	Maximum	Gait—level surfaces
Mod/severe	Auditory	assistance	Community	assistance	Gait—uneven terrain
Moderate	discrimination	Moderate	activities	Moderate	Joint mobility
Mild/mod	Cognitive-	assistance	Dressing	assistance	Physical restraints
Mild	linguistics	Minimal assistance	Emergency	Minimal	Sitting balance
Independent	Expressive	Standby	response/safety	assistance	Skin integrity
	language	assistance	procedures	Standby	Stair climbing
	Reading	Modified	Feeding	assistance	Standing balance
	comprehension	independence	Functional	Modified	Transfers
	Speech production	Total	communication	independence	Wheelchair mobility
	Swallowing	independence	Grooming/hygiene	Independent	
	Voice		Home		
	Written expression		management		
			Joint mobility		
			Meal preparation/ cleanup		
			Medication routine		
			Physical restraints		
			Toilet hygiene		

Courtesy of Sun Systems, Inc., Aliso Viejo, California.

IMPLEMENTATION/TRAINING OF THE ROM-II

SCRS trained 40 of its managers/associates in preparation for rolling out the ROM-II to staff and later PPT clients. Upon completion, the users were trained in the manner described below.

Train-the-Trainer

The Train-the-Trainer program was a two-day session. The ROM core training team (made up of original ROM developers) trained designated clinicians within their discipline to become ROM users as well as ROM trainers. On the first day, participants became certified to use the ROM and learned how to train users of the ROM. The second day consisted of a mock training session in which participants had the opportunity to practice and apply what was learned on day one. Trainers became certified ROM users upon successful completion of the ROM Skills Assessment taken after the user training. Training certification was awarded following successful completion of the mock training.

Train-the-User

The Train-the-User program was a half-day session. Certified ROM trainers trained clinicians within their discipline to become ROM users. These facility-based clinicians learned how to use the ROM and became certified upon successful completion of the ROM Skills Assessment.

In total, rollout of the ROM for SCRS took two to three months, given the operational logistics that had to be considered and planned for prior to the associates receiving the ROM scales on their facility-based computers. Feedback regarding the contents of the scales as well as the rollout itself was excellent, based on the course evaluation forms completed by every ROM Train-the-Trainer and Train-the-User participant. Users particularly liked the fact that the measured areas were specific enough to capture the unique characteristics of their patient population.

CURRENT STUDY

For the purpose of this report, a subsection of the existing database was analyzed across selected diagnosis groups for length of stay and amount of change in selected treatment (deficit areas). The selected data encompassed 6,625 patients receiving SLP services in LTC facilities across the nation. A total of 8,737 separate rehabilitation programs (having distinct admission and discharge dates) was tracked from this patient population. Since each patient could have more than one treatment (deficit area) addressed during a rehabilitation program, there were 11,740 deficit area treatments analyzed for LOS and amount of change (improvement).

COLLECTION AND USE OF DATA

The current OMS version collects data in the individual LTC facilities. The data are entered by the therapist or his or her designee at the facility upon the patient's admission (following an evaluation procedure). Data entered include name, date of birth, payer source with identifying numbers or status, ICD-9, DRG (often not available), and onset date. ROM information is recorded for up to three treatment areas (deficit areas) for each patient, in each discipline. Treatment information is entered daily, collecting time of treatment in units (15 minutes = 1 unit) and number of visits (QD, BID × weekly, etc.). This information is used at the facility for generation of report forms (including Medicare forms) and to initiate billing procedures. Upon discharge, the patient is again rated using the ROM for each deficit area. The discharge location is also collected. This information is polled weekly and collected at a central location, forming a growing repository of outcomes and treatment data. To analyze the collected data, this extract was prepared using SQL syntax operating against a Microsoft™ SQL Server. The subset of data is summarized on geographical, discipline, and DRG keys throughout a Crystal Reports template. Charts are generated into the summary report and distributed electronically as Adobe-Acrobat™ PDF (portable document format) objects. The data were then converted to a spreadsheet (Excel 7.0). Counts, averages, and display charts were generated from this spreadsheet. As this process is still in the early discovery stages, no statistical analysis has been done. Data use is limited to averages and trends extracted from repeated analysis over time.

DATA ANALYSIS: RESULTS

For the purpose of demonstrating our data collection to date for this article, a portion of data was extracted from the current database. The data were collected over a two-year period of time in various LTC facilities throughout the United States of America. This extract was selected based on most frequently used ICD-9 codes by SLPs in the LTC rehabilitation programs. The diagnoses reviewed included acute strokes (436.0), Alzheimer's dementia (331.0), Parkinson's disease (332.0), dysphagia (787.2), other symbolic dysfunction (784.6), and stroke–late effects (438.0). The internationally recognized

ICD-9 is currently the system used for classifying primary disease for each patient record.

The data were then reviewed for deficit area (see Table 2) categories and averaged for length of stay (number of days enrolled in the rehab program), average admission level, average discharge level, and average amount of change (using ROM scales). Table 3 summarizes the data. Figure 1 depicts the proportional breakdown of this particular population. Patients seen over the two-year study period may have had more than one course of rehabilitation with SLP services. Each patient counted in this population may have had up to three deficit areas recorded for each rehabilitation program. Acute stroke patients made up 13 percent of the population; symbolic dysfunction, 19 percent; stroke–late effects, 4 percent; Parkinson's, 1 percent; Alzheimer's, 2 percent; and dysphagia, 61 percent. Patients were divided into the respective diagnosis groups based on the primary diagnosis code (ICD-9) extracted from the medical record of each patient.

Special note: Patients seen under the primary medical diagnosis of dysphagia had difficulty swallowing as their main area of need (for SLP services) while those treated for swallowing problems under other diagnostic codes most likely had other deficits of equal or greater significance to that patient. Diagnoses are assigned by the treating physician.

Deficit Areas

The treating certified SLP chooses from one to three primary treatment areas for each patient (see Table 1 for a complete listing of the nine available treatment deficit areas). The patient is then rated according to level of function from profound to independent (see Table 1). Each SLP, a certified ROM user, rated the patient in the selected deficit areas. Figure 2 depicts the percentage of patient programs in each deficit area. Swallowing was treated most frequently across all diagnoses (51.76 percent).

LOS

The average length of stay on a rehab program for SLP services was 12.02 days. The range was 6.3 to 21.67. This LOS indicates the number of days the therapist is actively involved in case management for this patient. Results depicted in Figure 3 indicate that patients with acute stroke were seen for the longest time in this setting, followed by patients with late effects of stroke. Patients with Alzheimer's disease were seen for the briefest time (average of 9.84 days per treatment program).

Admission Level

The average admission level for all deficit areas was 0.797, which places the average level of function upon ad-

Table 2. Population Diagnosis and Treatment Deficit Areas

ICD-9	Description	# of Treated deficit areas	# of Patients	LOS	Deficit area	Admit level	Discharge level	Improvement
331.00	Alzheimer's	58	55	14.28	CogLing	0.81	1.08	0.267
331.00	Alzheimer's	34	32	7.00	Swallowing	1.058	1.441	0.382
331.00	Alzheimer's	25	24	6.80	Aud Comp	0.760	0.840	0.080
331.00	Alzheimer's	24	22	6.33	Verb Exp	0.771	0.791	0.021
332.00	Parkinson's	62	41	10.73	Swallowing	1.411	1.75	0.339
332.00	Parkinson's	39	28	10.85	Spch Intlblty	1.32	1.564	0.244
332.00	Parkinson's	29	29	10.66	CogLing	1.155	1.35	0.19
332.00	Parkinson's	18	13	11.39	Verb Exp	1.027	1.278	0.25
332.00	Parkinson's	14	14	10.57	Aud Comp	1.393	1.540	0.143
436.00	Stroke (acute)	393	296	17.48	Swallowing	1.066	1.439	0.373
436.00	Stroke (acute)	333	252	19.65	Verb Exp	0.76	1.1502	0.391
436.00	Stroke (acute)	286	162.5	18.80	Aud Comp	0.864	1.247	0.383
436.00	Stroke (acute)	280	259	17.28	CogLing	0.982	1.429	0.446
436.00	Stroke (acute)	165	128	17.56	Spch Intlblty	1.2	1.5	0.3
438.00	Stroke (late effects)	87	66	12.44	Swallowing	1.276	1.615	0.339
438.00	Stroke (late effects)	84	89	17.46	CogLing	1.375	1.679	0.303
438.00	Stroke (late effects)	74	61	21.68	Verb Exp	0.804	1.08	0.277
438.00	Stroke (late effects)	60	44	15.90	Spch Intlblty	1.059	1.317	0.259
438.00	Stroke (late effects)	56	51	21.50	Aud Comp	1.04	1.38	0.339
784.60	Sym. dysfunc.	1,301	1,085	15.09	CogLing	1.11	1.471	0.359
784.60	Sym. dysfunc.	345	254	13.42	Aud Comp	0.958	1.206	0.248
784.60	Sym. dysfunc.	216	191	15.00	Verb Exp	1.139	1.481	0.342
784.60	Sym. dysfunc.	178	140	15.43	Swallowing	1.326	1.693	0.368
784.60	Sym. dysfunc.	66	58	16.77	Spch Intlblty	1.485	1.621	0.136
787.20	Dysphagia	5,299	3,373	10.64	Swallowing	1.291	1.695	0.404
787.20	Dysphagia	1,133	831	13.95	CogLing	0.946	1.211	0.264
787.20	Dysphagia	771	547	13.78	Verb Exp	0.743	0.941	0.197
787.20	Dysphagia	740	534	14.85	Aud Comp	0.882	1.089	0.207
787.20	Dysphagia	429	318	15.89	Spch Intlblty	1.261	1.591	0.33

This table reflects the five most frequently reported treated deficit areas for this study's population. One category, Alzheimer's, has only four areas reported because all other deficit areas in this category had only one patient indicated. Each patient in this study could have up to three deficit areas reported. An admission and deficit level of function are reported for each area. Please refer to Table 1 for further explanation.

mission at the severe level. For a CVA patient seen for expressive language, that would indicate that the patient could complete 10 percent of the task and expresses basic or simple needs and wants either verbally or nonverbally and may be able to imitate single sounds or syllables. This patient would have the ability to use automatic language only. Table 2 gives average admission levels for all deficit areas and primary diagnoses.

Discharge Level

The average discharge level for all deficit areas was 1.040, which places the average level of function upon admission at the moderate to severe level. The range was from 0.840 to 1.695 for all diagnostic categories. For a patient seen for swallowing, this would indicate that the patient tolerates an oral diet, but may require an alternate feeding source. This patient requires a modified diet consistency with a consistent need for cueing and compensatory strategies. Swallowing is safe in a highly structured setting (see Table 2).

Amount of Change

Amount of change is generated by subtracting discharge level of function (using the ROM scale) from the admission level of function. The average amount of change, weighted for number of programs, was 0.384. The range was 0.021 to 0.426.

For stroke patients the average amount of change for swallowing (deficit treatment area) was 0.373, and 0.446 for cognitive linguistics (deficit treatment area) (see Figure 4).

Table 3. Most Frequently Treated Deficit Areas

Primary diagnosis	Dysphagia	Symbolic dysfunction	Stroke (acute)	Stroke (late effects)	Alzheimer's	Parkinson's
Swallowing	5299	178	393	87	34	62
Cognitive linguistics	1133	1301	280	84	58	29
Verbal expression	771	216	233	74	24	18
Auditory comprehension	740	345	286	56	25	29
Speech intelligibility	429	69	165	60	1	39

This table lists the number of deficit areas treated within each diagnostic category. Only the five most frequently treated areas are listed for each diagnosis.

Other Results

There are additional data available for future analyses. The purpose of this article was to share the preliminary review of outcomes data. This data collection method is unique in that it combines standard measures of outcome such as length of stay and diagnosis with a new functional measurement system that was designed specifically for this population. Future data analysis will attempt to detail significance of these findings as well as report trends within the data.

INTERPRETING THE DATA

While data analysis at the present time is limited to averages and trends, we can begin to use these data to manage and direct our clinical programs.

There are several trends apparent in this sample of the data that have implications for field management and clinical training. These data can assist our managers and their customers in estimating resource utilization for staffing purposes and managed care contracting. The purpose of this discussion is to demonstrate a sampling of these trends and how they might be used in the management of services in the setting of LTC.

LOS

The average number of days that a patient is on program in the LTC setting is influenced by patient goals, caregiver support, discharge plans, and payer constraints. Under typical guidelines a patient must demonstrate the ability to participate in the physician-approved rehabilitation program; have sufficient positive prognostic factors to predict a positive outcome; and demonstrate continuous improvement in order to continue on the program. Working with the mostly geriatric population in the LTC, we know that progress is affected by medical stability, caregiver support from within and outside of the setting, aging process, and mental health of the patient. All of these factors are considered in clinician judgment and the determination of services.

An additional factor is the knowledge base of the treating rehabilitation team. In the case of SLP services, the clinician may have had limited experience with diagnoses such as dementia or depression. Use of the LOS information can help the manager determine areas for improvement for a clinician's program. LOS data will indicate clinicians who need further support in managing specific patients. The same data can be used to estimate admission expectations as well. If we know that the average LOS of patients treated for swallowing is 12.02 days (as reflected in this data), then the facil-

Figure 1. Reflected is the number of different patients who received SLP services during the two-year study. Each patient may have been seen more than once and each patient had up to three deficit areas tracked during the course of this study for each rehabilitation program.

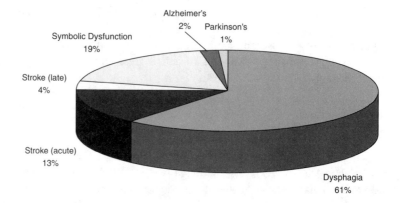

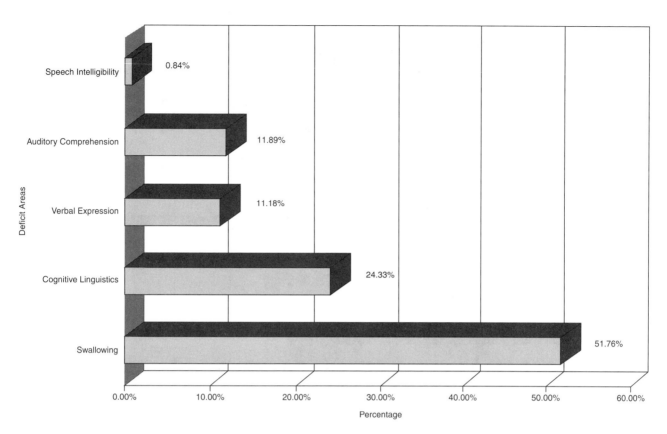

Figure 2. This diagram reflects the percentage of treatment areas chosen for all diagnoses in this study (taken from ROM deficit areas). Each patient could have from one to three deficit areas reflected per treatment program. Overall, swallowing and cognitive linguistics were the most frequently treated areas (total of 76.09 percent) for this study's population.

ity staff can better predict for the patient, the patient's family, and payers the length of stay in the facility, particularly if this is the primary reason for LTC placement.

The length of stay for the indicated SLP services is reducing. The exact reduction cannot be ascertained without earlier periods of data collection. LOS is shortening due in part to changing health care trends, an increase in use of home health services, and evolving referral patterns by physicians. Another use of outcomes data will be to measure and demonstrate treatment efficiency for payers of health care services.

Amount of Change

At the present time, no psychometric review or statistical analyses of the ROM scale measurement have been completed. The purpose of this preliminary article is to demonstrate the type of data available on this system and explain the potential applications.

As reflected in Figure 3, new acute stroke patients appear to be gaining increased functional levels more so in the area of cognitive linguistics than in the area of swallowing. This trend appears to be the opposite of the other diagnostic groups. A

clinical manager may be able to use the trend observations to specify clinical training for the therapists and/or decide to study in more detail the patient population.

Presently, these preliminary data are suggestive of trends only. Until statistical analyses are completed, including, but not limited to, validity and reliability assessment, the data must be viewed as suggestive only.

More Questions

The information from the database begs more questions than it answers at the present time. There is the potential to describe and learn more about clinician practice using new measures. Health care providers are striving to clearly define additional outcome measures and reach consensus on a standardized dataset with utility within the continuum of provider services.

BENEFITS OF THE ROM

ROM-generated information affords many benefits to the health care community. The ROM has been designed to

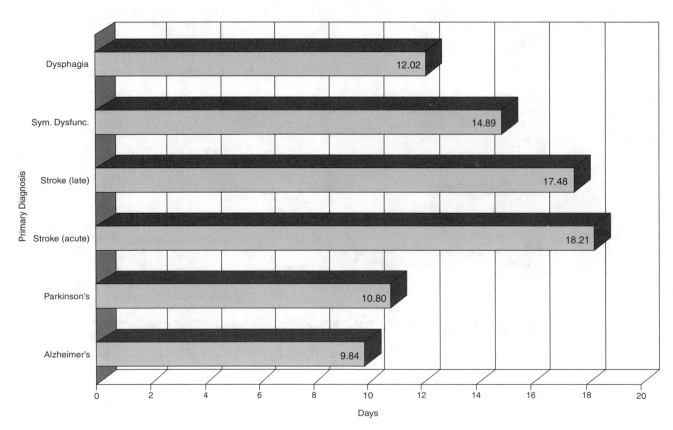

Figure 3. Displayed is the average number of days a patient was on caseload for skilled SLP services in the SNF setting. The number of days was measured from start of treatment (including evaluation day) through discharge from SLP services. Nontreatment days, such as weekends, were included in the day count. Patients were seen longest in the new stroke classification and seen for the shortest period of time for the Alzheimer's classification.

complement existing discipline-free scales, such as the functional independence measure (FIM), and to present a comprehensive view of patients' progress from both the intra- and interdisciplinary frames of reference. Access to this information enables clinicians, managers, and payers to make additional decisions regarding patient care and utilization of services.

For clinicians, the ROM is an easy-to-use diagnostic tool, which eases the reporting of patient progress to physicians, case managers, fellow clinicians, and payers. It simplifies communications with nonclinicians, such as patients and their family members. Further, the ability to consistently track progress in a measurable manner facilitates decision support for treatment and discharge planning. Collection of outcome information provided by the ROM enables clinicians to begin establishing their own standards for rehabilitative care.

Administrative and clinical managers also benefit from ROM-generated information. Collection of ROM data enables managers to conduct trend analysis for new program development, program enhancement, and service delivery modifications and improvements. The ROM also provides

managers with the ability to make real-time decisions based on the analysis of outcome information that is descriptive and measurable.

Lastly, payers benefit from access to outcome data the ROM provides. By furnishing measurable, descriptive, patient-specific information, the ROM simplifies the treatment authorization process, ultimately benefiting the patient.

FUTURE DEVELOPMENT OF THE ROM

Self-study Certification Program

SCRS will continue to enhance the ROM-II in the evolving world of health care. Most recently, a self-study certification method for training was piloted successfully in the southeast. Unlike the formalized training in which a certified trainer trains clinicians of the same discipline, the self-study method involves the participant receiving the same discipline-specific material he or she would have been given had he or she participated in the former method. The participant is given one week to review the materials alone, then takes the same skills assessment. The manager scores the assessment, and should the participant pass, he or she is allowed to begin using the ROM-II. As in the formal training method, should he or she receive less than 75 percent accuracy (passing criteria), the manager reviews the responses and then a second, different assessment is given.

Results of the self-study method for training in the southeastern United States have been very favorable. One hundred percent of all participants in the self-study passed their skills assessment. The continued use of this new method will be evaluated to determine test viability and rater reliability.

Predictability

Payers are demanding justification for rehabilitation services. In order to provide this, clinicians must understand both the impact of their treatment plan and the associated costs. New skills will be necessary to decrease LOS for patients from providers whose outcomes are outside of expected ranges. The SCRS system provides this data through

reporting of units of services, treatment modalities, and ROM outcomes. Then this information loop is complete, SCRS will be able to begin predicting outcomes with inclusion of a method for risk adjustment, further enhancing the clinical product. The industry, as a whole, will benefit from real-time data that capture resource utilization, treatment planning/documentation, and functional outcomes.

Future Development

At the current time, SCRS and Pulse Point are planning the introduction of the Documentation Assistant,[4] which is a PC-based software application that automates the documentation process for PT, OT, and SLP. It also adds to the ability to collect more patient information such as multiple ICD-9 codes (including primary, secondary, and treatment diagnosis). This will allow for greater accuracy in patient classification. Once fully linked, the Documentation Assistant will allow OMS to extract and analyze information about treatment areas, effect on patient status, and discharge status. Information re-

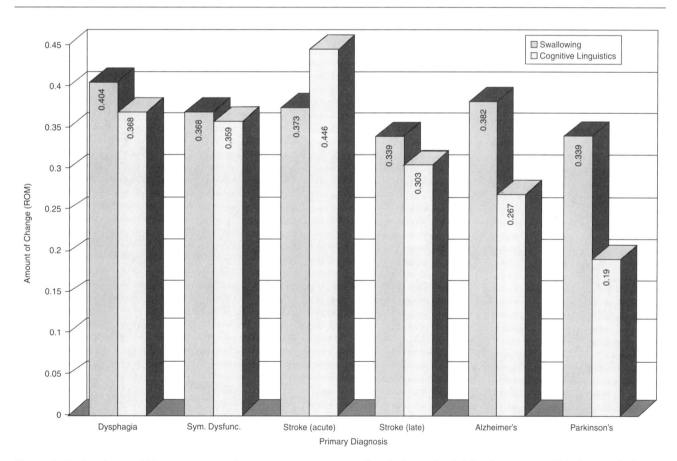

Figure 4. Each patient could have as many as three treatment areas reported on during each rehabilitation program. This diagram depicts the two most frequently chosen treatment areas (ROM deficit areas) for the listed diagnoses. Overall, they made up a total of 76.09 percent (swallowing 51.76 percent, cognitive linguistics 24.33 percent) of the treated deficit areas (see Figure 1). The amount of change demonstrated reflects ROM scale measurements. Significance has not yet been determined.

garding the effects of cognitive status on treatment and the delineation of treatment areas most affected by intervention will be readily available and linked to resources utilized.

The next version of OMS/ROM/DA will link all current data collection systems within the context of a relational database. The eventual goal is to provide for a system that reflects real-time events. In addition to units, minutes of treatment will be collected for treatment procedures and modalities.

Planned changes on the management side will focus on roles of individuals and how they can change in the course of the day at multiple sites, if necessary.

Comprehensive information regarding the results of patient interventions will permit refining of services, expansion of management strategies, and response to customers (patients, associates, and clients). Instead of questioning the eventual outcomes of our patients, we will be increasingly able to predict a rehabilitation unit LOS and level of resource utilization, including costs. By informing our patients and payers of projected outcomes at the initiation of care, clinicians will make more informed decisions. By increasing our knowledge and detail of our health care processes and outcomes, we will meet the challenges of a fast-paced and changing health care delivery system.

REFERENCES

1. Granger, C.V., et al. "Functional Assessment Scales: A Study of Persons after Stroke." *Archives of Physical Medicine and Rehabilitation* 74, no. 2 (1993): 133–38.

2. South Coast Rehabilitation Services & Communicology of Ohio, Inc. *Rehabilitation Outcomes Measures.* Laguna Hills, CA, 1994.

3. South Coast Rehabilitation Services & Communicology of Ohio, Inc. *OMS Network*, Laguna Hills, CA, 1994.

4. South Coast Rehabilitation Services & Communicology of Ohio, Inc. *Documentation Assistant*, Laguna Hills, CA, 1996.

PART VI

Cardiac Rehabilitation Outcomes

31

Outcomes Measurement in Cardiopulmonary Disease and Rehabilitation: A Minnesota Approach

Barbara Tate Unger

IMPLEMENTING RELEVANT GOALS

The health environment in the state of Minnesota has been transitioning to managed care, case management, community involvement, and integration of care throughout the continuum of care for the past several years. As a member of the Minnesota Nurses Association for Healthcare Reform and a member of the American Association of Cardiovascular and Pulmonary Rehabilitation (AACVPR), I often obtained early access to information on strategic initiatives and activities. The purpose of this article will be to discuss the process of outcomes management in cardiopulmonary disease and rehabilitation, through the sharing of successful ideas and insights gleaned from over three years of experience at Itasca Medical Center (IMC), located in Grand Rapids, Minnesota.

The department of cardiovascular services at IMC was monitoring the environmental factors related to health care reform. With the ardent support of local physicians who advocated case management of cardiopulmonary disease, the department began development work towards patient lifestyle management. Our attempt to provide case management for patients began with the multidisciplinary team approach, and the recommendations of national health care organizations such as the AACVPR and the American Heart Association. These organizations provided valuable information for patient care and the importance of accountability for patient outcomes within specified time frames.

A process of outcomes management was planned and implemented to measure results. The past three years (1994–1996) have been extremely educational for our clinical team, through the delineation of which outcomes to measure and the process for data collection. In the preliminary discus-sions and determination of which outcomes to measure, we discovered that an essential goal of cardiac rehabilitation was risk factor reduction. The simple part was agreement on cholesterol management and smoking cessation. The more difficult aspect was the measurement of retention and comprehension of educational information by patients and their families, and if the use of the knowledge subsequently impacted patient risk factors and prevented future visits to the hospital.

In 1995, we placed our department "indicators" for quality assurance on a spreadsheet program. Using Microsoft Works (Microsoft Corporation), we used database and spreadsheet applications to record and monitor information. We initially measured patient risk factors, length of stay, and exercise compliance. One of our first reports featured patients by physician and risk factors. An example of this early report listed each of our physicians and the percentage of their patients with the risk factors of smoking and hypercholesterol levels. As a result of observations made from this report, a pattern emerged and resulted in more aggressive management of cholesterol as a risk factor. We initiated an energetic campaign to provide patient education in the physician offices for prevention as well as after onset of a cardiovascular event in our program. Our efforts resulted in the establishment of standing orders for cholesterol assessment in patient management, and provided for physician education in newer techniques for cholesterol management.

By early 1996, we became more sophisticated in the determination and use of outcome measurement parameters by the addition of a staff member experienced in research. At this time, we were made aware of one of the first cardinal rules for outcome measurement:

J Rehabil Outcomes Meas, 1997, 1(3), 48–57
© 1997 Aspen Publishers, Inc.

Use nationally established definitions, guidelines, and parameters.

Following the American Heart Association definition of risk factors, we clarified and operationally defined each of our outcome measures. It is important to inform all providers and staff in your facility of national guidelines and developing processes for outcomes measurement. Our guidelines were shared with physicians, the coronary care staff, the cardiovascular staff, and patients. Billfold-size cards were printed and laminated that listed the parameters for cholesterol, exercise, blood pressure, and smoking as support for secondary prevention. Staff encouraged patients to carry their card with them, and to review the cards with each physician appointment, in order to encourage discussion and to spark involvement by the patients in their own care and recovery.

The second cardinal rule for outcomes measurement slowly became apparent:

Disease management occurs over time.

Even if we were able to gather and record initial outcomes information, we would need to record and monitor results periodically thereafter. The book *Lifestyle Management,* by Nancy Houston Miller,[1] was most informative and mirrored this approach. Another source of critical information was an article "A Case Management System for Coronary Risk Factor Modification after Acute Myocardial Infarction."[2] Each of these sources became invaluable references. Both publications reveal methods for effective consultation and counseling of patients via telephone, which can be extremely effective in assisting patients to make the necessary lifestyle changes. Our facility was confident in our success during cardiac rehabilitation, but what was our outcome durability? We determined that measurements of our program effectiveness were necessary one year after discharge from rehabilitation.

A follow-up procedure was established, and patients were contacted by telephone approximately one year following the conclusion of their rehabilitation. For example, data was obtained on smoking cessation and exercise frequency to ascertain the impact of our education efforts. The results showed that smoking was resuming at a less than desirable rate. Following clinician training in instructional programs for smoking cessation by the American Lung Association, our staff began calling patients each quarter to (1) reinforce no smoking, and (2) counsel patients and notify their physicians if smoking had been resumed. This team approach between the cardiovascular services staff and physicians has worked extremely well and has met with a great deal of success. We are now able to report the rates of smoking cessation on a quarterly basis (patients are monitored for seven consecutive quarters following discharge from rehabilitation). This type of approach fulfills the second cardinal rule,

with a monitoring of lifestyle management through an effective process of case management.

The third cardinal rule of outcomes measurement is:

Measure only what you need to know in the simplest manner possible.

I have seen many health care providers fail at outcome measurement because they were overwhelmed by the sheer volume and complexity of measures. IMC has a four-bed Cardiovascular Care Unit (CCU) and provides cardiac rehabilitation for approximately 160 patients annually. Our resources do not include a sizable information system nor a support staff to support outcomes measurement. My experiences on the national outcomes committee for AACVPR and elsewhere indicated that recording outcome measures "on paper" is the preferred early method. There are generally productivity implications of staff to consider, and we did not wish to impact negatively our professionals' time with their patients.

We were indeed fortunate to be able to add a secretary to our staff, with skills in both documentation transcription and database management. The creation of a database and spreadsheet using Microsoft Access and Microsoft Excel (Microsoft Corporation) respectively for input of information is a high priority in the initial design stages of outcomes management. The process includes the definition of uniform parameters and providing for ease in use. A carefully designed paper-based system, including evaluation and assessment tool, care plan, and education sheet, facilitates data entry into the database. Our secretary established an intake questionnaire and automated notification system for follow-up contact. This process organized our time well. We were able to put our parameters together on a single piece of paper, minimizing the use of paper and redundancy of data collection. Our database is organized such that a list of follow-up contacts is generated each month with minimum effort. The database is capable of printing address labels as well, greatly saving time for the process of follow-up mailings and support group notification.

The health environment and managed care penetration was indicating that the measurement of patient health-related quality of life and patient satisfaction was becoming more essential, and would be influential in future reimbursement paradigms. However, our patient population was not accustomed to the completion of health questionnaires. After a search of the available questionnaires, we selected the Dartmouth COOP.[3] This tool has worked extremely well in our facility. The Dartmouth COOP is a series of nine questions with scoring intervals of 1–5. The questionnaire is completed at the initiation and conclusion of rehabilitation, and at one year after discharge. Patients can complete the questionnaire in about two or three minutes. One of our tertiary care (referral) centers is currently distributing the questionnaire before discharge and forwarding scores to IMC.

One of the best examples of our successful use of the Dartmouth COOP is the assessment of patient "social support." If the patient rates this area low, it immediately triggers early intervention through the case manager. Our experience has shown that patients with minimal social support have a high rate of readmission and death within the first year post onset of their condition. We believe we have a mechanism in place to assist in the identification of "risk" patients early in the intervention process, which will ultimately improve our outcome success.

IMC began use of the Dartmouth COOP in January of 1996. Patients are asked to complete the form at the entry point into our system, whether it begins at the local hospital or at our tertiary center. If a patient self-scores at the dysfunctional end of the scale (4 or 5), it immediately triggers our intervention. Our experience has shown a high rate of readmission and mortality for those patients with a depression or isolation in the first year after a myocardial infarction (MI) or coronary artery bypass graft (CABG). With over one year of experience now, we can now share with the cardiologists and cardiac centers (Abbott Northwestern and the Minneapolis Heart Institute, both of Minneapolis) in their search for answers to the question: "Did cardiac procedures completed improve the patient's subsequent quality of life?" We also view this as an integral process of the continuum of care concept, and meeting the vision of the Joint Commission on Accreditation of Healthcare Organizations. The effectiveness of cardiology, surgery, and rehabilitation is measured and monitored through combined efforts in a comprehensive outcomes management approach.

We have not seen the determination of a consensus patient satisfaction instrument nationally, and therefore elected to create our own questionnaire consisting of ten items (yes/no responses). Although our instrument has not been fully validated, it provides us with valuable information on patient satisfaction.

The fourth cardinal rule for outcomes measurement is:

Be open to constant change.

A valuable lesson learned has been that health care providers must be receptive to change, and not remain rigidly convinced that there is only one way or one tool to measure outcomes. Since instituting the database for measurement, we have changed and expect to modify our approach in the future. If a patient satisfaction instrument becomes nationally recognized and accepted, we expect to begin use of the instrument.

One of the reasons that change continues to occur is the rapid expansion of outcome measures that are becoming available, adding to the complexity in assimilation of outcomes information and methodologies. I have met many providers who state that "I'll wait until *they* tell me what, how, and when to measure." From my experiences with the

AACVPR outcomes committee, I have learned some valuable lessons. I have begun advocating a key message: "One needs to get started, follow AACVPR guidelines on which domains to measure, set parameters of measurement within national guidelines, and measure over time."

Outcomes are needed in both the short term, or immediately after discharge from the rehabilitation program, and the long term, secondary to case management for one year following discharge. Our measurement system was developed from the viewpoint of the typical patient goals upon admission, and the available nationally recognized guidelines. The AACVPR, an organization of professionals spanning several disciplines in cardiovascular and pulmonary rehabilitation, has indicated three domains to follow in outcome measurements: *clinical, behavioral, and health.*[4] Clinical domains include mortality, morbidity, quality of life, and satisfaction. Behavioral domains include smoking and exercise. Health domains cover lipids, functional capacity, return to work, and recurring emergency room visits. Each of these domains may be interrelated with each other. The categorization of outcome measures into domains eases the identification and final selection of specific measures.

EXAMPLES

Behavioral Outcome: Smoking

Each patient is counseled using the American Lung Association philosophy and approach to smoking cessation. The process of behavioral change begins at discharge, when patients are notified that they will be contacted each subsequent quarter by a staff member for a period of two years. A patient who resumes smoking is invited and encouraged to attend a complimentary smoking cessation class. If a patient declines to attend the class or prefers to try alone, our interviewers ask when the patient desires to be contacted again. These patients are managed under a different algorithm with more aggressive intervention. The patient's primary physician is given notice of his or her patient's status. Many physicians have chosen to contact the patient directly. Houston Miller's message that the more medical contact and reinforcement, the more patients quit smoking,[1] is clearly evident in our results. While this concerted effort appears to be a lot of work, our overriding philosophy is that the process of outcomes measurement is the key to secondary prevention and our long-term success.

Behavioral Outcome: Education

If a primary role of the health care provider in cardiopulmonary rehabilitation is to educate patients and their families, then the effectiveness of this intervention should be measured. There was interest from clinical and financial

PHYSICAL FITNESS

During the past 4 weeks . . .
What was the hardest physical activity you could do for at least 2 minutes?

Very heavy, (for example) • Run, fast pace • Carry a heavy load upstairs or uphill (25 lbs/10 kgs)		**1**
Heavy, (for example) • Jog, slow pace • Climb stairs or a hill moderate pace		**2**
Moderate, (for example) • Walk, medium pace • Carry a heavy load level ground (25 lbs/10 kgs)		**3**
Light, (for example) • Walk, medium pace • Carry light load on level ground (10 lbs/5 kgs)		**4**
Very light, (for example) • Walk, slow pace • Wash dishes		**5**

Figure 2. Test to assess physical fitness. *Source:* Copyright © Trustees of Dartmouth College/COOP Project, 1998.

CARDIAC REHAB DEPARTMENT PRE AND POST TEST

NAME: _____ DATE: _____

Please check the box with the correct answer(s)

1. All of the below are CONTROLLABLE risk factors except:
   a. obesity ☐
   b. sex (gender) ☐
   c. lack of exercise ☐
   d. stress ☐

2. A risk factor is a condition or characteristic that increases your chance of developing heart disease or progression of heart disease.
   a. True ☐   b. False ☐

3. Most people can feel when their blood pressure is high.
   a. True ☐   b. False ☐

4. Angina pain results in permanent damage to the heart muscle
   a. True ☐   b. False ☐

5. Regular aerobic exercise three times a week increases . . .
   a. HDL ☐
   b. LDL ☐
   c. VLDL ☐

6. Dietary modification is still needed even though your physician orders cholesterol reducing medicine for you.
   a. True ☐   b. False ☐

7. Even though a product is labeled "NO CHOLESTEROL" it may still contain fat.
   a. True ☐   b. False ☐

8. A general guideline following a coronary event is that if you can walk up two flights of stairs without symptoms, you may engage in sexual relations.
   a. True ☐   b. False ☐

9. Sex drive or sexual function may be decreased by
   a. medications (tranquilizers, antidepressants, high blood pressure medications)
   b. anxiety, depression
   c. both of the above

10. Take a second Nitroglycerin tablet after _____ minutes, if the first one has not given complete relief of anginal discomfort.
    a. 3 to 5 minutes
    b. 5 to 10 minutes
    c. 10 to 15 minutes

Figure 1. Test to assess comprehension of cardiac education. *Source:* Copyright © Trustees of Dartmouth College/COOP Project, 1998.

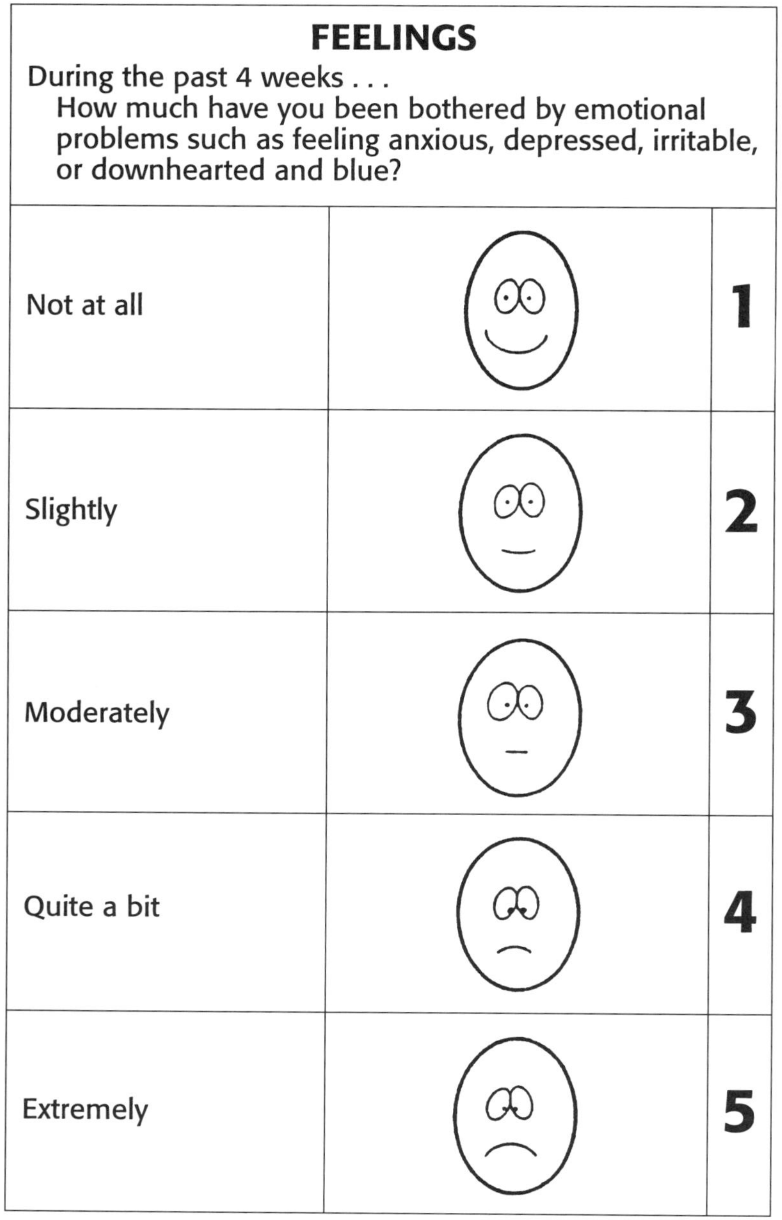

DAILY ACTIVITIES

During the past 4 weeks . . .
How much difficulty have you had doing your usual
activities or task, both inside and outside the house
because of your physical and emotional health?

1	No difficulty at all
2	A little bit of difficulty
3	Some difficulty
4	Much difficulty
5	Could not do

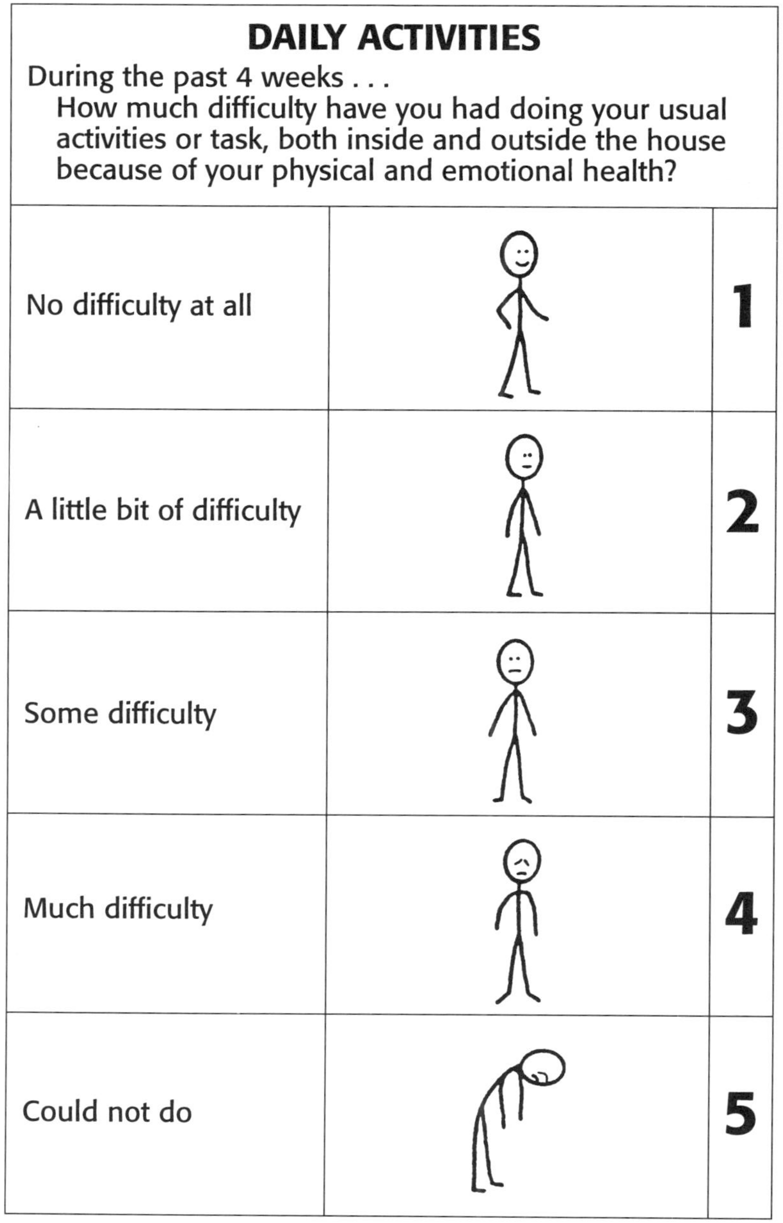

Figure 4. Test to assess ability to handle activities of daily living. *Source:* Copyright © Trustees of Dartmouth College/COOP Project, 1998.

FEELINGS

During the past 4 weeks . . .
How much have you been bothered by emotional
problems such as feeling anxious, depressed, irritable,
or downhearted and blue?

1	Not at all
2	Slightly
3	Moderately
4	Quite a bit
5	Extremely

Figure 3. Test to assess current emotional stability. *Source:* Copyright © Trustees of Dartmouth College/COOP Project, 1998.

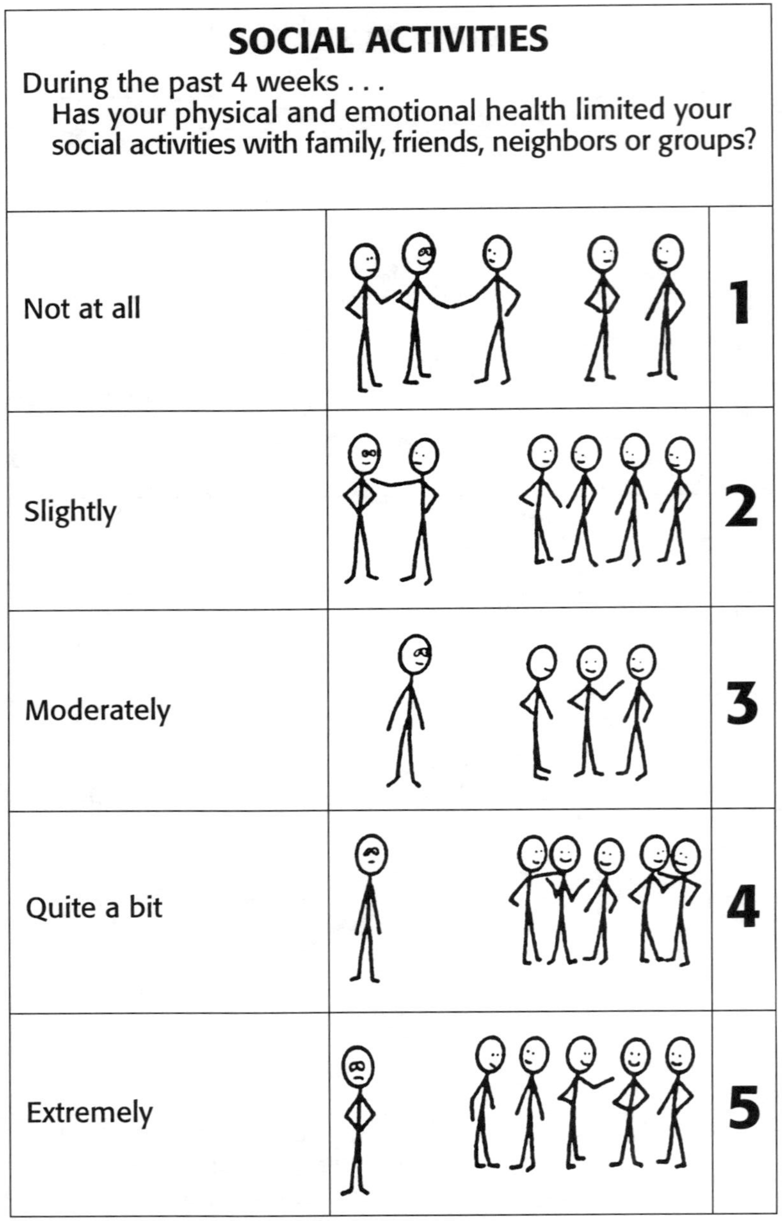

PAIN

During the past 4 weeks . . .
How much bodily pain have you generally had?

No pain		1
Very mild pain		2
Mild pain		3
Moderate pain		4
Severe pain		5

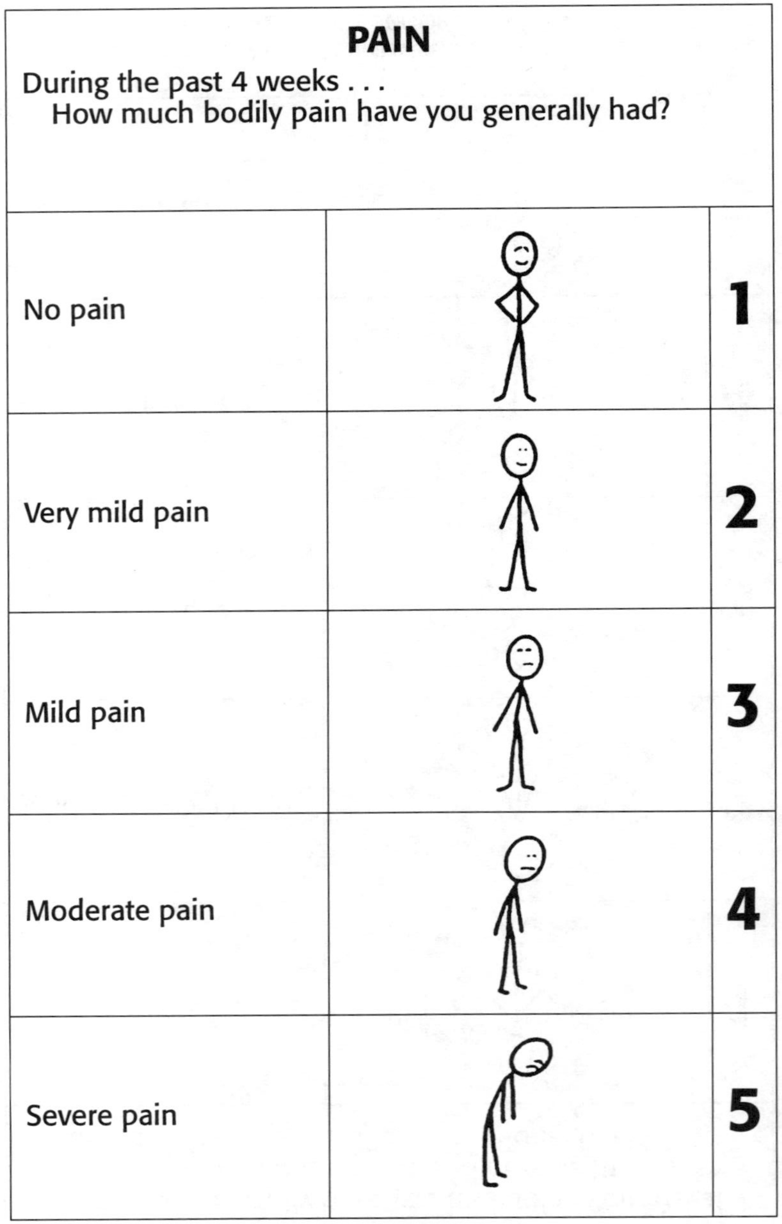

Figure 6. Test to evaluate degree of daily pain. *Source:* Copyright © Trustees of Dartmouth College/COOP Project, 1998.

SOCIAL ACTIVITIES

During the past 4 weeks . . .
Has your physical and emotional health limited your social activities with family, friends, neighbors or groups?

Not at all		1
Slightly		2
Moderately		3
Quite a bit		4
Extremely		5

Figure 5. Test to evaluate social functionability. *Source:* Copyright © Trustees of Dartmouth College/COOP Project, 1998.

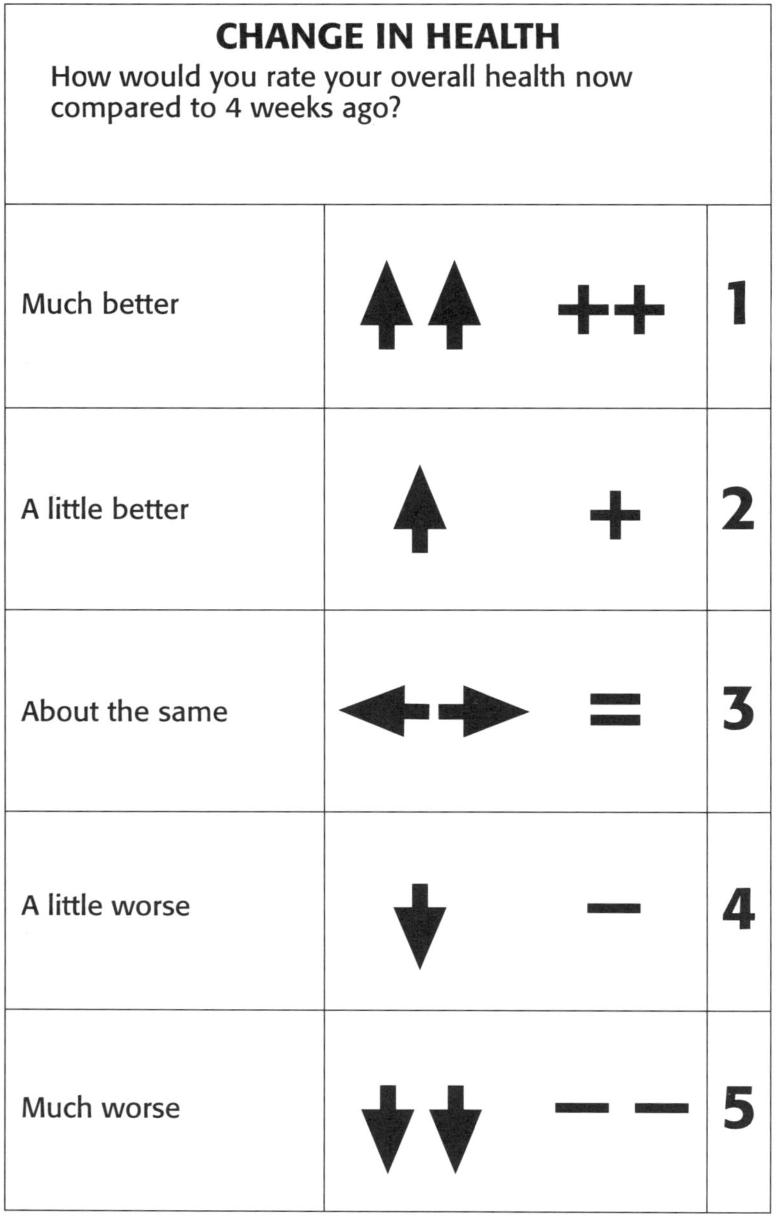

OVERALL HEALTH

During the past 4 weeks . . . .
How would you rate your health in general?

	Excellent	1
	Very good	2
	Good	3
	Fair	4
	Poor	5

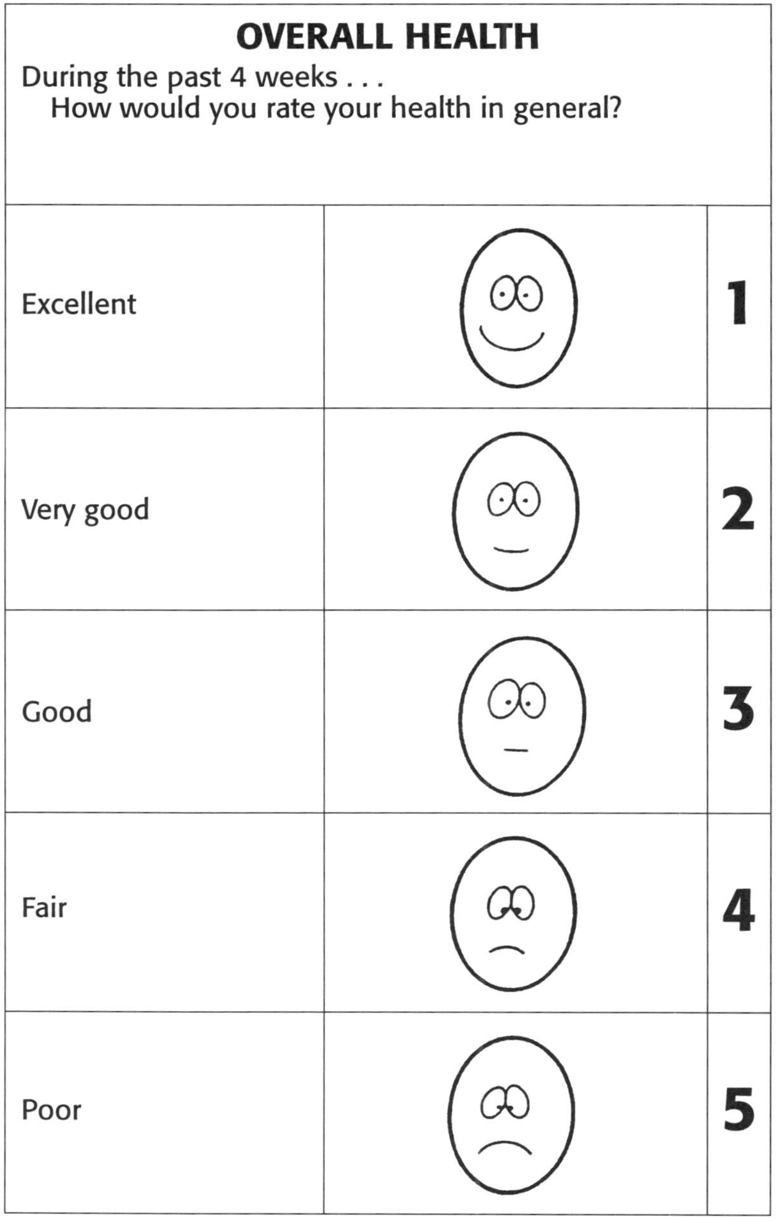

Figure 8. Test to assess current health overall. *Source:* Copyright © Trustees of Dartmouth College/COOP Project, 1998.

CHANGE IN HEALTH

How would you rate your overall health now compared to 4 weeks ago?

	Much better	1
	A little better	2
	About the same	3
	A little worse	4
	Much worse	5

Figure 7. Pictogram to compare current health with four weeks past. *Source:* Copyright © Trustees of Dartmouth College/COOP Project, 1998.

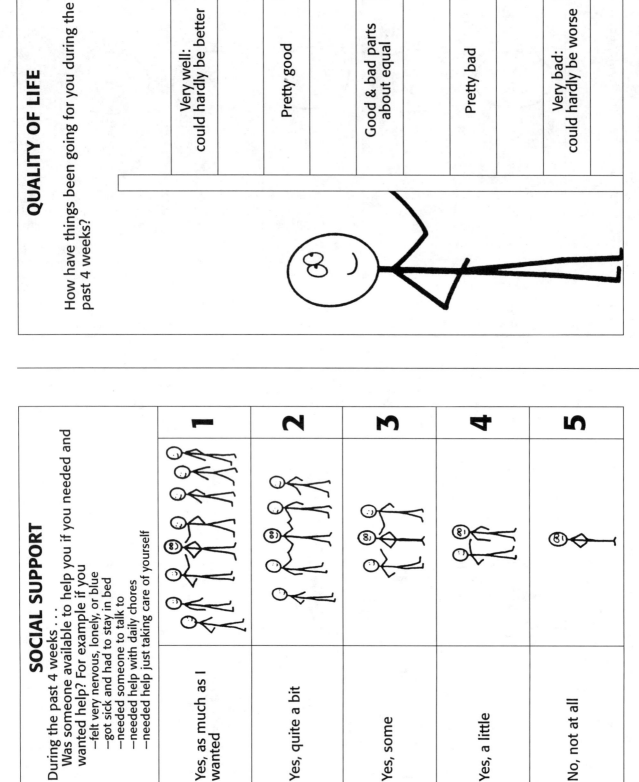

Figure 10. Test to rate overall quality of life. *Source:* Copyright © Trustees of Dartmouth College/COOP Project, 1998.

Figure 9. Questionnaire to determine availability of social support. *Source:* Copyright © Trustees of Dartmouth College/COOP Project, 1998.

Table 1. Outline of IMC's Cardiac Rehabilitation Outcomes Measurement Process

Outcome Domain			Timing of Measurement	
Quality of life	Admission	Discharge	None	At one year
Smoking	Admission	Discharge	3 mo. post d/c	Every 3 mo. × 7
MD/ER visit		Discharge	3 mo. post d/c	At one year
Rehospitalization		Discharge	3 mo. post d/c	At one year
Lipids	Admission		3 mo. post d/c	At one year
Education	Admission	Discharge		At one year

staff, as well as managed care organizations, in the content, process, and cost of patient education. The number of sessions and the cost was easily verified; comprehension by the patient over the long term was not. A test to assess comprehension of cardiac education was derived from several sources and assimilated into a ten-question format (see Figures 1–10). These ten questions were taken from several existing tests used in various rehabs. What it represents is a cross-section of educational objectives that are established for lifestyle change and management. Again, tools are just being developed and validated, and as they become available, we will utilize them in our comprehension evaluation.

Clinical Outcome: Lipids

Our management of outcomes in the continuum of care and prudent fiscal responsibility led to a process for periodic assessment of patient lipid levels, including the appropriate timing, where measures are taken, and the sharing of results. A large communication problem ensues with patients sharing providers among the tertiary care centers, physician clinics, and IMC. Fortunately, the willingness to gather and share information among the providers led to the establishment of the case manager at Itasca Medical Center assuming the responsibility for lipid rest results. The local clinics and Abbott Northwestern dedicated a "link" or care coordinator that we could contact for the information as well as to assist in the education of the patient. Lipid management, discharge needs, quality of life, and medical information was then shared for the best of care for patients and their families wherever they were in the system. (My point is, outcome data is useful not just for process improvement, but in the real care of individual patients.)

The management of lipid levels and results provides an opportunity to educate patients while in rehabilitation instead of simply passing on an awareness of this risk factor at discharge. With providers working in sync through more aggressive intervention, there has been an overall decrease in both total cholesterol and LDL levels. We have used these outcome results in planning for physician, nurse, and rehabilitation staff education.

Our process of outcomes management has been a focus on the minimum number of measures, using content domain suggested by AACVPR, and continuing to look for ways to decrease the impact on staff productivity. Our department now sends a questionnaire initially instead of calling each patient. A nurse assigned to follow-up reviews the returned questionnaires and determines if a call to the patient is warranted. Calls are assigned to staff each month. The physician is notified in instances where an intervention such as counseling is necessary or when the recommended follow-up visit schedule has been violated. Also, if a patient questionnaire is not returned, our computerized database system automatically triggers notice that a reminder phone call by the staff is necessary. If after three attempts we fail to contact the patient, they will be automatically recontacted in the next reporting period.

• • •

An outline of IMC's Cardiac Rehabilitation Outcomes Measurement process is described in Table 1.

The implementation of an outcomes management process required a great deal of receptivity to change on the part of the staff and physicians of IMC. We have seen improvement through our ability to benchmark outcome results with other institutions such as the Minneapolis Heart Institute (Abbott Northwestern Hospital), one of our primary referral centers. We are seeing outcomes data effectively "translated" into knowledge and information useful for identification of areas needing improvement and contributing to the success of rehabilitation and disease management over time. Our cooperative efforts will ultimately benefit patients, providers, and the payers of our services.

REFERENCES

1. Houston Miller, N., and Taylor, C.B. *Lifestyle Management for Patients with Coronary Heart Disease.* Champagne, IL: Human Kinetics, 1995.

2. "A Case Management System for Coronary Risk Factor Modification after Acute Myocardial Infarction." *Annals of Internal Medicine* 120, no. 9 (May 1994): 720–21.

3. Haskell, W., et al. "Effects of Intensive Multiple Risk Factor Reduction on Coronary Atherosclerosis and Clinical Cardiac Events in Men and Women with Coronary Artery Disease." *Circulation* 89, no. 3.

4. "Achieving Quality Patient Outcomes Across a Continuum of Care." *Cardiovascular Disease Management* 2, no. 3.

PART VII

Technology in Rehabilitation Outcomes Measurement

32

Information Technology for Medical Rehabilitation, Part 1: An Overview

Malcolm H. Morrison

APPROACHING THE INFORMATION TECHNOLOGY GOAL

A recent article on managed care case management stated, "An online, integrated, demographic and clinical information software system that contains data on baseline health status, approved treatment plan, service utilization (planned versus actual services and related costs), specific quality and clinical indicators to measure improvements and optional outcomes, established treatment standards, clinical pathways and consumer and provider satisfaction will be vital to the success of all health care providers. . . . Computer technology will enable us, as well as payers, to see where the dollars are going and what the relationship is between cost and care."[1] In one form or another, this kind of *information* is the goal of most health care providers, many payers, and informed consumers. And, it is generally recognized that this goal can only be achieved using information technology (IT).

The computer revolution has raised the expectations of the health care sector (as indicated above), sometimes beyond their capability or willingness to invest the resources required to achieve the growing benefits available from information technology. In addition, many health care providers (especially in specialty areas), continue to seek inexpensive "plug and play" software solutions that *they believe* will provide the comprehensive information they need. This is particularly true in such areas as outcomes, case management, patient satisfaction, and quality monitoring systems. When it is discovered that these existing software "solutions" are not comprehensive and do not have the capability to integrate data on costs, quality, effectiveness, and patient satisfaction (for example), providers sometimes purchase partial systems and/or conclude that integrated information technology solutions either do not exist or are not affordable.

While the "on-line, integrated demographic and clinical information software system" does not yet exist, this does not mean that information technology cannot be used to begin building such systems. On the contrary, appropriate use of technology and decision-support capabilities can in fact achieve some of the goals of an integrated system. To accomplish this practical objective requires understanding current health care information systems and how information technology is used in health care. This knowledge can then be used to evaluate and select technology options that will in fact improve the operations of health care providers focused on medical rehabilitation and care of chronic illness.

BASIC PRINCIPLES

The two most important fundamental principles to understand initially are related to the management of information technology:

- The use of information technology usually requires a significant capital investment and requires training and retraining of administrative and clinical staff. Both financial and staff resources must be provided to obtain the benefits of this investment. An important corollary of this principle is that trying to minimize this investment, for example, by purchasing software products "just-in-time" to satisfy customer requirements, often ends up costing more even in the short run because these solutions are quickly out of date.
- The best results of information technology will be achieved using a planning cycle approach. Information technology planning and updating is a continuous process, requiring an ongoing organizational commitment.

J Rehabil Outcomes Meas, 1997, 1(3), 44–47

The debate about the return-on-investment (ROI) for information technology is almost always resolved favorably when a continuous planning cycle approach is used. A positive ROI often occurs because sound initial investment decisions reduce the need and expense for purchasing new systems (or expensive systems upgrades) later on. This can only occur through ongoing continuous technology planning.

Two other important points regarding information technology relate to what comprises "IT" and its uses. Information technology, in fact, consists of information systems (administrative, clinical, data), hardware (computers and peripherals), telephone and video systems, networking of computers, and applications software programs. The information so much desired by health care organizations is produced using all of this technology. Obviously, unless an organization is willing to invest in this technology, it cannot obtain the benefits available. These benefits include both the traditional administrative and financial systems applications and the new use of IT for financial risk analysis, case management and patient tracking (including pathways), contract management, outcomes analysis, electronic medical records, and so on.

Finally, there is a need for realism on the part of executives and managers involved in technology planning and implementation. Existing systems (and even new systems designed for specific applications such as hospital information systems), cannot always be adapted to meet needs for which they were not designed. This is particularly important in designing information systems that collect and analyze data for patients receiving treatment in multiple venues of care. Few if any major health information systems available today were designed for postacute care venues, and this has led to a proliferation of more limited software products for these settings. New systems may be required for integrated health care and managed care, and the limitations of existing systems should be recognized as IT decisions are made.[2]

TYPES OF INFORMATION TECHNOLOGY

IT consists of:

- *Applications software,* which automates major financial, administrative, and clinical functions of an organization;
- *Hardware and peripherals,* which run the applications software;
- *Communications and networks,* which link hardware, peripherals, and software, sometimes including linking multiple organizations with computer networking;
- *Systems integration,* which connects hardware and software systems together so that data is shared and transmitted within or between systems.

Each of these functional areas of IT is supported by a growing group of vendors who provide the various technologies. In general, most vendors have concentrated their efforts on acute care hospital organizations and, more recently, integrated health systems. While theoretically, the systems and software that has been developed could be used in the postacute care environment, few successful applications have been developed and therefore it has been difficult for postacute care to adopt "whole systems solutions" that provide integrated financial, clinical, and administrative data. Postacute care software applications that can be linked to hospital systems are in early stages of development, but are clearly feasible and will increase in the future. Because of current systems integration capabilities, postacute care providers and payers should carefully consider their need for financial and clinical data in multiple venues of care before making IT design and purchasing decisions. That is, making cost-effective IT decisions requires clarification of an organization's business objectives and the specific benefits (functions) that information will provide for business operations.[2]

MAJOR INFORMATION SYSTEMS APPLICATIONS

While in the past, clinical and administrative systems applications were often considered separately, this is changing significantly. Today, primarily because of managed care, the capability to "integrate" financial, clinical, and administrative data is a major goal of most health care organizations. Few executives want to design or purchase any systems that do not have the capability for data integration; and the need for "decision-support" applications to support financial and clinical decisions is growing rapidly. Thus, while individual software applications for case management, outcomes, and patient satisfaction reporting are still used, their ultimate value depends on their capability to be integrated into more complete IT solutions that provide integrated information based on multiple types of data.

With this in mind, there are several general types of systems applications that are being used in health care organizations.

- *Administrative and general financial management systems,* including patient billing and accounts receivable, accounts payable, materials management, payroll, human resources, general ledger, budgeting, admission, discharge, transfer and patient registration, scheduling, medical records, quality assurance, outcomes, productivity/staffing management, contract management, and utilization review.
- *Clinical support systems,* including: nursing care, order entry/results, critical pathways/patient protocols, case management, electronic patient records, outcomes management, patient tracking, and patient satisfaction.

- *Decision support applications,* including cost accounting and budgeting, case-mix analysis, market analysis, reimbursement models, clinical process improvement/pathway analysis, utilization review analysis, cost effectiveness analysis, patient classification/cost analysis, patient tracking and disease management systems.
- *Ancillary clinical systems,* including pharmacy, radiology, laboratory, and supplies.

These systems are being supported and enhanced with several developing technological improvements that are enabling new forms of data integration, leading to significantly improved information for management. Data storage improvements are enabling the development of data repositories, electronic data exchange, and improved data integration. Improved presentation tools are resulting in better data analyses, graphical presentations, and report generation. And, improved data integration tools now enable faster data storage in relational databases, and more rapid data analyses and use of decision-support programs.

These technological improvements are important because they permit multiple points of access to patient care records, enable case management across multiple venues of care, and establish a more complete record of patient treatment over time. Therefore, they encourage more of a continuum-of-care approach, which is of value in treating chronic illness and impairment. In addition, these technologies and the information systems they support have multiple uses in managed care, which seeks optimal results at lower cost.[2]

• • •

Use of information technology is fundamental in today's postacute health care environment.[3-5] Knowledge of information systems functions and support applications is essential to improve financial and clinical management with the evolution of managed care. Through improved use of IT, executives and managers improve their understanding and use information to make informed decisions. Technology functions to continuously improve the cost effectiveness of care, both short- and long-term patient outcomes, and the ability to manage patients with chronic illness. For this reason, the use of technology is a requirement for medical rehabilitation and postacute care.

REFERENCES

1. Chmielski, M. "Network Connect." *Case Review* (Fall 1992): 73, 75.
2. DeLuca, J.M., and Cagan, R.E. *The CEO's Guide to Health Care Information Systems.* Chicago: American Hospital Publishing, pp. 1–7.
3. Austin, C.J. *Information Systems for Health Services Administration.* Chicago: Health Administration Press, 1992.
4. Tan, J.K.H. *Health Management Information Systems, Theories, Methods, and Applications.* Gaithersburg, MD: Aspen Publishers, Inc.
5. Wolper, L.F., ed. *Health Care Administration, Principles, Practices, Structure, and Delivery.* 2nd ed. Gaithersburg, MD: Aspen Publishers, Inc.

33

Information Technology for Medical Rehabilitation, Part 2: Requirements

Malcolm H. Morrison

Improved information technology (IT) will continue to be a necessity in health care delivery systems. But, the ongoing cost and complexity of information systems, combined with its staff resource requirements, result in continuing questions about the value of IT investments.

Some of the confusion and concern about the value of IT results from limitations in knowledge and understanding of technology, while additional difficulties arise because of misinformation and misinterpretation about IT's actual capabilities to improve business and clinical operations. Also, many providers and payers continue to view IT as a solution that will rapidly improve efficiency and effectiveness of service delivery. When the improvement does not occur, executives question the payback for the investment in IT, rather than recognize the fact that its effectiveness depends on using functional software applications to support changes and/ or redesign of clinical and business processes.

Under these circumstances, the best approach is for organizations to decide what redesign is required in business and clinical processes, implement management control of the redesign, measure the changes (including financial and program performance) and use *information technology applications* to support and maintain the redesigned system. By using this approach, it will become readily apparent that the most significant value will be achieved through developing an integrated information system linking financial, clinical process, and outcomes data. The challenge to information technology, then, is to develop applications to accomplish this goal.

This article addresses some of the most fundamental issues related to IT and its use in medical rehabilitation settings. The article is based on the view that medical rehabilitation must be viewed as part of the continuum of care, and that its use of IT should be broadly defined in terms of the technology used in health care as a whole, that is, information technology is treated objectively in terms of its functionality for both medical rehabilitation and health care overall. This view limits the attention given to niche technology products designed solely for rehabilitation, and instead recommends that such products (where required) be "imbedded" in larger and more generic information systems. This is consistent with the development of integrated delivery networks, large health care conglomerates, and managed care organizations. However, this comprehensive approach may not be as useful for smaller stand-alone health care providers. Nevertheless, as major systems vendors continue to grow and new vendors develop, their products will conform more and more to common systems standards, platforms, and software criteria, to enable significantly improved communication with the broader health care environment (physicians, providers, payers, and patients). Thus, a comprehensive view of IT is justified in addressing the current and future needs of rehabilitation providers.

IMPORTANCE OF IT PLANNING AND SYSTEMS INTEGRATION

The one area of IT that cannot be overemphasized is planning. This planning is not necessarily typical in that it is not undertaken solely to meet a current need or solve a current problem. IT planning is and must be a continuous process in the organization. This usually begins with strategic planning (long-range and short-term) and is developed using a systems life-cycle concept, which includes developing system requirements, selecting vendors, contracting, implementing

J Rehabil Outcomes Meas, 1997, 1(4), 10–14

systems, monitoring and updating systems, and then returning to strategic planning.

In addition to proper planning, use of IT usually requires major financial investments over a sustained time period. In the past, often only 2–4 percent of an organization's budget would be allocated for information systems. Under today's conditions and in the foreseeable future, this low level of investment will not be sufficient to assure even minimal compliance with IT requirements. In general (and especially if introducing major IT improvements), organizations should be prepared to invest 5–10 percent of their budget in IT over a multiyear period. This is not simply because of the costs of software products or integrated systems. The IT investment also covers the expense of new hardware, networking and communications, standard software, staff training, and professional consultation, to assure that the expenditures are appropriate and that the deliverables will perform as expected. As most organizations have discovered, IT requires a sustained major commitment on a continuous basis.

There are many advantages to the new IT environment that are highly significant for organization operations. Potentially the most significant advantage available is using "integrated systems," which provide information by linking financial, administrative, and clinical data, analyzed using decision-support technology. This capability allows providers to evaluate costs, efficiency, and effectiveness of their services, including outcomes, client satisfaction, and quality improvement. As health care payers continue to limit reimbursement, the need for information that can assist in reducing costs while maintaining quality becomes very important. Use of IT through integrated systems can provide this information and therefore is a necessity in health care. Additional advantages of IT include:

- network communications for multisite operations,
- electronic medical records,
- improved case management systems for managed care,
- improved cost-accounting systems that merge financial and patient data (clinical programs), and
- newly emerging decision-support applications that enhance managed care contracting, clinical efficiency, quality improvement, and patient tracking.

These types of improvements are being developed and introduced very rapidly, which is creating both volatility and rapid IT product obsolescence. This makes management of IT extremely challenging for organizations that must invest in technology to remain competitive. Under these conditions, strategic IT planning becomes critical, not only to assure reasonable return on investment but, more importantly, to obtain the correct technology to respond to market requirements.

KEYS TO UNDERSTANDING: THE CURRENT SOFTWARE APPLICATION DILEMMA

One of today's major difficulties with information systems is their limited integration. Most software applications in existing systems have limited functions often focused on financial and/or accounting data/analysis, with either no or very limited *integrated* clinical data on patients. Alternatively, clinical data applications (few of which are designed for rehabilitation or other postacute care settings), including electronic medical records, quality management, outcomes, case management, productivity, critical pathways, utilization review, and so forth; are not linked in a seamless way to the financial systems. This creates major difficulty in accomplishing functions such as marketing, contract negotiations, patient management, accreditation, productivity and efficiency improvement, and cost-effectiveness analysis. These functions are extremely important in a competitive, managed care environment, where demonstrating both cost and quality management is decisive for obtaining contracts.

The multiple software applications used today came about primarily because of a logical focus on acute care hospital operations (and operating information requirements) by software development firms as they began building software "legacy" systems for acute hospitals in the late 1960s. Larger scale development of these systems—"a new generation"—occurred in the mid-1980s, and it is frequently this technology that is in use today, albeit with many enhancements, the latest of which is desktop, client-server technology based on Windows™ products.

Even though few postacute medical rehabilitation providers have adopted hospital legacy information systems, they face similar "systems integration" problems and usually have great difficulty in linking financial, clinical, and outcomes data. Various IT strategies are being used to address this problem, with the most prevalent being establishing a data repository to store data from the various existing financial, administrative, clinical, and outcomes systems and then using various "decision support" analytical tools to analyze the data and provide intelligible reports for decision makers. This is not a true systems integration strategy, but it can provide meaningful reports that use linked data.

What this means is that there are few completely integrated information systems available today, and frequently what is "integrated" are certain financial, scheduling, ordering, productivity, and limited clinical data functions, which do not always generate useful reports for decision making. This problem has led to the conclusion that the main issue facing providers is to improve integration of their information systems so as to produce a seamless information technology environment. But, in fact, this is not the most important IT issue. Instead, organizations must focus on, seek out, and participate in the development of *software applications* that will improve processes such as clinical treatment, marketing, outcomes and cost effectiveness, productivity, and quality—that is, define how information technology and information systems can be used to change or reengineer the processes used by the organization to improve efficiency and effectiveness for the customer. What is required for medical rehabilitation to adopt this approach to IT?

USE OF MAJOR IT SYSTEMS BY MEDICAL REHABILITATION

The most fundamental factors that medical rehabilitation should consider are:

- that the emerging health care environment will continue to evolve toward multiple venues of care with an increasing emphasis on postacute treatment settings (including outpatient, rehabilitation, subacute, transitional, assisted living, and home health),
- that improved capability to manage care efficiently, reduce cost, and produce good patient outcomes will become the most important competitive advantage of health care providers, and
- that in the future, it will be necessary to communicate (exchange data and information) with numerous other organizations and groups to sustain and develop business.

These factors have major implications for the IT approach of medical rehabilitation providers.

First, before investing in any major "hospital" type legacy systems (even with accompanying modules designed for postacute care), providers should review their strategic business plans to decide on the venues in which they will be operating and the organizations/groups with whom they will be interacting (e.g., acute hospitals, physician groups, integrated delivery networks, different payers). If "older" legacy systems cannot meet strategic business requirements, their expense will not be justifiable unless vendors are willing to provide substantial systems redesign. This is very unusual. To address the need for IT systems for multiple venues, a better strategy is to consider adapting existing systems using customized technology to produce needed applications using a data repository and report generation software. As time goes on, new integrated software systems will be produced that will collect, process, analyze, and report data from multiple treatment venues. These can be considered once they have an established performance record.

And second, to more completely respond to the information requirements of managed care, integrated delivery networks, insurers, workers' compensation carriers, and physician groups, providers should seek out (and participate in developing) managed information systems that clearly link clinical with financial, resource use, and outcomes data. Systems that include automated case management functions are preferable, although difficult to locate for postacute care. In selecting such systems, providers should keep in mind both their strategic business plan and the need for communicating with a variety of other organizations. This means that new software applications must be designed to run on networks that have the capability to communicate with outside organizations. Despite recent development of Internet communication technology, this is still new and lacks the reliability required for most network health care data transfers. Therefore, more comprehensive and reliable communication technology is a requirement for new IT and software applications for managed care.

The third requirement that providers need to address is the extent and quality of the "decision support technology" that software vendors in fact provide in their information systems. This technology is what performs the analysis of data and produces reports from which decisions can be reached. Decision support technology is often overly complex, requires a great deal of user sophistication, and produces reports that are difficult for staff to understand and use. This technology often requires either a substantial additional software investment for the organization or a large amount of staff training to operate the software. Frequently, therefore, the executives who are supposed to benefit from the technology never do so, because it is too complex and does not produce actionable reports. Here again, unless an "off-the-shelf" package can be located to satisfy the needs of medical rehabilitation, it is better to have a customized application developed that will meet the needs of the organization.

GUIDELINES

There are numerous descriptions of health information systems now available.[1–3] These identify major information systems and their functions and describe their uses in hospitals, integrated delivery systems, physician practices, and managed care organizations. Also, these same resources usually contain background on IT strategic planning and development, selection of hardware and software vendors, and management of information systems in organizations. Knowledge of an organization's strategic business requirements is crucial to developing an effective IT plan.

For medical rehabilitation, general background information on IT should lead to a review of current IT capabilities, defining new requirements, and formulating an overall IT strategy for meeting requirements. It is critical to recognize that the documentation of existing capabilities and the identification of needs are not the same as a practical IT plan. And, to correctly prepare such a plan, the involvement of key financial, clinical, and administrative staff is essential.

In formulating the IT plan, the following types of information systems applications should be considered:

- general ledger/general financial,
- cost accounting/budgeting,
- admission, discharge, transfer (ADT),
- scheduling,
- order entry,
- medical records,
- utilization review,
- quality measurement standards,
- outcomes/patient tracking,
- patient acuity/productivity,
- marketing/referral,
- case mix/critical pathways,
- human resource,
- claims/reimbursement (managed care),
- contract management (managed care),
- case management,
- central data repository,
- patient documentation (electronic medical record),
- ancillary clinical systems, and
- applications for home health treatment.

In considering these applications, the actual requirements of the provider's operations (finance, administration, and clinical) and strategic direction should determine the specific applications to be reviewed, the establishment of priorities, and the defining of needed data elements to be collected.

There are few information systems designed for medical rehabilitation and it continues to be difficult to obtain *functional* applications, particularly for clinical patient management, quality, outcomes, contract management, and case management. In addition, it is difficult to locate integrated financial and clinical systems, and multivenue systems are only in early stages of development. For these reasons, it is usually imperative to focus on (1) obtaining or upgrading integrated applications that are available and that are required for business operations, (2) reviewing available clinical systems (including electronic patient records systems) to evaluate suitability for clinical management, and (3) contracting for the development of systems integration, decision support, and reporting applications. For most providers and payers, a combination IT strategy is the only way to achieve integrated data and information that can provide decision support assistance for management. It should be recognized that outcomes and quality management/reporting systems can almost always be included in clinical systems data collection and reporting using current technology.

In addition to applications, all organizations must now develop networking and telecommunications plans so that there can be both internal and external communication with referral sources, other providers, payers, and health networks. These functions are critically important for organizations and therefore investment in networking/communications must be planned and carefully managed.

• • •

IT is a major continuing investment for medical rehabilitation, postacute care providers, and payers. Managing this investment to obtain value is a challenge that must be fulfilled. To manage IT effectively, medical rehabilitation providers must recognize that IT is broadly applied in health care and must be adapted to their needs. IT must be planned and designed to support business and clinical processes, and the focus must be on technology applications that link financial, clinical, and outcomes data. Providers should be prepared to accept certain existing health information systems that only partially meet their requirements, and to either purchase or develop applications that they need and are not available in larger scale systems. All systems must be designed to operate on networks, and telecommunication planning must be a fundamental part of the overall IT strategy and implementation. In working with IT, the most practical approach is usually to focus on the key applications needed for operating the organization and obtaining up-to-date and flexible technology to satisfy these applications.

REFERENCES

1. DeLuca, J.M., and Cagan, R.E. *The CEO's Guide to Health Care Information Systems.* Chicago: American Hospital Publishing, 1996.
2. Johns, M.L. *Information Management for Health Professions.* Albany, NY: Delmar Publishers, 1997.
3. Shortliffe, E.H., Perreault, L., Wiederhold, A., and Fagan, L.M., eds. *Medical Informatics Computer Applications in Health Care.* Reading, MA: Addison-Wesley, 1990.

PART VIII

Rehabilitation Outcome Measures

34

The Pediatric Evaluation of Disability Inventory (PEDI)

Stephen M. Haley

The Pediatric Evaluation of Disability Inventory (PEDI) was developed to provide a comprehensive clinical assessment of key functional capabilities and performance in children between the ages of six months and seven years. The PEDI was designed primarily for the functional evaluation of young children; however, it can also be used for the evaluation of older children if their functional abilities fall below those expected of seven-year-old children with disabilities. The assessment was designed to serve as a descriptive measure to assist with goal-setting and outcome documentation, as a discriminative measure to identify functional delay, and as a method to track change across time.

The PEDI measures functional activities and the performance of complex functional tasks in three content domains: (1) self-care, (2) mobility, and (3) social function. Functional activities are measured by the identification of skills for which the child has demonstrated mastery and competence. Item selection for this scale was directed by the criterion of identification of meaningful functional units within complex functional tasks. Functional performance is measured by the level of caregiver assistance needed to accomplish major functional tasks such as eating or outdoor locomotion. A modifications scale provides a measure of environmental modifications and equipment used by the child in routine daily activities.

RELIABILITY

Internal consistency coefficients (Cronbach alpha) on the normative sample for the three domains range from 0.95–0.99. Range of inter-interviewer reliability coefficients (ICC [2,1]) was 0.96–0.98 for the normative standardization sample; 0.84–

0.99 for the clinical standardization sample.[1] Additional reliability data have been reported.[2,3]

VALIDITY

Concurrent validity has been reported with the Battelle Developmental Inventory Screening Test ($r = 0.73$ to 0.91) and the Functional Independence Measure for Children (Wee-FIM) ($r = 0.89$ to 0.97). Discriminant analysis reveals that the PEDI differentiates between children with and without disabilities better than the Battelle Developmental Inventory Screening Test. Additional validity data have been reported. [3–6]

SCORING

The PEDI has been standardized on a normative sample of children, which enables the clinician or educator to calculate normative standard scores and scaled performance scores.

Scores are recorded in a booklet containing a summary score sheet that can be used to construct a profile of the child's performance across the different domains and scales. A software program for data entry, scoring, and generation of individual summary profiles is also available for IBM-compatible computers. Scoring utilizes the Rasch Item-Response Theory methodology, which yields interval level data. The computer program calculates a goodness-of-fit score.

BURDEN

The PEDI can be administered by professional judgment of clinicians and educators who are familiar with the child, or by structured interview of the parent. The amount of time required for the parent interview is about 45 minutes. Administration guidelines, criteria for scoring each item, and

J Rehabil Outcomes Meas, 1997, 1(1), 61–69
© 1997 Aspen Publishers, Inc.

examples are given in the manual. The manual also contains information on instrument development and validation, including normative information as well as data from several clinical samples. Cost of the manual is $75; manual score forms and software can be purchased for $185.

REFERENCES

1. Haley, S.M., et al. *Pediatric Evaluation of Disability Inventory: Development, Standardization, and Administration Manual.* Boston: New England Medical Center Hospitals, 1992.

2. Reid, D.T., Boschen, K., and Wright, V. "Critique of the Pediatric Evaluation of Disability Inventory (PEDI)." *Physical & Occupational Therapy in Pediatrics* 13, no. 4 (1996): 15–24.

3. Nichols, D.S., and Case-Smith, J. (1996). "Reliability and Validity of the Pediatric Evaluation of Disability Inventory." *Pediatric Physical Therapy* 8 (1996): 15–24.

4. Coster, W.J., Haley, S.M., and Baryza, M.J. "Functional Perfomance of Young Children after Traumatic Brain Injury: A 6-Month Follow-up Study." *American Journal of Occupational Therapy* 48 (1994): 211–18.

5. Dudgeon, B.J., et al. "Prospective Measurement of Functional Changes after Selective Dorsal Rhizotomy." *Archives of Physical Medicine and Rehabilitation* 75 (1994): 46–53.

6. Haley, S.M., Coster, W.J., and Faas, R. "A Content Validity Study of the Pediatric Evaluation of Disability Inventory." *Pediatric Physical Therapy* 3 (1991): 177–84.

Pediatric Evaluation of Disability Inventory

VERSION 1.0

Stephen M. Haley, Ph.D., P.T., Wendy J. Coster, Ph.D., OTR/L, Larry H. Ludlow, Ph.D.,
Jane T. Haltiwanger, M.A., Ed.M., Peter J. Andrellos, Ph.D.

Score Form

ABOUT THE CHILD

ID# _____

Name _____

Sex M ❑ F ❑   Ethnic group or race _____

Age	Year	Month	Day
Interview Date	_____	_____	_____
Birth Date	_____	_____	_____
Chronological Age	_____	_____	_____

Diagnosis (if any) _____

ICD-9 code(s) _____ _____ _____
            primary   additional

CURRENT STATUS OF CHILD

❑ hospital inpatient   ❑ lives at home

  ❑ acute care   ❑ lives in residential facility

  ❑ rehabilitation

other (specify) _____

School of other facility _____

Grade placement _____

ABOUT THE RESPONDENT (Parent or Guardian)

Name _____

Sex M ❑ F ❑

Relationship to child _____

Type of work (be specific) _____

Years of education _____

ABOUT THE INTERVIEWER

Name _____

Position _____

Facility _____

ABOUT THE ASSESSMENT

Referred by _____

Reason for the assessment _____

_____

_____

_____

Notes _____

_____

GENERAL DIRECTIONS

Below are the general guidelines for scoring. All the items have specific descriptions. Consult the Manual for individual item scoring criteria.

PART I Functional Skills:
197 discrete items of functional skills

Self-care, Mobility, Social Function

0 = unable, or limited in capability, to perform item in most situations

1 = capable of performing item in most situations, or item has been previously mastered and functional skills have progressed beyond this level

PART II Caregiver Assistance:
20 complex functional activities

Self-care, Mobility, Social Function

5 = Independent

4 = Supervise/Prompt/Monitor

3 = Minimal Assistance

2 = Moderate Assistance

1 = Maximal Assistance

0 = Total Assistance

PART III Modifications:
20 complex functional activities

Self-care, Mobility, Social Function

N = No Modifications

C = Child-oriented (non-specialized) Modifications

R = Rehabilitation Equipment

E = Extensive Modifications

PLEASE BE SURE YOU HAVE ANSWERED ALL ITEMS.

PEDI Research Group, c/o Stephen M. Haley, Department of Rehabilitation Medicine, New England Medical Center Hospital, #75K/R, 750 Washington St, Boston, MA 02111-1901 • Phone (617) 956-5031, Fax (617) 956-5353

Part I: Functional Skills

SELF-CARE DOMAIN Place a check corresponding to each item:
Item scores: 0 = unable; 1 = capable

UNABLE / CAPABLE

A. Food Texture   0 1
1. Eats pureed/blended/strained foods
2. Eats ground/lumpy foods
3. Eats cut up/chunky/diced foods
4. Eats all textures of table food

B. Use of Utensils   0 1
5. Finger feeds
6. Scoops with a spoon and brings to mouth
7. Uses a spoon well
8. Uses a fork well
9. Uses a knife to butter bread, cut soft foods

C. Use of Drinking Containers   0 1
10. Holds bottle or spout cup
11. Lifts cup to drink, but cup may tip
12. Lifts open cup securely with two hands
13. Lifts open cup securely with one hand
14. Pours liquid from carton or pitcher

D. Toothbrushing   0 1
15. Opens mouth for teeth to be brushed
16. Holds toothbrush
17. Brushes teeth; but not a thorough job
18. Thoroughly brushes teeth
19. Prepares toothbrush with toothpaste

E. Hairbrushing   0 1
20. Holds head in position while hair is combed
21. Brings brush or comb to hair
22. Brushes or combs hair
23. Manages tangles and parts hair

F. Nose Care   0 1
24. Allows nose to be wiped
25. Blows nose into held tissue
26. Wipes nose using tissue on request
27. Wipes nose using tissue without request
28. Blows and wipes nose without request

G. Handwashing   0 1
29. Holds hands out to be washed
30. Rubs hands together to clean
31. Turns water on and off, obtains soap
32. Washes hands thoroughly
33. Dries hands thoroughly

H. Washing Body & Face   0 1
34. Tries to wash parts of body
35. Washes body thoroughly, not including face
36. Obtains soap (and soaps washcloth, if used)
37. Dries body thoroughly
38. Washes and dries face thoroughly

I. Pullover/Front-Opening Garments   0 1
39. Assists, such as pushing arms through shirt
40. Removes T-shirt, dress or sweater (pullover garment without fasteners)
41. Puts on T-shirt, dress or sweater
42. Puts on and removes front-opening shirt, not including fasteners
43. Puts on and removes front-opening shirt, including fasteners

J. Fasteners   0 1
44. Tries to assist with fasteners
45. Zips and unzips, doesn't separate or hook zipper
46. Snaps and unsnaps
47. Buttons and unbuttons
48. Zips and unzips, separates and hooks zipper

K. Pants   0 1
49. Assists, such as pushing legs through pants
50. Removes pants with elastic waist
51. Puts on pants with elastic waist
52. Removes pants, including unfastening
53. Puts on pants, including fastening

L. Shoes/Socks   0 1
54. Removes socks and unfastened shoes
55. Puts on unfastened shoes
56. Puts on socks
57. Puts shoes on correct feet; manages velcro fasteners
58. Ties shoelaces

M. Toileting Tasks (clothes, toilet management, and wiping only)   0 1
59. Assists with clothing management
60. Tries to wipe self after toileting
61. Manages toilet seat, gets toilet paper and flushes toilet
62. Manages clothes before and after toileting
63. Wipes self thoroughly after bowel movements

N. Management of Bladder (Score = 1 if child has previously mastered skill)   0 1
64. Indicates when wet in diaper or training pants
65. Occasionally indicates need to urinate (daytime)
66. Consistently indicates need to urinate with time to get to toilet (daytime)
67. Takes self into bathroom to urinate (daytime)
68. Consistently stays dry day and night

O. Management of Bowel (Score = 1 if child has previously mastered skill)   0 1
69. Indicates need to be changed
70. Occasionally indicates need to use toilet (daytime)
71. Consistently indicates need to use toilet with time to get to toilet (daytime)
72. Distinguishes between need for urination and bowel movements
73. Takes self into bathroom for bowel movements, has no bowel accidents

Self-Care Domain Sum

PLEASE BE SURE YOU HAVE ANSWERED ALL ITEMS.

Comments

MOBILITY DOMAIN   Place a check corresponding to each item:
Item scores: 0 = unable; 1 = capable

UNABLE CAPABLE

A. Toilet Transfers   0 1
1. Sits if supported by equipment or caregiver
2. Sits unsupported on toilet or potty chair
3. Gets on and off low toilet or potty
4. Get on and off adult-sized toilet
5. Gets on and off toilet, not needing own arms

B. Chair/Wheelchair Transfers   0 1
6. Sits if supported by equipment or caregiver
7. Sits unsupported on chair or bench
8. Gets on and off low chair or furniture
9. Gets in and out of adult-sized chair/wheelchair
10. Gets in and out of chair, not needing own arms

C. Car Transfers   0 1
11. Moves in car; scoots on seat or gets in and out of car seat
12. Gets in and out of car with little assistance or instruction
13. Gets in and out of car with no assistance or instruction
14. Manages seat belt or chair restraint
15. Gets in and out of car and opens and closes car door

D. Bed Mobility/Transfers   0 1
16. Raises to sitting position in bed or crib
17. Comes to sit at edge of bed; lies down from sititng at edge of bed
18. Gets in and out of own bed
19. Gets in and out of own bed, not needing own arms

E. Tub Transfers   0 1
20. Sits if supported by equipment or caregiver in a tub or sink
21. Sits unsupported and moves in tub
22. Climbs or scoots in and out of tub
23. Sits down and stands up from inside tub
24. Steps/transfers into and out of an adult-sized tub

F. Indoor Locomotion: Methods (Score = 1 if mastered)   0 1
25. Rolls, scoots, crawls, or creeps on floor
26. Walks, but holds onto furniture, walls, caregivers or uses devices for support
27. Walks without support

G. Indoor Locomotion: Distance/Speed (Score = 1 if mastered)   0 1
28. Moves within a room but with difficulty (falls; slow for age)
29. Moves within a room with no difficulty
30. Moves between rooms but with difficulty (falls; slow for age)
31. Moves between rooms with no difficulty
32. Moves indoors 50 feet; opens and closes inside and outside doors

H. Indoor Locomotion: Pulls/Carries Objects   0 1
33. Changes physical location purposefully
34. Moves objects along floor
35. Carries objects small enough to be held in one hand
36. Carries objects large enough to require two hands
37. Carries fragile or spillable objects

I. Outdoor Locomotion: Methods   0 1
38. Walks, but holds onto objects, caregiver, or devices for support
39. Walks without support

J. Outdoor Locomotion: Distance/Speed   0 1
(Score = 1 if mastered)
40. Moves 10–50 feet (1–5 car lengths)
41. Moves 50–100 feet (5–10 car lengths)
42. Moves 100–150 feet (35–50 yards)
43. Moves 150 feet and longer, but with difficulty (stumbles; slow for age)
44. Moves 150 feet and longer with no difficulty

K. Outdoor Locomotion: Surfaces   0 1
45. Level surfaces (smooth sidewalks, driveways)
46. Slightly uneven surfaces (cracked pavement)
47. Rough, uneven surfaces (lawns, gravel driveway)
48. Up and down incline or ramps
49. Up and down curbs

L. Upstairs (Score = 1 if child has previously mastered skill)   0 1
50. Scoots or crawls up partial flight (1–11 steps)
51. Scoots or crawls up full flight (12–15 steps)
52. Walks up partial flight
53. Walks up full flight, but with difficulty (slow for age)
54. Walks up entire flight with no difficulty

M. Downstairs (Score = 1 if child has previously mastered skill)   0 1
55. Scoots or crawls down partial flight (1–11 steps)
56. Scoots or crawls down full flight (12–15 steps)
57. Walks down partial flight
58. Walks down full flight, but with diffuclty (slow for age)
59. Walks down full flight with no difficulty

Mobility Domain Sum

PLEASE BE SURE YOU HAVE ANSWERED ALL ITEMS.

SOCIAL FUNCTION DOMAIN   Place a check corresponding to each item: Item scores: 0 = unable; 1 = capable

UNABLE CAPABLE

A. Comprehension Word Meanings   0 1
1. Orients to sound
2. Responds to "no"; recognizes own name or that of familiar people
3. Understands 10 words
4. Understands when you talk about relationships among people and/or things that are visible
5. Understands when you talk about time and sequence of events

B. Comprehension of Sentence Complexity   0 1
6. Understands short sentences about familiar objects and people
7. Understands 1-step commands with words that describe people or things
8. Understands directions that describe where something is
9. Understands 2-step commands, using if/then, before/after, first/second, etc.
10. Understands two sentences that are about the same subject but have a different form

C. Functional Use of Communication   **UNABLE** 0 **CAPABLE** 1

11. Names things
12. Uses specific words or gestures to direct or request action by another person
13. Seeks information by asking questions
14. Describes an object or action
15. Tells about own feelings or thoughts

D. Complexity of Expressive Communication   0 1

16. Uses gestures with clear meaning
17. Uses single word with meaning
18. Uses two words together with meaning
19. Uses 4–5 word sentences
20. Connects two or more thoughts to tell a simple story

E. Problem-resolution   0 1

21. Tries to show you the problem or communicate what is needed to help the problem
22. If upset because of a problem, child must be helped immediately or behavior deteriorates
23. If upset because of a problem, child can seek help and wait if it is delayed a short time
24. In ordinary situations, child can describe the problem and his/her feelings with some detail (usually does not act out)
25. Faced with an ordinary problem, child can join adult in working out a situation

F. Social Interactive Play (Adults)   0 1

26. Shows awareness and interest in others
27. Initiates a familiar play routine
28. Takes turn in simple play when cued for turn
29. Attempts to imitate adult's previous action during a play activity
30. During play child may suggest new or different steps, or respond to adult suggestion with another idea

G. Peer Interactions (Child of similar age)   0 1

31. Notices presence of other children, may vocalize and gesture toward peers
32. Interacts with other children in simple and brief episodes
33. Tries to work out simple plans for a play activity with another child
34. Plans and carries out cooperative activity with other children; play is sustained and complex
35. Plays activities or games that have rules

H. Play with Objects   0 1

36. Manipulates toys, objects or body with intent
37. Uses real or substituted objects in simple pretend sequences
38. Puts together materials to make something
39. Makes up extended pretend play routines involving things the child knows about
40. Makes up elaborate pretend sequences from imagination

I. Self-Information   **UNABLE** 0 **CAPABLE** 1

41. Can state first name
42. Can state first and last name
43. Provides names and descriptive information about family members
44. Can state full home address; if in hospital, name of hospital and room number
45. Can direct an adult to help child return home or back to the hospital room

J. Time Orientation   0 1

46. Has a general awareness of time of mealtimes and routines during the day
47. Has some awareness of sequence of familiar events in a week
48. Has very simple time concepts
49. Associates a specific time with actions/events
50. Regularly checks clock or asks for the time in order to keep track of schedule

K. Household Chores   0 1

51. Beginning to help care for own belongings if given constant direction and guidance
52. Beginning to help with simple household chores if given constant direction and guidance
53. Occasionally initiates simple routines to care for own belongings; may require physical help or reminders to complete
54. Occasionally initiates simple household chores; may require physical help or reminders to complete
55. Consistently initiates and carries out at least one household task involving several steps and decisions; may require physical help

L. Self-Protection   0 1

56. Shows appropriate caution around stairs
57. Shows appropriate caution around hot or sharp objects
58. When crossing the street with an adult present, child does not need prompting about safety rules
59. Knows not to accept rides, food or money from strangers
60. Crosses busy street safely without an adult

M. Community Function   0 1

61. Child may play safely at home without being watched constantly
62. Goes about familiar environment outside of home with only periodic monitoring for safety
63. Follows guidelines/expectations of school and community setting
64. Explores and functions in familiar community settings without supervision
65. Makes transactions in neighborhood store without assistance

Social Function Domain Sum

PLEASE BE SURE YOU HAVE ANSWERED ALL ITEMS.

Comments

Parts II and III: Caregiver Assistance and Modification

Circle the appropriate score for Caregiver Assistance and Modification for each item.

Caregiver Assistance Scale: Independent, Supervision, Minimal, Moderate, Maximal, Total
Modification Scale: None, Child, Rehab, Extensive

SELF-CARE DOMAIN

Item	5	4	3	2	1	0	N	C	R	E
A. **Eating:** eating and drinking regular meal; do not include cutting steak, opening containers or serving food from serving dishes	5	4	3	2	1	0	N	C	R	E
B. **Grooming:** brushing teeth, brushing or combing hair and caring for nose	5	4	3	2	1	0	N	C	R	E
C. **Bathing:** washing and drying face and hands, taking a bath or shower; do not include getting in and out of a tub or shower, water preparation, or washing back or hair	5	4	3	2	1	0	N	C	R	E
D. **Dressing Upper Body:** all indoor clothes, not including back fasteners; include help putting on or taking off splint or artificial limb; do not include getting clothes from closet or drawers	5	4	3	2	1	0	N	C	R	E
E. **Dressing Lower Body:** all indoor clothes; include putting on or taking off brace or artificial limb; do not include getting clothes from closet or drawers	5	4	3	2	1	0	N	C	R	E
F. **Toileting:** clothes, toilet management or external device use, and hygiene; do not include toilet transfers, monitoring schedule, or cleaning up after accidents	5	4	3	2	1	0	N	C	R	E
G. **Bladder Management:** control of bladder day and night, clean-up after accidents, monitoring schedule	5	4	3	2	1	0	N	C	R	E
H. **Bowel Management:** control of bowel day and night, clean-up after accidents, monitoring schedule	5	4	3	2	1	0	N	C	R	E

Self-Care Totals — SELF-CARE SUM ☐ — Self-Care Modification Frequencies

MOBILITY DOMAIN

Item	5	4	3	2	1	0	N	C	R	E
A. **Chair/Toilet Transfers:** child's wheelchair, adult-sized chair, adult-sized toilet	5	4	3	2	1	0	N	C	R	E
B. **Car Transfers:** mobility within car/van, seat belt use, transfers, and opening and closing doors	5	4	3	2	1	0	N	C	R	E
C. **Bed Mobility/Transfers:** getting in and out and changing positions in child's own bed	5	4	3	2	1	0	N	C	R	E
D. **Tub Transfers:** getting in and out of adult-sized tub	5	4	3	2	1	0	N	C	R	E
E. **Indoor Locomotion:** 50 feet (3–4 rooms); do not include opening doors or carrying objects	5	4	3	2	1	0	N	C	R	E
F. **Outdoor Locomotion:** 150 feet (15 car lengths) on level surfaces; focus on physical ability to move outdoors (do not consider compliance or safety issues such as crossing streets)	5	4	3	2	1	0	N	C	R	E
G. **Stairs:** climb and descend a full flight of stairs (12–15 steps)	5	4	3	2	1	0	N	C	R	E

Mobility Totals — MOBILITY SUM ☐ — Mobility Modification Frequencies

SOCIAL FUNCTION DOMAIN

Item	5	4	3	2	1	0	N	C	R	E
A. **Functional Comprehension:** understanding of requests and instructions	5	4	3	2	1	0	N	C	R	E
B. **Functional Expression:** ability to provide information about own activities and make own needs known; include clarity of articulation	5	4	3	2	1	0	N	C	R	E
C. **Joint Problem Solving:** include communication of problem and working with caregiver or other adult to find a solution; include only ordinary problems occurring during daily activities (for example, lost toy; conflict over clothing choices)	5	4	3	2	1	0	N	C	R	E
D. **Peer Play:** ability to plan and carry out joint activities with a familiar peer	5	4	3	2	1	0	N	C	R	E
E. **Safety:** caution in routine daily safety situations, including stairs, sharp or hot objects and traffic	5	4	3	2	1	0	N	C	R	E

Social Function Totals — SOCIAL FUNCTION SUM ☐ — Social Function Modification Frequencies

Pediatric Evaluation of Disability Inventory

VERSION 1.0

Name _____ Test Date _____ Age _____

ID # _____ Respondent/Interviewer _____

Score Summary

Composite Scores

Domain		Raw Score	Normative Standard Score	Standard Error	Scaled Score	Standard Error	Fit Score*
Self-Care	Functional Skills						
Mobility	Functional Skills						
Social Function	Functional Skills						
Self-Care	Caregiver Assistance						
Mobility	Caregiver Assistance						
Social Function	Caregiver Assistance						

*Obtainable only through use of software program

Modification Frequencies

Self-Care (8 Items)				Mobility (7 Items)				Social Function (5 Items)			
None	Child	Rehab	Extensive	None	Child	Rehab	Extensive	None	Child	Rehab	Extensive

Score Profile

Domain		Normative Standard Scores	Scaled Scores
Self-Care	Functional Skills	10 30 50 70 90	0 50 100
Mobility	Functional Skills	10 30 50 70 90	0 50 100
Social Function	Functional Skills	10 30 50 70 90	0 50 100
Self-Care	Caregiver Assistance	10 30 50 70 90	0 50 100
Mobility	Caregiver Assistance	10 30 50 70 90	0 50 100
Social Function	Caregiver Assistance	10 30 50 70 90	0 50 100

± 2 standard errors

Pediatric Evaluation of Disability Inventory

VERSION 1.0

Name _____ Case 1 (Jane) _____	Test Date _____ Age _____ 2.0 yr. _____
ID # _____	Respondent/Interviewer _____

Score Summary

Composite Scores

Domain		Raw Score	Normative Standard Score	Standard Error	Scaled Score	Standard Error	Fit Score*
Self-Care	Functional Skills	32	42.8	2.3	50.3	1.7	
Mobility	Functional Skills	46	40.3	3.5	66.2	2.5	
Social Function	Functional Skills	29	36.8	3.3	47.9	1.2	
Self-Care	Caregiver Assistance	15	52.8	3.8	49.8	3.7	
Mobility	Caregiver Assistance	26	45.8	4.9	65.0	4.3	
Social Function	Caregiver Assistance	6	39.7	4.3	39.6	6.0	

*Obtainable only through use of software program

Modification Frequencies

Self-Care (8 Items)				Mobility (7 Items)				Social Function (5 Items)			
None	Child	Rehab	Extensive	None	Child	Rehab	Extensive	None	Child	Rehab	Extensive
3	5	0	0	4	3	0	0	5	0	0	0

Score Profile

Domain		Normative Standard Scores	Scaled Scores
Self-Care	Functional Skills		
Mobility	Functional Skills		
Social Function	Functional Skills		
Self-Care	Caregiver Assistance		
Mobility	Caregiver Assistance		
Social Function	Caregiver Assistance		

± 2 standard errors

35

The Functional Independence Measure
(FIM^SM Instrument)

Anne Deutsch, Susan Braun, and Carl V. Granger

In 1984, the Department of Rehabilitation Medicine of the State University of New York at Buffalo was awarded a grant by the National Institute on Disability and Rehabilitation Research to develop a system to measure severity of disability and the outcomes of medical rehabilitation. The resulting Uniform Data Set for Medical Rehabilitation includes the Functional Independence Measure (FIM^SM instrument), which is currently the most widely used functional assessment scale throughout the world. The FIM instrument and its copyrights are owned and maintained by the Uniform Data System for Medical Rehabilitation (UDS_MR^SM), a division of U B Foundation Activities, Inc. Subscribers to UDS_MR are licensed to use the FIM System™, including the FIM instrument, for data collection and research purposes.[1,2]

PURPOSE

The FIM instrument describes an individual's functional abilities and limitations in terms of activities required to support the physical aspects of daily living. The purpose of the data set is to document the severity of a person's disability, functional abilities and limitations, and the effectiveness and efficiency of the outcomes of medical rehabilitation.[1–3] The FIM instrument is a principal component of program evaluation models for rehabilitation services in the U.S.[4–6] and an essential element to the Penn Ability System® (PAS™) FIM–Function-Related Groups (FIM-FRGs), a severity-adjusted model that predicts average length of stay and average discharge functional status for inpatient comprehensive rehabilitation care.[7]

POPULATION

The FIM instrument may be used to describe the functional abilities of persons seven years and older. A pediatric version of the FIM instrument, the WeeFIM® scale, may be used to assess the function of children six months to seven years of age. The FIM instrument is currently used in inpatient comprehensive medical rehabilitation, subacute rehabilitation, long-term care, and home care. It has been administered to persons who are disabled from a variety of impairments including stroke, brain injury, orthopedic, spinal cord dysfunction, arthritis, debility, cancer, and acquired immunodeficiency syndrome (AIDS).[8–10] The scale is also used in over a dozen countries outside of the United States.

ADMINISTRATION

The FIM instrument may be administered by any rater trained through a process of self-study, training videos, or training workshop. Clinician raters include occupational therapists, nurses, physical therapists, speech/language pathologists, physicians, and program evaluation/quality improvement coordinators. Credentialing, which includes an examination that assesses a rater's knowledge of the FIM item definitions and the functional levels, is required for facilities submitting data to UDS_MR.[4]

UDS_MR^SM and FIM^SM are service marks and WeeFIM® is a registered service mark of the Uniform Data System for Medical Rehabilitation, a division of U B Foundation Activities, Inc. Penn Ability System® (PAS™) is a registered trademark of the Trustees of the University of Pennsylvania.

J Rehabil Outcomes Meas, 1997, 1(2), 67–71

The FIM score is to reflect the person's *usual* performance rather than the person's *best* performance. Direct observation of a person's functional status is preferred, but interviews with the person, other staff/team members, and family members may be appropriate.

The time required for administration of the FIM instrument is 20–40 minutes the first time a clinician uses it. Depending on the interviewer's familiarity with the FIM instrument and the functional status of the person, the time may be reduced to 10–20 minutes.

DESCRIPTION

The FIM instrument is an 18-item, seven-level ordinal scale that assesses severity of disability. Disability is operationally defined in terms of the *need for assistance (burden of care)*, the type and amount of assistance required for a disabled person to perform basic life activities effectively. The FIM instrument measures a minimum number of key activities in the areas of self-care, sphincter control, transfers, communication, and cognition.[4]

1. Motor items
   - Self-Care (eating, grooming, bathing, dressing—upper body, dressing—lower body, toileting)
   - Sphincter control (bladder management, bowel management)
   - Transfers (bed, chair, wheelchair, toilet, tub or shower)
   - Locomotion (walk/wheelchair, stairs)
2. Cognitive items
   - Communication (comprehension, expression)
   - Social cognition (social interaction, problem solving, memory)

The seven-level scoring scale includes two independent levels and five helper levels.

The FIM item scores for each of the 18 items may be summed and the result is referred to as the *Total FIM* or *FIM-18* score. Total FIM scores range from 18 to 126, with 126 representing the highest level of independence. FIM data may also be reported in terms of *Motor FIM*, the sum of the first 13 FIM item scores, and *Cognitive FIM*, the sum of the last five scores. Motor FIM scores range from 13 to 91 and Cognitive FIM scores range from 5 to 35.

APPLICATION

The FIM instrument is used in clinical settings as a tool for program evaluation and quality management. Typically, FIM assessments are completed within 72 hours of admission, and discharge assessments are administered within 72 hours prior to discharge. In addition, follow-up assessments (usually completed over the phone) 80 to 180 days after discharge from rehabilitation may be done. Functional improvement, the difference between discharge and admission scores, provide a gauge of the effectiveness of the rehabilitation program.

RELIABILITY

Internal consistency, interrater, intrarater, intermodal, and proxy agreement of the seven-level FIM instrument have been reported in the literature.[11–15] Researchers have found the instrument to be reliable, and FIM training and credentialing to be useful in increasing interrater agreement. Proxy agreement was less reliable than clinician reporting, primarily in the assessment of cognitive level.[16]

VALIDITY

Face validity has been rated as better than average.[2,6] In the assessment of concurrent validity, a strong relationship was found with the Barthel Index[17,18] and to a lesser extent, the Patient Evaluation Conference System (PECS).[19] Construct validity of the FIM instrument has been evaluated and demonstrated in several situations describing how FIM scores would change based on various clinical scenarios.[11,20–23] The FIM instrument has demonstrated predictive validity, including such outcomes as the level of assistance needed, discharge functional status, length of stay and discharge setting.[24–38]

RESPONSIVENESS

Responsiveness, or a scale's sensitivity to show change that is clinically relevant, is essential. The responsiveness of the FIM instrument has been described in several articles, particularly to age, diagnosis, and treatment setting.[11,20,22] Functional improvement in terms of FIM gain during inpatient rehabilitation stay has been reported in numerous articles.[11,39–42]

LIMITATIONS

Limitations of the FIM instrument identified in the literature include the ordinal nature of FIM data,[43,44] and "floor" and "ceiling" effects.[45] However, the more recent use of Rasch analysis, which transforms raw scores into interval measures, has helped reduce the impact of some limitations.[44] Other limitations include lower sensitivity for persons with brain injury and persons with high-level spinal cord injuries.[6,45,46] The FIM instrument does not measure the speed and ease of task completion or quality of task execution.

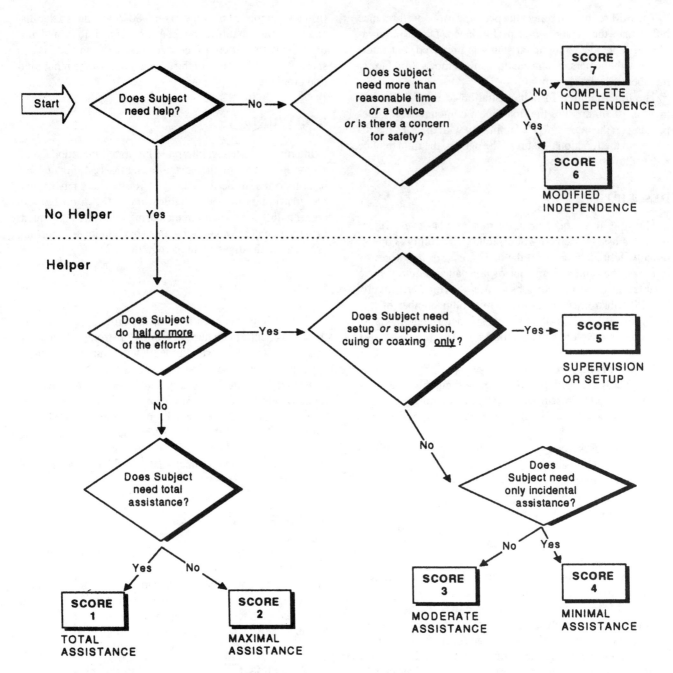

Figure 1. General description of FIM instrument levels of function and their scores. Copyright © 1996. Reprinted with permission of the Uniform Data System for Medical Rehabilitation, a division of U B Foundation Activities, Inc.

STRENGTHS

The FIM instrument has been extensively studied and has been shown to have acceptable reliability, validity, and responsiveness. Reliability studies suggest training and testing (credentialing) are necessary, and that training should be completed prior to use of the FIM instrument in the clinical setting.

In terms of validity, the FIM instrument has been shown to have acceptable face validity, construct validity, and concurrent validity. The ability of the FIM instrument to predict rehabilitation outcomes such as average length of stay, average discharge functional status, and the likelihood of discharge to the community has broadened its utility. The FIM instrument has been increasingly viewed as a universal measure of disability. Also, the FIM instrument may be used in a variety of rehabilitation settings, and is increasingly used to demonstrate the impact of changes in care provided at the program and treatment level.

REFERENCES

1. Granger, C.V., et al. "Advances in Functional Assessment for Medical Rehabilitation." *Topics in Geriatric Rehabilitation* 1, no. 3 (1986): 59–74.

2. Hamilton, B.B., et al. "A Uniform National Data System for Medical Rehabilitation," in *Rehabilitation Outcomes: Analysis and Measurement,* ed. M.J. Fuhrer. Baltimore: Paul H. Brookes Publishing Co., 1987, 137–47.

3. Keith, R.A., et al. "The Functional Independence Measure: A New Tool for Rehabilitation," in *Advances in Clinical Rehabilitation,* vol. 1, eds. W.G. Eisenberg and R.C. Grzesiak. New York: Springer, 1987, 6–18.

4. *Guide to the Uniform Data Set for Medical Rehabilitation* (FIM^SM Instrument) Version 5.0. Buffalo, NY: State University of New York at Buffalo, 1996.

5. Fiedler, R.C., and Granger, C.V. "The Functional Independence Measure: A Measurement of Disability and Medical Rehabilitation," in *Functional Evaluation of Stroke Patients,* eds. N. Chino and J.L. Melvin. Tokyo: Springer-Verlag Tokyo, 1996, 75–92.

6. Watson, A.H., et al. "Use of Standardized Activities of Daily Living Rating Scales in Spinal Cord Injury and Diseases Services." *American Journal of Occupational Therapy* 49, no. 3 (1995): 229–34.

7. Stineman, M.G., et al. "A Case-mix Classification System for Medical Rehabilitation." *Medical Care* 32, no. 4 (1994): 366–79.

8. Fucile, J. "Functional Rehabilitation Cancer Care." *Seminars in Oncology Nursing* 8, no. 3 (1992): 186–89.

9. Marciniak, C.M., et al. "Functional Outcome Following Rehabilitation of the Cancer Patient." *Archives of Physical Medicine and Rehabilitation* 77, no. 1 (1996): 54–7.

10. O'Dell, M.W., et al. "Disability in Persons Hospitalized with AIDS." *American Journal of Physical Medicine and Rehabilitation* 70, no. 2 (1991): 91–5.

11. Dodds, T.A., et al. "A Validation of the Functional Independence Measurement and Its Performance among Rehabilitation Inpatients." *Archives of Physical Medicine and Rehabilitation* 74, no. 5 (1993): 531–6.

12. Hamilton, B.B., et al. "Interrater Reliability of the 7-level Functional Independence Measure." *Scandinavian Journal of Rehabilitation Medicine* 26 (1994): 115–19.

13. Chau, N., et al. "Inter-rater Agreement of Two Functional Independence Scales: The Functional Independence Measure (FIM) and a Subject Uniform Continuous Scale." *Disability and Rehabilitation* 16, no. 2 (1994): 63–71.

14. Fricke, J., Unsworth, C., and Worrell, D. "Reliability of the Functional Independence Measure with Occupational Therapists." *The Australian Occupational Therapy Journal* 40, no. 1 (1993): 7–15.

15. Ottenbacher, K.J., et al. "Inter-rater Agreement and Stability of Functional Assessment in the Community-based Elderly." *Archives of Physical Medicine and Rehabilitation* 75, no. 12 (1994): 1297–1301.

16. Segal, M.E., Gillard, M., and Schall, R.R. "Telephone and In-person Proxy Agreement between Stroke Patients and Caregivers for the Functional Independence Measure." *American Journal of Physical Medicine and Rehabilitation* 75, no. 3 (1996): 208–12.

17. Kidd, D., et al. "The Functional Independence Measure: A Comparative Validity and Reliability Study." *Disability and Rehabilitation* 17, no. 1 (1995): 10–14.

18. Roth, E., "Functional Assessment in Spinal Cord Injury: A Comparison of the Modified Barthel Index and the 'Adapted' Functional Independence Measure." *Clinical Rehabilitation* 4 (1995): 277–85.

19. Fisher, W.P., Jr., et al. "Rehabits: A Common Language of Functional Assessment." *Archives of Physical Medicine and Rehabilitation* 76, no. 2 (1995): 113–22.

20. Menter, R.R., et al. "Impairment, Disability, Handicap and Medical Expenses of Persons Aging with Spinal Cord Injury." *Paraplegia* 29, no. 9 (1991): 613–19.

21. Linacre, J.M., et al. "The Structure and Stability of the Functional Independence Measure." *Archives of Physical Medicine and Rehabilitation* 75, no. 2 (1994): 127–32.

22. Heinemann, A.W., et al. "Relationships between Impairment and Physical Disability as Measured by the Functional Independence Measure." *Archives of Physical Medicine and Rehabilitation* 74, no. 6 (1993): 566–73.

23. Granger, C.V., et al. "Performance Profiles of the Functional Independence Measure." *American Journal of Physical Medicine and Rehabilitation* 72, no. 2 (1993): 84–9.

24. Alexander, M.P. "Stroke Rehabilitation Outcome: A Potential Use of Predictive Variables to Establish Levels of Care." *Stroke* 25, no. 1 (1994): 128–34.

25. Falconer, J.A., et al. "The Critical Path Methods in Stroke Rehabilitation: Lessons from an Experiment in Cost Containment and Outcome Improvement." *Quality Review Bulletin* 19, no. 1 (1993): 8–16.

26. Granger, C.V., et al. "Functional Assessment Scales: A Study of Persons with Multiple Sclerosis." *Archives of Physical Medicine and Rehabilitation* 71 (1990): 870–75.

27. Granger, C.V., et al. "Functional Assessment Scales: A Study of Persons after Stroke." *Archives of Physical Medicine and Rehabilitation* 74, no. 2 (1993): 133–8.

28. Granger, C.V., Divan, N., and Fiedler, R.C. "Functional Assessment Scales: A Study of Persons after Traumatic Brain Injury." *American Journal of Physical Medicine and Rehabilitation* 74, no. 2 (1995): 107–13.

29. Disler, P.B., Roy, C.W., and Smith, B.P. "Predicting Hours of Care Needed." *Archives of Physical Medicine and Rehabilitation* 74, no. 2 (1993): 139–43.

30. Corrigan, J.D., Smith-Knapp, K., and Granger, C.V. "Validity of the Functional Independence Measure for Persons with Traumatic Brain Injury." Unpublished manuscript, 1996.

31. Mauthe, R.W., et al. "Predicting Discharge Destination of Stroke Persons Using a Mathematical Model Based on Six Items from the Functional Independence Measure." *Archives of Physical Medicine and Rehabilitation* 77, no. 1 (1996): 10–13.

32. Granger, C.V., Hamilton, B.B., and Fielder, R.C. "Discharge Outcome after Stroke Rehabilitation." *Stroke* 23, no. 7 (1992): 978–82.

33. Wilson, D.B., Houle, D.M., and Keith, R.A. "Stroke Rehabilitation: A Model Predicting Return Home." *Western Journal of Medicine* 154, no. 5 (1991): 587–90.

34. Oczkowski, W.J., and Barreca, S. "The Functional Independence Measure: Its Use to Identify Rehabilitation Needs in Stroke Survivors." *Archives of Physical Medicine and Rehabilitation* 74, no. 12 (1993): 1291–94.

35. Werner, R.A. "Predicting Outcome after Acute Stroke with the Functional Independence Measure." *Topics in Stroke Rehabilitation* 1, no. 3 (1994): 30–9.

36. Muecke, L., et al. "Functional Screening of Lower-limb Amputees: A Role in Predicting Rehabilitation Outcome?" *Archives of Physical Medicine and Rehabilitation* 73, no. 9 (1992): 851–8.

37. Stineman, M.G. "Function-based Classification for Stroke Rehabilitation and Issues of Reimbursement: Using Person Classification Systems to Scale Payment to Person Complexity." *Topics in Stroke Rehabilitation* 1, no. 3 (1994): 40–50.

38. Heinemann, A.W., et al. "Prediction of Rehabilitation Outcomes with Disability Measures." *Archives of Physical Medicine and Rehabilitation* 75, no. 2 (1994): 133–43.

39. Fielder, R.C., Granger, C.V., and Ottenbacher, K.J. "The Uniform Data System for Medical Rehabilitation: Report of First Admissions for 1994." *American Journal of Physical Medicine and Rehabilitation* 75, no. 2 (1996): 125–9.

40. Whitlock, J.A., and Hamilton, B.B. "Functional Recovery after Rehabilitation for Severe Traumatic Brain Injury." *Archives of Physical Medicine and Rehabilitation* 76, no. 12 (1995): 1103–12.

41. Hamilton, B.B., and Granger, C.V. "Disability Outcomes Following Inpatient Rehabilitation for Stroke." *Physical Therapy* 74, no. 5 (1994): 494–503.

42. Stineman, M.G., et al. "Functional Gain and Length of Stay for Major Rehabilitation Impairment Categories." *American Journal of Physical Medicine and Rehabilitation* 75 (1996): 68–78.

43. Merbitz, C., Morris, J., and Grip, J.C. "Ordinal Scales and Foundations of Misinference." *Archives of Physical Medicine and Rehabilitation* 70, no. 4 (1989): 308–12.

44. Heinemann, A.W., et al. "Measurement Characteristics of the Functional Independence Measure." *Topics in Stroke Rehabilitation* 1, no. 3 (1994): 1–15.

45. Marino, R.J., et al. "Assessing Selfcare Status in Quadriplegia: Comparison of the Quadriplegia Index of Function (QIF) and the Functional Independence Measure (FIM)." *Paraplegia* 31, no. 4 (1993): 225–33.

46. Davidoff, G.N., et al. "Cognitive Dysfunction in Spinal Cord Injury Patients: Sensitivity of the Functional Independence Measure Subscales vs. Neuropsychological Assessment." *Archives of Physical Medicine and Rehabilitation* 71, no. 5 (1990): 326–9.

36

The Functional Assessment Measure (FAM)

Karyl Hall

DESCRIPTION OF THE FUNCTIONAL ASSESSMENT MEASURE

The Functional Assessment Measure (FAM) was developed as an adjunct to the functional independence measure (FIM[SM]) to specifically address the major functional areas key to brain injury that are relatively less emphasized in the FIM, including cognitive, behavioral, communication, and community functioning measures. There are 12 items intended for use as an addition to the 18-item FIM. The total 30-item scale combination is referred to as the "FIM + FAM." The FAM utilizes a 7-point ordinal scale similar to the FIM. The FAM is considered part of the public domain, and may be used by a trained rater.

Clinically, the FAM has demonstrated utility for outcomes measurement in patients with traumatic and nontraumatic brain injury, stroke, and other disorders that affect cognition and reasoning.

RELIABILITY

FAM items involving abstract concepts such as "attention" tend to be less reliable than directly observable behaviors.[1] As a test of the FAM items interrater reliability, FAM training and testing vignettes (which also included the FIM items) were completed by trained raters including a physical therapist (PT), occupational therapist (OT), certified occupational therapy assistant (COTA), data analyst, and researcher. Each item's three vignettes were written to cover low, intermediate, and high functioning levels within the 1 to 7 scale. The percentage of rating agreement for the three lev-

els of FAM function were 86, 86, and 92 percent respectively. For FIM items, the percentage of rating agreement was 89 percent. The Kappa score for the FAM was .85, and for the FIM, .87.

In another interrater reliability training endeavor, the four TBI Model Systems (Medical College of Virginia, Richmond, VA; Rehabilitation Institute of Michigan, Detroit, MI; Santa Clara Valley Medical Center, San Jose, CA; Institute of Rehabilitation and Research, Houston, TX) staff were given the vignettes to train and test several raters from different disciplines at each center. Each of the centers passed with an overall accuracy hovering just above 80 percent for the FIM + FAM.

VALIDITY

FAM items contribute significantly to the overall proportion of disability in all categories and in the total score for the ratings 2–6. The FAM may be an even greater contributor to a valid measure of disability during the follow-up period, as many of the items relate to community functioning: car transfers, employability, community mobility, adjustment to limitations.[2]

FAM items have undergone Rasch analyses at both rehabilitation admission and discharge.[3] The results demonstrated that FAM items rated at admission correlated significantly with indices of injury severity in similar patterns to the FIM. The FAM does not appear to contribute beyond the FIM in predicting length of inpatient stay or costs. The FAM does appear to have increased sensitivity beyond the FIM alone for inpatient rehabilitation discharge and postacute rehabilitation functional assessment. There is evidence that the FAM at rehabilitation discharge has less "ceiling effect" than the FIM and is more strongly related to rehabilitation charges than the FIM.[4]

J Rehabil Outcomes Meas, 1997, 1(3), 63–65

Definitions of FAM Items

Swallowing: ability to safely eat regular diet by mouth.

Car transfers: the activity includes approaching the car, managing the car door and lock, getting on or off the car seat, and managing the seat belt. If a wheelchair is used for mobility, the activity includes loading and unloading the wheelchair.

Community access: ability to manage transportation, including planning a route, time management, paying fares, and anticipating access barriers (excluding car transfers).

Reading: ability to understand nonvocal written material.

Writing: includes spelling, grammar, and completeness of written communication.

Speech intelligibility: includes articulation, rate, volume, and quality of vocal communication.

Emotional status: includes frequency and severity of depression, anxiety, frustration, ability, unresponsiveness, agitation, interference with general life functioning, ability to cope with and take responsibility for emotional behavior.

Adjustment to limitations: includes denial/awareness, acceptance of limitations, willingness to learn new ways of functioning, compensating, taking appropriate safety precautions, and realistic expectations for long-term recovery.

Employability: the term *employed* or *employability* as used in this scale represents involvement in one or more of the following categories: in the work force; as a student; as a homemaker. If a person is of retirement age and retired, score should reflect the person's potential for employment. If the person is a student and/or homemaker, score should reflect how well the person is functioning in that capacity, in determining potential for employment. If the person is in a sheltered workshop, he or she will score a 2, 3, or 4, depending on the level of functioning. The disability may be physical, cognitive, or psychosocial.

Orientation: includes consistent orientation to person, place, time, and situation.

Attention: defined as the length of time able to concentrate on a task, taking into consideration distractibility, level of responsiveness, and the difficulty and length of task.

Safety judgment: includes orientation to one's situation, awareness of one's deficits and their implications, ability to plan ahead, ability to understand the nature of situations involving potential danger and to identify risks involved, freedom from impulsivity, ability to remember safety-related information, and ability to respond appropriately if danger arises.

The Rating Scale

The 7-point Rating Scale is as follows:
Independent: Another person is not required for the activity (NO HELPER).

7 **Complete independence:** all of the tasks described as making up the activity are typically performed safely without modification, assistive devices, or aids, and within reasonable time.

6 **Modified independence:** activity requires any one or more of the following: an assistive device, more than reasonable time, or there are safety (risk) considerations.

Dependent: Another person is required for either supervision or physical assistance in order for the activity to be performed, or it is not performed (REQUIRES HELPER).

Modified dependence: the subject expends half (50 percent) or more of the effort. The levels of assistance required are:

5 **Supervision or setup:** subject requires no more help than standby, cueing, or coaxing, without physical contact. Or, helper sets up needed items or applies orthoses.

4 **Minimal contact assistance:** with physical contact the subject requires no more help than touching, and subject expends 75 percent or more of the effort.

3 **Moderate assistance:** subject requires more help than touching, or expends half (50 percent) or more (up to 75 percent) of the effort.

Complete dependence: the subject expends less than half (less than 50 percent) of the effort; maximal or total assistance is required, or the activity is not performed. The levels of assistance required are:

2 **Maximal assistance:** subject expends less than 50 percent of the effort, but at least 25 percent.

1 **Total assistance:** subject expends less than 25 percent of the effort.

SCORING

The FAM utilizes the same 7-point rating scale as the FIM, and therefore scoring is completed using the same methods as the FIM. The total FIM + FAM composite score ranges from 30 to 210 (7 × 30 items = 210), rather than 18 to 126 for the FIM (7 × 18 items = 126). If scoring separately for motor and cognitive subscales, which is recommended, all FAM items are included in the cognitive subscale, with the exception of three items: swallowing, car transfers, and community access, which are motor items, as determined by Rasch analysis.

TIME INPUT REQUIRED

The time required to administer the FIM + FAM is approximately 35 minutes, but varies substantially, depending on how familiar the rater is with the subject. Training for the FAM can be completed through self-study, which requires approximately three hours. There is a fee of $20.00 for obtaining the worksheet, definitions of terms (including syllabus and decision trees for each item), and training materials. The syllabus and decision trees can be obtained free of charge at the FAM website: *http://members.aol.com/ KHallVMC/FAMTOC.html.*

REFERENCES

1. Hall, K.M. "Overview of Functional Assessment Scales in Brain Injury Rehabilitation." *NeuroRehabilitation* 2, no. 4 (1992): 97–112.
2. Marosszeky, J. "UDS and Australia: An International Perspective." Presented at the Conference on Progress in Medical Rehabilitation: Issues in Measurement, June 19, 1992, Buffalo, NY.
3. Hall, K.M., et al. "Characteristics and Comparisons of Functional Assessment Indices: Disability Rating Scale, Functional Independence Measure, and Functional Assessment Measure." *Journal of Head Trauma Rehabilitation* 8, no. 2 (1993): 60–74.
4. Hall, K.M., et al. "Functional Measures After Traumatic Brain Injury: Ceiling Effects of FIM, FIM + FAM, DRS, and CIQ." *Journal of Head Trauma Rehabilitation* 11, no. 5 (1996): 27–39.

SUGGESTED READING

Hall, K.M. "Functional Assessment and Outcome Measurement." In *Rehabilitation of the Adult and Child with Traumatic Brain Injury,* 3rd ed., eds. Rosenthal et al. F.A. Davis Company, accepted for publication.

Hall, K.M., and Johnston, M.V. "Outcomes Evaluation in Traumatic Brain Injury Rehabilitation. Part I: Overview and System Principles." *Archives of Physical Medicine and Rehabilitation* 75, no. 12 (suppl.) (1994): SC-2–9.

Hall, K.M., and Johnston, M.V. "Outcomes Evaluation in Traumatic Brain Injury Rehabilitation. Part II: Measurement Tools for a Nationwide Data System." *Archives of Physical Medicine and Rehabilitation* 75, no. 12 (suppl.) (1994): SC-10–18.

Johnston, M.V., et al. "Functional Assessment and Outcome Evaluation for Traumatic Brain Injury Rehabilitation." In *Medical Rehabilitation of Traumatic Brain Injury,* eds. L.J. Horn and N.D. Zasler. Philadelphia, PA: Hanley & Belfus, 1996.

37

The Rehabilitation Institute of Chicago Functional Assessment Scale

Kristine C. Cichowski

DESCRIPTION

The Rehabilitation Institute of Chicago Functional Assessment Scale (RIC-FAS) was developed to comprise a comprehensive set of outcome measures pertinent to physical rehabilitation. The RIC-FAS is a set of 98 items that utilize a 7-point ordinal scale. The data set includes the 18 items of the Functional Independence Measure (FIM[SM]).[1] (FIM[SM] is a service mark of the Uniform Data System for Medical Rehabilitation—UDS[MR™]—UB Foundation Activities, Inc., Buffalo, NY.) The additional 80 RIC-FAS items extend the FIM[SM] items for measurement of a broader range of skills acquired in physical rehabilitation. The non–FIM[SM] items further describe status or progress in medical management, health maintenance, psychosocial, cognition, community integration, and vocational rehabilitation. The data set was designed to complement the FIM[SM] domains of self-care, mobility, communication, and cognition.

The RIC-FAS is intended to measure what a patient *actually does,* versus what he or she *ought to* be able to do. Outcomes are collected for patients who are a minimum of 16 years of age, whose length of stay was greater than three days, who have complete admission and discharge ratings, and who are not deceased at the time of discharge. Goal ratings are assigned for each item in order to provide query of results based on the goals set. The RIC-FAS has had four revisions since development in 1987.

RELIABILITY

Assessment of interrater reliability was completed in the first year of implementation using 30 adult patients repre-

senting a variety of conditions typical of the RIC inpatient population. Correlations reported, at a minimum were: 93 percent for communicative disorders; 66 percent for nursing items; 85 percent for occupational therapy items; 62 percent for physical medicine; 87 percent for physical therapy; 72 percent for psychology; and 78 percent for social work.

VALIDITY

The RIC-FAS, comprising FIM[SM] items and items measuring medical management, health maintenance, psychosocial, social work, community integration, and vocational, has good construct validity. With its detailed and extensive 90-day postdischarge follow-up questionnaire, the instrument aptly assesses the impact of a patient's disability in the community.

SCORING

The RIC-FAS utilizes virtually the same 7-point rating scale as the FIM[SM], and scoring is completed using the same methods as the FIM[SM]. Differences in operational definitions pertaining primarily to the degree of verbal cueing have existed in the application of ratings with the RIC-FAS and the FIM[SM] items until early 1995 when terminology was aligned more closely.

In contrast to scoring for the FIM[SM] (7×18 items = 126), which provides for a composite score, the RIC-FAS was designed to rate each item individually. Clinicians rate patient functioning based on the goals of treatment. Results are analyzed by item, reflecting improvement, goal attainment, and maintenance of skills.

BURDEN

The time required to administer the RIC-FAS is approximately one hour, but varies substantially, depending on how

J Rehabil Outcomes Meas, 1997, 1(4), 66–71
© 1997 Aspen Publishers, Inc.

282

familiar the rater is with the subject. Some disciplines have more rating items, such as nursing. Training for the RIC-FAS can be completed through self-study, which requires approximately four hours. There is a fee of $30 for obtaining a copy of the instrument.

●   ●   ●

For further information regarding the RIC-FAS instrument, contact :

Kristine C. Cichowski, MS
Director, Outcomes Management
Rehabilitation Institute of Chicago
345 E. Superior St.
Chicago, IL 60611

PH: 312-908-7835
FAX: 312-908-5925

To acquire a copy of the RIC-FAS instrument, contact :

Ellie Wydeven
Education and Training
Rehabilitation Institute of Chicago
345 E. Superior St.
Chicago, IL 60611
PH: 312-908-2859

REFERENCE

1. Deutsch, A., Braun, S., and Granger, C.V. "The Functional Independence Measure (FIM^{SM} Instrument)." *Journal of Rehabilitation Outcomes Measurement* 1, no. 2 (1997): 67–71.

APPENDIX A

RIC-FAS Rating Items

MEDICAL MANAGEMENT

Medical status
Respiratory management
Skin status
Skin management
Skin pressure tolerance
Muscle tone
Bladder management (FIM^{SM})
Bowel management (FIM^{SM})
Chewing/swallowing
Hearing
Endurance
Nutritional status
G/U dysfunction-alteration
Urinary retention
Vision status

HEALTH MAINTENANCE

Patient/caregiver education
Financial resources
Housing
Transportation
Community placement
Support network
Guardianship and relevant legal
  issues
Caregiver requirements
Continuity of care

SELF-CARE

Eating (FIM^{SM})
Grooming (FIM^{SM})
Bathing (FIM^{SM})
Dressing upper body (FIM^{SM})
Dressing lower body (FIM^{SM})
Toileting (FIM^{SM})

MOBILITY

Bed mobility
Wheelchair propulsion

Ambulation distance
Ambulation equipment
Locomotion: walk/wheelchair
  (FIM^{SM})
Stair climbing (FIM^{SM})
Transfers: bed, chair, wheelchair
  (FIM^{SM})
Transfer: toilet (FIM^{SM})
Transfers: tub or shower (FIM^{SM})
Car transfers

COMMUNICATION

Auditory comprehension
Oral expression
Reading comprehension
Written expression
Speech production
Pragmatics
Comprehension (FIM^{SM})
Expression (FIM^{SM})
Alternative/augmentative communi-
  cation

COGNITIVE

Cognitive status
Problem solving (FIM^{SM})
Memory (FIM^{SM})
Alertness/attention/concentration
Orientation
Visual–spatial abilities
Behavior control
Learning potential

PSYCHOSOCIAL

Social interaction (FIM^{SM})
Anxiety
Depression
Interpersonal skills
Adjustment to the rehabilitation
  setting
Adjustment to disability

Family understanding of disability
Anxiety + phobias
Hostility + anger
Emotional control
Sexuality understanding
Insight/awareness of disability
Self-esteem
Pain control
Compliance
Patient/staff interaction

COMMUNITY INTEGRATION

Leisure skill
Recreation resource awareness
Community recreation reintegration
Money management
Writing/phone use
Meal preparation and clean-up
Clothing care
Household maintenance
Emergency procedures
Financial management
Community skill
Care of others
Leisure abilities
Leisure time management
Initiation of leisure/recreation
  participation
Community activity status

VOCATIONAL

Vocational discharge plan
Vocational participation
Vocational goal setting
Work behavior
Physical tolerance of work
Family vocational support
Employability
Driving readiness
Vocational activities

Examples of RIC-FAS Items

DOMAIN: Medical Management

ITEM NAME: Skin Management

DEFINITION: Skin management is the extent to which an individual carries out and directs a program for maintaining healthy, intact skin, and the assistance required to do so. A skin care program includes skin checks and maintenance of sitting and turning tolerances.

SCALE POINTS

NO HELPER

7   Complete Independence   Totally independent and consistent in performing skin program. Can be left alone to perform the program safely and within a reasonable length of time OR skin program NOT needed.

6   Modified Independence   Uses specialized equipment (e.g., McCormick loops, mirror) or requires more than reasonable time for quality performance.

HELPER

5   Supervision or Set-up   Requires supervision, frequent cueing demonstrating, "hands off" guarding, or "standby" to complete the program. Cannot be left alone to perform program.

4   Minimal Physical Assistance   Patient performs 75% or more of the task. May require "hands on" or "contact" guarding.

3   Moderate Physical Assistance   Patient performs 50% to 74% of the task. Only one person is required for physical assistance.

2   Maximum Physical Assistance   Patient performs 25% to 49% of the task. Only one person is required for physical assistance or patient may direct care.

1   Total Assistance   Requires total assistance. Patient performs less than 25% of the task. One or more persons may be required for performance of the activity.

DOMAIN: Communication

ITEM NAME: Auditory Comprehension

DEFINITION: Understanding linguistic information via spoken word. Reasons for difficulty in auditory comprehension will vary depending on communication diagnosis. May be due to a symbolic linguistic disorder, reduced processing rate, and/or deficits in underlying cognitive processes such as attention, perception, memory, organization, reasoning, and problem solving. Auditory comprehension is assessed independent of hearing acuity.

SCALE POINTS

7   Normal   In all situations, subject understands directions and conversation that are complex or abstract. A subject may receive this rating if auditory comprehension is functional with no assistance required and is at pre-morbid level.

6   Minimal Impairment   In most situations, subject understands complex or abstract directions and conversation readily or with only mild difficulty (e.g., self-initiates request for repetition or responses may be delayed).

5   Mild Impairment   Subject understands directions and simple conversation about a variety of topics more than 90% of the time. May require occasional (less than 10% of the time) repetition or rephrasing to aid comprehension. Breakdown may occur when content is complex, abstract, inferential, or lengthy.

4   Mild to Moderate Impairment   Subject understands directions and conversation about basic daily needs and activities 75% to 90% of the time. May require some assistance (e.g., repetition, rephrasing) to aid comprehension.

3   Moderate Impairment   Subject understands directions and conversation about basic daily needs 50% to 74% of the time. May require moderate assistance (e.g., repetition, rephrasing) to aid comprehension.

2   Moderate to Severe Impairment   Subject inconsistently (25% to 49%) understands simple directions and brief statements about basic daily needs. Requires prompting more than half the time.

1   Severe Impairment   May not comprehend any auditory stimuli or responds inappropriately or inconsistently (less than 25% of the time) to brief statement about basic daily needs.

0   Not Applicable (e.g., deaf, non–English speaking).

DOMAIN: Psychosocial

ITEM NAME: Adjustment to Disability (RIC-FAS IV)

DEFINITION: The cognitive recognition and emotional "working through" of disability and its potential implications. This includes acceptance of limitations, appropriate expression of grief, and reinvestment in life goals in accordance with current disability status.

SCALE POINTS

7	No Problem	Patient clearly recognizes the reality of his/her disability and its implications. Patient shows genuine signs of reinvestment by making plans or lifestyle modifications that are congruent with current disability status (e.g., appreciates and accepts the need to quit driving, sees the necessity of making home modifications, modifies vocational goals in accordance with current functional status). Patient may experience grief reactions that do not interfere with functioning or engagement in treatment.
6	Minimal Problem	Patient clearly recognizes the reality of his/her disability and its potential implications, but shows limited evidence of reinvestment (e.g., patient passively accepts lifestyle modifications recommended by others). Patient may continue to experience grief reactions that do not interfere with functioning or engagement in treatment.
5	Mild Problem	Patient generally recognizes the reality of his/her disability but does not fully appreciate its potential implications (e.g., the patient recognizes the permanency of his/her inability to ambulate, but talks periodically about resuming activities that require ambulation). Patient shows no evidence of reinvestment. Grief reactions may interfere minimally with functioning or engagement in treatment.
4	Mild to Moderate Problem	Patient has some recognition of the reality of his/her disability (e.g., patient recognizes physical but not cognitive changes) but significantly underestimates its implications (e.g., patient does not believe memory deficits will preclude a return to work). Grief reactions interfere with functioning (e.g., patient has difficulty with some aspects of treatment because they confront or highlight deficits).
3	Moderate Problem	Patient has minimal recognition of his/her disability and its potential implications. Patient may demonstrate appropriate grief (e.g., talks fleetingly of negative impact current losses will have on future, or makes occasional comments about frustration secondary to inability to perform activities of daily living). Inappropriate expression of negative effect is likely when treatment activities highlight deficits (e.g., patient acts in a hostile way toward staff or family when frustrated; patient is resistant to treatment and does not understand the need for it).
2	Moderate to Severe Problem	Patient does not recognize his/her disability and its potential implications. She/he may demonstrate signs of emotional distress, but does not associate distress with current losses (e.g., patient sees no need for and refuses treatment).
1	Severe Problem	Patient does not recognize his/her disability and its potential implications. The patient shows minimal or no evidence of emotional distress related to disability. Patient passively complies or withdraws from participation in treatment.
0	Not Applicable	

38

Child Health Questionnaire

Edward A. Dobrzykowski

The Child Health Questionnaire (CHQ) was developed from research conducted at the New England Medical Center's Health Institute (Boston, MA), which began in 1990. The primary mission was to develop and validate a family of generic tools for the measurement of functional status and well-being of children in pediatric health care settings, traditional academic research efforts, and clinical trials. Private sponsorship has resulted in the availability of the CHQ instrument to the public, through completion of a User's Agreement.[1,p.534]

DESCRIPTION

The Child Health Questionnaire is a valid, comprehensive assessment tool developed for the measurement of physical and psychosocial well-being of children five years of age or older.[1,p.30] Development work is under way on a parent-reported instrument for children ages younger than five years.

The original research resulted in the construction of a 98-item version (CHQ-PF98), reported by the parent or guardian. Two short-form versions of the CHQ have been derived from the original 98-item instrument: one consisting of 50 items (CHQ-PF50) and one consisting of 28 items (CHQ-PF28), which are also completed by the parent or guardian. Each of the parent forms yields a health concept profile score for 14 health concepts (see box) and two summary component scores.[1,p.32] An 87-item instrument (CHQ-CF87) is available, and is completed by children 10 years of age and older. The instruments have norms available and are constructed for use among children with and without chronic conditions.[1,p.31]

The CHQ in the United States may be used with parents and children who speak or read English. A Spanish-American version is in development. The CHQ has been translated in 13 languages (Spanish, Canadian-French, Finnish, French, German, Dutch, Italian, Greek, Honduran, Mexican, Norwegian, Portuguese, and Swedish).[2]

RELIABILITY/VALIDITY

Extensive work has been completed to estimate reliability (Cronbach's alpha coefficient) for both parent/guardian completed versions (CHQ-PF50 and CHQ-P28); two summary measures for these instruments; and the child-completed questionnaire (CHQ-CF87). Studies have been completed to assess reliability with populations of both boys and girls; five age groups (5–7, 8–10, 11–12, 13–15, and 16–18); maternal and paternal respondents; and parent ethnicity, education, and work status.[1,p.250]

The CHQ has had its measures' psychometric properties evaluated in child populations that include asthma, attention deficit hyperactivity disorder (ADHD), cystic fibrosis, epilepsy, juvenile rheumatoid arthritis, and psychiatric problems. The minimum criteria for item internal consistency (.40) of the CHQ-PF50 was exceeded on average by 91 percent of all item tests performed for U.S. samples and related

---

The Child Health Questionnaire has been approved for distribution by the Medical Outcomes Trust, 20 Park Plaza, Suite 1014, Boston, MA 02116-4313. Phone: 617-426-4046. Internet address: http://www.outcomes-trust.org.

Child Health Questionnaire (CHQ): A User's Manual, authored by Jeanne M. Landgraf, Linda Abetz, and John E. Ware, Jr., is available through the Health Institute, New England Medical Center, Boston, MA, phone 800-572-9394. Direct queries to the principal developer at (617) 245-7800.

J Rehabil Outcomes Meas, 1997, 1(5), 62–65
© 1997 Aspen Publishers, Inc.

CHQ Health Concepts

Physical Functioning
Role/Social Limitations—Physical
General Health Perceptions
Bodily Pain/Discomfort
Parental Impact—Time
Parental Impact—Emotional
Role/Social Limitations—Emotional
Role/Social Limitations—Behavioral
Mental Health
Self Esteem
General Behavior
Family Activities
Family Cohesion
Change in Health

subgroups, and by 84 percent of all test items performed for the clinical samples. The average success rate for tests of item discriminant validity of the CHQ-PF50 for these samples was a minimum of 94 percent.[1,p.53]

In testing of the CHQ in the specific conditions previously noted, overall scale score means were highest for the representative U.S. sample of children relative to the clinical samples; scale scores were lower for children with more debilitating conditions; scores for physical functioning were lowest in children with active rheumatoid arthritis; and in children with ADHD, significant morbidity was observed in the psychosocial health component.[1,p.295] Other findings demonstrated consistency in standard errors across the samples; and F-statistics for all scales, which were statistically very significant at $p < 0.000$.[1,p.295]

Factor analysis has been conducted to evaluate the construct validity of the CHQ-PF50 and validity of each of the CHQ scales in relation to a two-dimensional order structure of physical and psychosocial dimension of health. These two components accounted for 59.2 percent of the total measured variance in the CHQ scales in the general U.S. population.[1,p.284] For a more comprehensive description of reliability and validity research performed with this instrument, the reader is encouraged to refer to results published in *Child Health Questionnaire (CHQ): A User's Manual.*[1]

ADMINISTRATION/BURDEN

The CHQ is designed for self-completion by parent/guardian or child, and can also be used in telephone and face-to-face administration. The instrument can be completed in homes, schools, and clinics. It is meant to be a freestanding instrument or a component of a longer questionnaire, interview, or other data collection instrument.[1,p.41] The time for completion by parent/guardian or child will depend upon the actual instrument(s) selected, the reading ability of the respondent, and whether the information is collected through self-report or interview. The time for completion of the instruments is six to seven questions per minute (i.e., the time for completion of the CHQ-PF28 is four to five minutes).[3] Scoring algorithms and software code are available.[1,p.175]

REFERENCES

1. Landgraf, J.M., Abetz, L., and Ware, J.E. Jr. *Child Health Questionnaire (CHQ): A User's Manual.* 1st ed. Boston, MA: The Health Institute, New England Medical Center, 1996.
2. "The Child Health Questionnaire: Design and Application." *Medical Outcomes Trust Bulletin* 5, no. 3 (1997): 1.
3. Personal correspondence, June 1997.

List of Items[a] and Response Options[b] Found in the CHQ-PF50

1. In general, would you say your child's health is:

2. Has your child been limited in any of the following activities due to health problems?
   a. Doing things that take a lot of energy, such as playing soccer or running?
   b. Doing things that take some energy such as riding a bike or skating?
   c. Ability (physically) to get around the neighborhood, playground, or school?
   d. Walking one block or climbing one flight of stairs?
   e. Bending, lifting, or stooping?
   f. Taking care of him/herself, that is, eating, dressing, bathing, or going to the toilet?

3. Has your child's school work or activities with friends been limited in any of the following ways due to EMOTIONAL difficulties or problems with his/her BEHAVIOR?
   a. limited in the KIND of schoolwork or activities with friends he/she could do
   b. limited in the AMOUNT of time he/she could spend on schoolwork or activities with friends
   c. limited in PERFORMING schoolwork or activities with friends (it took extra effort)

4. Has your child's school work or activities with friends been limited in any of the following ways due to problems with his/her PHYSICAL health?
   a. limited in the KIND of schoolwork or activities with friends he/should could do
   b. limited in the AMOUNT time he/she could spend on schoolwork or activities with friends

5a. How much bodily pain or discomfort has your child had?

5b. How often has your child had bodily pain or discomfort?

6. How often did each of the following statements describe your child?

   a. argued a lot
   b. had difficulty concentrating or paying attention
   c. lied or cheated
   d. stole things inside or outside the home
   e. had tantrums or a hot temper
   f. Compared to other children your child's age, in general would you say his/her behavior is:

7. How much of the time do you think your child:
   a. felt like crying?
   b. felt lonely?
   c. acted nervous?
   d. acted bothered or upset?
   e. acted cheerful?

8. How satisfied do you think your child has felt about:
   a. his/her school ability?
   b. his/her athletic ability?
   c. his/her friendships?
   d. his/her looks/appearance?
   e. his/her family relationships?

9. How true or false is each of these statements for your child?
   a. My child seems to be less healthy than other children I know.
   b. My child has never been seriously ill.
   c. When there is something going around my child usually catches it.
   d. I expect my child will have a very healthy life.
   e. I worry more about my child's health than other people worry about their children's health.
   f. Compared to one year ago, how would you rate your child's health now.

10. How MUCH emotional worry or concern did each of the following cause YOU?
   a. Your child's physical health
   b. Your child's emotional well-being or behavior
   c. Your child's attention or learning abilities

11. Were you LIMITED in the amount of time YOU had for your own needs because of,

a. Your child's physical health
b. Your child's emotional well-being or behavior
c. Your child's attention or learning abilities

12. <u>How often</u> has your child's <u>health or behavior</u>:
   a. limited the types of activities you could do as a family?
   b. interrupted various everyday family activities (eating meals, watching tv)?
   c. limited your ability as a family to "pick up and go" on a moment's notice?

d. caused tension or conflict in your home?
e. been a source of disagreements or arguments in your family?
f. caused you to cancel or change plans (personal or work) at the last minute?

13. Sometimes families may have difficulty getting along with one another. They do not always agree and they may get angry. In general, how would you rate your family's ability to get along with one another?

[a]A four week recall period is used for all scales except for the Change in Health (CH) and Family Cohesion (FC) items and the General Health (GH) scale. The scale for Change in Health is "compared to last year."

[b]Options include the following: Excellent; Very good; Good; Fair; Poor—Yes, limited a lot; Yes, limited some; Yes, limited a little; No, not limited—None; Very mild; Mild; Moderate; Severe; Very severe—None of the time; Once or twice; A few times; Fairly often; Very often; Every/almost every day—Very often; Fairly often; Sometimes; Almost never; Never—All of the time; Most of the time; Some of the time; A little of the time; None of the time—Very satisfied; Somewhat satisfied; Neither satisfied nor dissatisfied; Somewhat dissatisfied—Definitely True; Mostly True; Don't Know; Mostly False; Definitely False—Much better now than 1 year ago; Somewhat better now than 1 year ago; About the same now as 1 year ago; Somewhat worse now than 1 year ago; Much worse now than 1 year ago—None at all; A little bit; Some; Quite a bit; A lot.

Index